From Horror to Hope

From Horror to Hope

Recognizing and Preventing the Health Impacts of War

Barry S. Levy

WITH THE ASSISTANCE OF
Heather L. McStowe

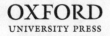

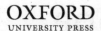

Oxford University Press is a department of the University of Oxford. It furthers
the University's objective of excellence in research, scholarship, and education
by publishing worldwide. Oxford is a registered trade mark of Oxford University
Press in the UK and certain other countries.

Published in the United States of America by Oxford University Press
198 Madison Avenue, New York, NY 10016, United States of America.

Library of Congress Cataloging-in-Publication Data
Names: Levy, Barry S., author.
Title: From horror to hope : recognizing and preventing the health impacts
of war / Barry S. Levy.
Description: New York, NY : Oxford University Press, 2022. |
Includes bibliographical references and index.
Identifiers: LCCN 2021051123 (print) | LCCN 2021051124 (ebook) |
ISBN 9780197558645 (paperback) | ISBN 9780197645970 (hardback) |
ISBN 9780197558669 (epub) | ISBN 9780197558676 (other)
Subjects: MESH: Public Health | Warfare—prevention & control | Weapons of
Mass Destruction | Military Health
Classification: LCC RA418 (print) | LCC RA418 (ebook) | NLM WA 295 |
DDC 362.1—dc23/eng/20220106 (digital-online)
LC record available at https://lccn.loc.gov/2021051123
LC ebook record available at https://lccn.loc.gov/2021051124

DOI: 10.1093/oso/9780197558645.001.0001

9 8 7 6 5 4 3 2 1

Paperback printed by Marquis, Canada
Hardback printed by Bridgeport National Bindery, Inc., United States of America

To Nancy

Contents

Profiles*

*   The individuals featured in profiles in this book and the institutions and organizations with which they are or have been affiliated are independent of other content in this book. The people who are profiled do not necessarily agree with any statements in the book.

Preface

I have written this book for three reasons: to broaden your understanding of the health impacts of war, to enable you to recognize and prevent these impacts, and to engage you in preventing war and promoting peace.

I first witnessed the health impacts of armed conflict and genocide many years ago when I worked in a "holding camp" in Thailand for displaced Cambodians. They had suffered under the brutal Khmer Rouge regime and fled to Thailand when the regime was overthrown and the border was opened. Many of their family members had died. And these survivors had been physically and psychologically traumatized. How could this have happened? Why hadn't the United States or the United Nations intervened? What were the roles of health professionals and others in addressing the needs of these people, documenting these horrors, and preventing them from happening again?

Today, most wars are civil wars, fought in distant countries unfamiliar to most Americans: Ethiopia, South Sudan, Yemen. These wars are not civil. Women are raped. Children starve. Young men are "forcibly disappeared." Families are uprooted and separated. Civil society is destroyed. Hospitals and water treatment plants are bombed. The environment is damaged. Many people die. And the survivors are scarred for life.

Recent and current developments may increase the likelihood of war. Nationalism is increasing in many countries. The international arms trade is making lethal weapons more easily available throughout the world. Massive displacement of people is causing political and socioeconomic instability. And climate change is contributing to the risk of war.

Two comments before going further: First, I am acutely aware that when governments and their agents brutally oppress people and systematically violate their human rights, victims sometimes see no alternative but to develop armed resistance and fight back. Second, I am a citizen of the United States, which has not experienced war within its own borders in 150 years—a country that has done much to promote peace, but has also engaged in activities that have directly and indirectly contributed to war.

We Americans are often blind to the horrors of war affecting other countries. News outlets sanitize war, such as by describing brutal attacks as "hostilities." Official reports use acronyms, such as "GBV" for gender-based violence and "WMDs" for weapons of mass destruction, to create distance from the realities of war. Academics and policymakers use statistics that are detached from human suffering. Meanwhile, the U.S. military budget soars—now greater than the next 11 countries combined. Massive amounts of financial and human resources that could be used for improving public health, education, and the social safety net are allocated to the military. And militarism influences our daily lives.

At the same time, there are reasons to hope. Disputes between and within countries are being settled without resorting to violence. Human rights continue to motivate grassroots actions for peace and justice. Gender-based violence is increasingly recognized and addressed. Researchers are learning more about recognizing and preventing war-related mental disorders. Epidemiology, psychology, and other scientific disciplines are being applied to document, assess, and prevent the health impacts of war. New treaties restrict the arms trade and nuclear weapons. Humanitarian assistance is becoming more systematic and evidence-based. And, as reflected in the profiles of individuals throughout this book, many people have chosen—and are choosing—to devote a significant proportion of their lives to preventing the health impacts of war and promoting peace.

B. S. L.

January 17, 2022

Acknowledgments

I greatly appreciate the excellent work of Heather McStowe, my longtime administrative assistant, who assisted me in developing and revising the manuscript, performing literature searches, and obtaining journal articles, books, photographs, and other materials.

I am grateful for the helpful comments and suggestions of Robert Gould, Robert Lawrence, Leonard Rubenstein, and Patrice Sutton, who reviewed the entire manuscript; Paula Braveman, Richard Garfield, Timothy Holtz, Howard Hu, William Schulz, and Paul Walker, who reviewed chapters; and Daryl Kimball and Martha Davis, who reviewed descriptions of selected international treaties and conventions.

I thank the individuals profiled for their willingness to be interviewed and included in this book. I thank Susannah Sirkin for her helpful advice on these profiles, and Emily Warne for her assistance with the profile of Denis Mukwege.

I deeply appreciate the wisdom and assistance of Sarah Humphreville, Senior Editor for Public Health, Epidemiology, Genetics, and Tech Studies at Oxford University Press, who guided me through the entire process of developing this book, and the assistance during the production process of Emma Hodgdon, Editorial Assistant at Oxford University Press; Prabha Karunakaran, Production Editor at Newgen KnowledgeWorks; and Wendy Walker, Copy-editor.

I acknowledge my colleagues in public health who have shared their observations and insights, provided helpful critiques of my work, and assisted and encouraged me. I especially acknowledge my longtime colleague in this work, the late Victor (Vic) Sidel, who opened my eyes to the horror of war and provided much hope to me and many others for a better future. And I acknowledge my colleagues in the Department of Public Health and Community Medicine at Tufts University School of Medicine and in the Peace Caucus of the American Public Health Association.

Finally, I acknowledge my wife, Nancy, for many years of love, encouragement, and support, without whom I would not have been able to write this book.

B. S. L.

About the Author

Barry S. Levy, M.D., M.P.H., is a physician, epidemiologist, and an Adjunct Professor of Public Health in the Department of Public Health and Community Medicine at Tufts University School of Medicine. He has written and spoken extensively on the public health impacts of war, terrorism, social injustice, climate change, and environmental and occupational hazards. He has edited 20 previous books, including two editions each of *War and Public Health* and *Terrorism and Public Health* with Victor Sidel, M.D., and has authored more than 250 journal articles and book chapters. Dr. Levy has worked in several other countries, primarily Kenya, Thailand, China, Jamaica, and nations in Central and Eastern Europe. He is a Past President of the American Public Health Association and a recipient of its most prestigious award, the Sedgwick Memorial Medal.

Timespans of Wars Cited*

Afghanistan War (2001–2021)
American Revolution (1775–1783)
Angolan Civil War (1975–2002)
Bangladesh Liberation War, also known as the Bangladesh War of Independence (1971)
Bosnia and Herzegovina War (1992–1995)
Croatia War (1991–1995)
Darfur armed conflict (2003–2012)
Eritrea–Ethiopia War (1998–2000)
First World War, U.S. participation in (1917–1918)
Gaza War (2014)
Guinea Bissau Civil War (1998–1999)
Gulf War, also known as the Persian Gulf War (1990–1991)
Iraq War (2003–2013)
Iraq–Iran War (1980–1988)
Ivory Coast Civil War (2002–2007)
Korean War (1950–1953)
Lebanese Civil War (1975–1990)
Libyan Civil War (1989–1996)
Mozambican Civil War (1977–1992)
Nepalese Civil War (1996–2006)
Nigerian Civil War (1967–1970)
Second Congo War, also known as the Great War of Africa and the Democratic Republic of
the Congo Civil War (1998–2003)

* See Table 6-1 on page 107 for timespans of some genocides and mass killings in the 20th century.

Second Lebanon War (2006)
Second Liberian Civil War (1999–2003)
Second Sino-Japanese War (1937–1945)
Second World War, U.S. participation in (1941–1945)
Sierra Leone Civil War (1991–2002)
Spanish-American War (1898)
Sri Lankan Civil War (1983–2009)
Syrian Civil War (2011–present)
Ugandan Civil War (1986–2006)
United States Civil War (1861–1865)
Vietnam War, also known as the American War in Vietnam (1954–1975)
Yemeni Civil War (2015–present)

PART I

Introduction

A Public Health Perspective on War

What difference does it make to the dead, the orphans and the homeless,
whether the mad destruction is wrought under the name of totalitarianism or
in the holy name of liberty or democracy?
MAHATMA GANDHI

INTRODUCTION

War creates many individual and family tragedies. To a child, war may mean not having
enough to eat and feeling sick. To a woman, it may mean persistent threat of physical or
sexual assault. To an older person, it may mean there is no available medical care and no
available medicine to control diabetes and high blood pressure. To a displaced person, it may
mean separation from family members. To a military veteran, it may mean recurring night-
mares. And to those whose parents, spouse, siblings, children, or other family members or
friends were killed, it may mean eternal grief.

Public health is what we, as a society, do collectively to ensure the conditions in which
people can be healthy.[1] A healthy society meets basic human needs, ensures healthy and safe
environments, promotes equity, protects human rights, and provides health and social services, education, and employment opportunities. A healthy society also provides mechanisms
for citizens to participate in the governmental decisions that affect their lives.

In contrast, war creates conditions in which people cannot be healthy. It is anathema
to public health.

War causes injury, disease, and premature death. It adversely affects mental health. It
violates human rights. It forcibly displaces people. It damages essential elements of civilian
infrastructure. It contaminates the environment. It diverts resources to military uses from
health, education, and other services of social benefit. And it leads to more violence.

War causes civilian morbidity and mortality directly by indiscriminate and targeted
attacks. It also causes morbidity and mortality indirectly by mass displacement of people
and by damaging civilian infrastructure, including healthcare facilities, food supply systems,

From Horror to Hope. Barry S. Levy, Oxford University Press. © Oxford University Press 2022.
DOI: 10.1093/oso/9780197558645.003.0001

water treatment plants, and electrical grids. And war sometimes leads to import sanctions (embargoes) that restrict importation of food, medicine, and materials to repair war-related damage. The vast majority of deaths during most recent wars have resulted from these indirect causes.

War is a public health catastrophe.

DEFINITIONS

Before going further, it is useful to review some definitions and use of terms. *War* is "a state of armed conflict between different nations or states or different groups within a nation or state."[2] *Armed conflict* "involves the use of armed force between two or more states [countries] or non-state organized groups . . . causing 25 or more deaths in a given year."[3] Throughout this book, the terms *war*, *armed conflict*, and *conflict* are used interchangeably.

Armed conflicts can be categorized in a number of ways. They can be categorized by number of conflict-related deaths in a given year: *major conflicts*, 10,000 or more deaths; *high-intensity conflicts*, 1,000 to 9,999 deaths, and *low-intensity conflicts*, 25 to 999 deaths. They can also be categorized as *interstate conflicts*, which are fought between countries, and *intrastate conflicts*, which are fought within a country between the government and one or more non-state groups. Intrastate conflicts can be further categorized as *subnational conflicts*, which are confined to specific areas within a country, and *civil wars*, which involve most of a country and result in 1,000 or more deaths a year. (Because publications often overlook the distinction between the two last categories, the terms *civil war*, *intrastate conflict*, and *intrastate armed conflict* are used interchangeably throughout this book.) When there is substantial military or financial involvement in an intrastate conflict by one or more other countries or external entities, it is considered an *internationalized intrastate conflict*.[3] These internationalized conflicts are sometimes proxy wars between other countries.

A *state-based conflict* is "a contested incompatibility over government and/or territory, where at least one party is a state, and the use of armed force results in at least 25 battle-related deaths within a calendar year." A *non-state conflict* is "the use of armed force between organized groups, one of which is the government of a state, resulting in at least 25 annual battle-related deaths." An *extrastate conflict* is between a state (member of the international system) and an entity that is not a member of the international system. *One-sided violence* is "the use of armed force by the government of a state or by a formally organized group against civilians, which results in at least 25 deaths" (not including extrajudicial killings in custody). *Battle deaths* are "fatalities caused by the warring parties that can be directly related to combat, including civilian losses."[4]

War is a component of *collective violence*, which is defined by the World Health Organization as "the instrumental use of violence by people who identify themselves as members of a group . . . against another group or set of individuals in order to achieve political, economic, ideological, or social objectives."[5] Other components of collective violence are state-sponsored violence (such as genocide, repression, disappearances, and torture) and organized violent crime (such as gang warfare and banditry).

More broadly, war is part of a spectrum of violence that includes *structural violence*—"the ongoing and institutionalized harm done to individuals by preventing them from meeting their basic needs for survival, well-being, identity, and freedom." Norwegian sociologist Johan Galtung, who established this concept, observed that structural violence is built into the political system, the economy, and the sociocultural domination hidden in everyday life. Structural violence occurs not only within countries but also in the political, economic, and social relationships between the Global North and the Global South and within war-affected regions and countries. Structural violence can—and does—lead to physical violence, including war.[6,7]

THE EPIDEMIOLOGY OF WAR

Civilians (noncombatants) suffer a large proportion of deaths during war, although the exact proportion is difficult to determine.[8-10] Most of these are *indirect deaths*. For the 1990–2017 period, during which 1,118 armed conflicts occurred, Mohammed Jawad and colleagues estimated that 29.4 million *indirect* civilian deaths occurred as a result of war—approximately one million annually, on average. Of these indirect deaths, they estimated that 21.0 million were due to communicable, maternal, neonatal, and nutritional diseases; 6.0 million deaths were due to noncommunicable diseases; and 2.4 million deaths were due to injuries. The absolute increase in all-cause mortality associated with war was largest in children under age 5.[11]

In 2019, for the fifth consecutive year, the number of *recorded deaths* (almost 76,000) in all forms of organized violence—state-based armed conflicts, non-state armed conflicts, and one-sided violence—decreased, according to the Uppsala Conflict Data Program (UCDP) (Figure 1-1).[12] During the 1990–2017 period, the UCDP reported an annual average of approximately 47,000 recorded deaths in state-based armed conflicts[12]—much lower than the

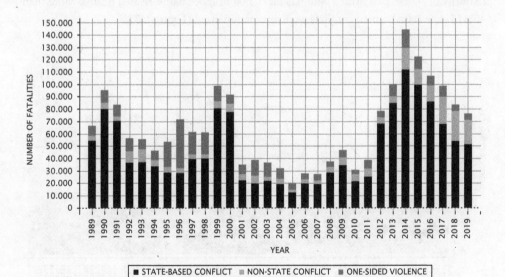

FIGURE 1-1 Number of fatalities in organized violence, by type (excluding Rwanda 1994), 1989–2019. (*Source*: Pettersson T, Magnus Ö. Organized violence, 1989–2019. Journal of Peace Research 2020; 57 [4].)

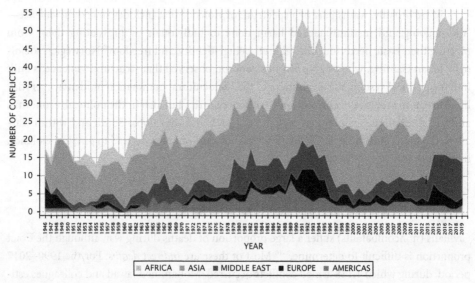

FIGURE 1-2 Number of state-based armed conflicts, by region, 1946–2019. (*Source*: Pettersson T, Magnus Ö. Organized violence, 1989–2019. Journal of Peace Research 2020; 57 [4].)

one million average war-related indirect civilian deaths per year during this same period estimated by Jawad and colleagues.[11] This difference is due to the high percentage of civilian deaths during many wars that occur indirectly as a result of damage to facilities for healthcare, the food supply, and water treatment and other critical infrastructure. These indirect deaths are typically not recorded as related to war. (See Chapters 2 and 14.)

The number of state-based armed conflicts in 2019 remained at a peak level—with the highest percentage in Africa, followed by Asia and the Middle East (Figure 1-2). The vast majority of state-based armed conflicts had 1,000 or more battle-related deaths. More than 40% of state-based armed conflicts were internationalized (Figure 1-3).[12]

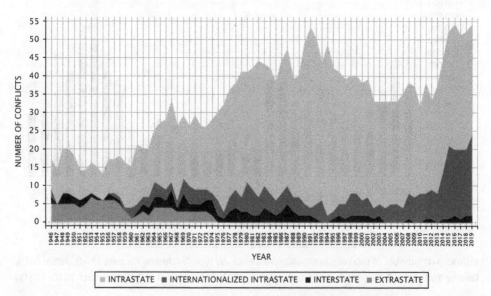

FIGURE 1-3 Number of state-based armed conflicts, by type, 1946–2019. (*Source*: Pettersson T, Magnus Ö. Organized violence, 1989–2019. Journal of Peace Research 2020; 57 [4].)

Active wars occurred in 32 countries during 2019: 15 in sub-Saharan Africa, seven in the Middle East and North Africa, seven in Asia and Oceania, two in the Americas, and one in Europe. Most were intrastate conflicts that occurred within low- and middle-income countries between government forces and one or more armed non-state groups. Only one of these wars was between countries (the border clashes between India and Pakistan). Two were waged between government forces and armed groups that aspired to statehood (between Israel and the Palestinians, and between Turkey and the Kurds).[3]

Three active wars during 2019 were major armed conflicts: in Afghanistan (with 41,900 reported deaths during the year, not including indirect deaths), in Yemen (with 25,900), and in Syria (with 15,300). And 15 wars were high-intensity armed conflicts, with 1,000 to 9,999 reported deaths—in Mexico, Nigeria, Somalia, the Democratic Republic of the Congo (DRC), Iraq, Burkina Faso, Libya, Mali, South Sudan, the Philippines, India, Myanmar, Cameroon, Pakistan, and Egypt. All three of the major armed conflicts and most of the high-intensity armed conflicts involved other countries.[3]

As of June 2021, the Syrian Civil War, which began in 2011, was the greatest humanitarian crisis related to war. By that time, more than 606,000 people had died and approximately 13 million Syrians had been displaced, about one-half internally and about one-half to other countries.[13] Overall, more than 22 million people were in need of humanitarian aid. As of November 2020, approximately half of the 113 public hospitals and more than half of almost 1,800 public health centers were partly functioning or not functioning at all. More than 900 health workers had died since the start of the war and many health workers had been detained and tortured.[14]

Civil wars often recur. Of all conflict episodes, 46% recur within the same conflict; of all conflicts between two armed actors, 33% recur within the same pair of actors. Recurrences of civil war frequently involve the same types of grievances and issues as in the previous war and often also involve participation by additional armed actors. In this sense, they could be described better as "continuously evolving," rather than "recurring."[15]

Civil wars are less likely to recur after a government victory or the deployment of peacekeepers (Chapter 15). The probability of recurrence of civil war is higher if the previous war was fought with rebels attempting to replace the government or if the warring parties were mobilized along ethnic lines.[16]

Some countries get caught in a "conflict trap" after a civil war. Armed conflict destroys the economy. Productive assets, ranging from factories to farmland, are damaged or destroyed. Workers are injured, killed, or forced to flee. These countries experience a reversal of economic development and an increased probability of recurrent war.[17]

During the past decade, non-state conflicts have more than doubled. There were 67 in 2019, representing about a 20% decrease from the previous 2 years. There have been few studies of these conflicts because they tend to occur in remote areas and governments have limited interest in or control over them, they occur in the midst of civil wars, and they are often associated with organized crime involving drugs or extraction and smuggling of resources.[4,18]

The number of people killed annually in one-sided violence is thought to be between 4,000 and 8,000. Most one-sided violence is committed by non-state actors, although reports do not include extrajudicial killings perpetrated by governments. Examples have included the mass killing of Muslim men in Srebrenica in 1995, violence perpetrated by non-state actors in the DRC in 2002, and one-sided violence perpetrated by the Islamic State in 2014 and 2015.[4]

CAUSES OF WAR

It is often difficult to determine all of the causes and contributing factors of a war, their relative importance, and their interaction. It is generally easier to identify the precipitating factors than the root causes.

Most causes of war involve greed or grievance. They include:

- Attempts to gain political power, territory, security, wealth, or control over resources
- Extreme poverty and socioeconomic inequities
- Militarism and availability of weapons
- Poor governance
- Intergroup animosity
- Environmental stress.

Poverty is strongly associated with civil war. An analysis of 127 civil wars between 1945 and 1999, each of which killed at least 1,000 people, found that low per-capita income was strongly associated with increased likelihood of civil war. Over the course of a decade, a country at the 10th percentile of income (among all countries) had an 18% probability of civil war, a country at the 50th percentile had an 11% probability of civil war, and a country at the 90th percentile had only a 1% probability of civil war. This analysis also found that, after controlling for per-capita income, more religiously or ethnically diverse countries were not more likely to experience civil war.[19]

Intrastate rebellion against a government requires both a motive and opportunities. The motive of grievance may be less of a factor in causing civil wars than opportunities. An analysis of data from 79 large civil conflicts over a 40-year period found that opportunities for rebellion better explained the onset of civil war than objective indicators of grievance. Opportunities included availability of financial support as well as military advantage conferred by a dispersed population.[20]

War may lead to more violence, in the form of intimate partner violence and gang warfare. And it may lead to recurrent armed conflicts because of political or socioeconomic instability, weak or corrupt government, continuing animosity between ethnic or religious groups, and revenge and unresolved issues from previous conflicts.[21] An historical context of peace in a region decreases the risk of future war, but an historical context of war greatly increases the risk of future war.[22]

More than 40 years ago, American political scientist Francis Beer observed that, once violence begins, it can spread exponentially through the susceptible part of the population. In the evolution of both world wars, there was rapid movement from peace to war, partly accelerated by the availability of military forces and weapons.[23]

Time and space patterns of war can sometimes explain which countries participate in war as well as the timing and location of armed conflict. Time and space patterns of war are often similar to the time and space patterns of infectious disease epidemics. If fighting starts in one region, there is a high probability that fighting will start in a nearby region soon afterward. In addition, traits or characteristics of countries that predispose them to war can diffuse to neighboring countries; for example, economic and political instability in one country may extend into a neighboring country.[24] A study in Darfur, Sudan, found that violence in one location increased the probability that violence would break out in a neighboring location within the next month.[25]

Several factors and their interaction can sustain wars. The civil war that took place in Côte d'Ivoire (Ivory Coast) is illustrative. It began with competition for power, but several factors sustained it: inflow of migrants, economic stagnation, high youth unemployment, regional inequalities, disputes over land ownership, resentment between ethnic groups, and availability of coffee and diamonds, which provided financial support for military forces.[26]

Resource wars are fought for control over valuable natural materials, such as oil, water, land, timber, animals or animal products, precious metals, diamonds, and other important minerals. Interstate resource wars occur when a country uses force to acquire land rich in resources, to access a critical resource deposit in another country, or to control a border region that has valuable resource deposits. Intrastate resource wars can occur when armed non-state groups that need more weapons exploit minerals or other natural resources and trade them for weapons. Additional factors that often contribute to the causation of resource wars include attempts to gain or increase power, border disputes, ethnic tensions, and socio-economic inequities.[27]

A frequent cause of or contributing factor to war is *militarism*—"a set of attitudes and social practices which regards war and the preparation for war as a normal and desirable social activity."[28] Militarism is based on the premise that war is an essential—and sometimes even desirable—part of life. It is often associated with large military budgets, which divert human and financial resources from health, social services, and education (Chapter 2). Militarism masks the inherent irrationality of war. It strips young men and women of their civilian identities, indoctrinates them in the concepts and behaviors of fighting, and places them in situations where they must kill others whom they do not know—or possibly be killed.[29]

Militarism can promote a mindset that makes people think that violence is an acceptable method for settling conflicts. Over the course of history, militarism has been normalized in many countries, including the United States, where military concepts are prevalent and military terminology pervades our language. Even in public health and medical care, we *wage war* against cancer and drugs, *target* vulnerable populations, and assign *frontline* workers to *battle* disease.

The military-industrial complex has played a central role in the U.S. economy. Americans were warned about its implications by the Farewell Address of President Dwight Eisenhower in 1961, when he said:

> [The] conjunction of an immense military establishment and a large arms industry
> is new in the American experience. The total influence—economic, political,
> even spiritual—is felt in every city, every state house, every office of the Federal
> government. We recognize the imperative need for this development. Yet we must not
> fail to comprehend its grave implications. . . . In the councils of government, we must

guard against the acquisition of unwarranted influence, whether sought or unsought, by the military-industrial complex. The potential for the disastrous rise of misplaced power exists and will persist. We must never let the weight of this combination endanger our liberties or democratic processes.[30]

Some analysts have observed that, in recent years, the U.S. military-industrial complex has morphed into a "national security state," in which functions of national security are integrated through much of the government. They assert that the national security state receives democratic legitimacy by providing national security and economic prosperity while shielding most Americans from the actual human and financial costs of war. As a result, they contend, there is "a widespread understanding that the proper function of federal government is continuous preparation for war."[31]

At the same time, there has also been increased concentration of ownership of the news media in the United States. Five conglomerates, which are linked directly or indirectly with the military and associated industries, own 90% of the news media. They control most news coverage and political messaging, which give them opportunities to promote perspectives favorable to the military, support deployment of U.S. forces, and disseminate sanitized accounts of war. And they tend not to investigate or air criticisms of the military. As a result, many Americans are not well informed about the military and armed conflict, making it difficult for them to hold the military or government accountable for deployment of U.S. forces, and unable to recognize nonviolent solutions to international disputes or other geopolitical problems.[32]

ROLES OF HEALTH PROFESSIONALS

We health professionals are well qualified and positioned to recognize and help prevent the health impacts of war. We provide healthcare and public health services in war zones, refugee camps, and countries that host war-displaced populations. We educate and raise awareness about the health impacts of war. We perform epidemiological studies and forensic investigations to assess, document, and research the impacts of war on health and human rights. We design, implement, and evaluate preventive measures. We advocate for policies to minimize the health impacts of war and to help prevent war. We promote respect, protection, and fulfillment of human rights. And we convene people and organizations to address the health impacts of war.[33,34] (See Chapter 15 and the profiles in this book of health professionals and the roles that they have played.)

However, the health impacts of war are rarely included in the curricula of schools of public health, medicine, nursing, and other health professions. A survey found that only 2% of more than 6,200 courses in 20 leading schools of public health, during the 2011–2012 academic year, focused on war-related topics and only 0.5% mentioned "war."[35] None of the foundational competencies in the accreditation criteria of the Council on Education for Public Health include war.[36] Relatively few faculty members teach or perform research on the health impacts of war. There are no endowed professorships to support academic work on this subject. There are very few academic journals that focus on war and its health impacts.[36] And a recent PubMed

TABLE 1-1 Numbers of Publications Found in a PubMed Search (on May 13, 2021), by Specific Keywords

Keyword	Number of Publications
Cancer	4,346,219
Heart disease	1,395,141
Diabetes mellitus	523,637
Stroke	369,704
Influenza	140,650
COVID-19	133,632
Armed conflict*	14,719

*The term *armed conflict* was used in this PubMed search instead of the term *war*, a term that is often used to mean something other than *armed conflict*, such as in the phrases "The War on Cancer" and "The War on Drugs."

search revealed that, compared to other major categories of morbidity and mortality, there have been far fewer journal articles on this subject (Table 1-1).

No component of public health practice at the federal, state, or local level in the United States focuses on the health impacts of war. Aside from military hospitals and the Veterans Health Administration, the health impacts of war are not the primary focus of any government health unit. There is no Center on War at the Centers for Disease Control and Prevention. There is no Institute on War at the National Institutes of Health. There is no Interagency Governmental Task Force on the Health Impacts of War. And, even though state and local public health departments serve populations that include people displaced from war-torn countries, military veterans and their families, and many other people who have been physically and psychologically affected by war, few public health departments have programs or even projects that address the health impacts of war.

This book aims to help place the health impacts of war in the mainstream of public health—in education, research, and public health practice. It is designed to improve the recognition of the health impacts of war in the course of healthcare; during rapid assessments, public health surveillance, and epidemiological studies in war zones; and by listening to the voices of people affected by war. It is designed to help prevent the health impacts of war. And it is designed to help prevent war and promote peace.

ORGANIZATION OF THIS BOOK

After this introductory chapter, Part I also includes Chapter 2, which describes the nature of war, focusing on damage to civilian infrastructure (including healthcare facilities), indirect civilian deaths, mass displacement, and diversion of human and financial resources. Part I also includes Chapter 3, which covers human rights, ethics, and international humanitarian law (including international covenants on human rights), Just War Theory, and ethical issues related to health and medical care.

Part II focuses on types of weapons. Chapter 4 describes conventional weapons, such as small arms and antipersonnel landmines, including the health and safety threats that these weapons pose; the international arms trade; and measures to control these weapons. Chapter 5 describes chemical, biological, and nuclear weapons—the history of their use, their adverse health effects, and international conventions and treaties regarding their production, testing, and use.

Part III focuses on major health impacts of war on civilians, the causes of these impacts, findings from illustrative epidemiological studies, and approaches to prevention of specific impacts of war. Chapter 6 describes morbidity and mortality from indiscriminate and targeted attacks on civilians, including gender-based violence and recruitment of child soldiers. Chapter 7 describes malnutrition and communicable diseases, including the epidemiology of these diseases and their long-term consequences. Chapter 8 describes the causes and manifestations of mental disorders and their prevention. Chapter 9 focuses on the adverse effects of war on reproductive health. Chapter 10 describes noncommunicable diseases associated with war, their causes, access to healthcare, and preventive measures. And Chapter 11 discusses populations vulnerable to the health impacts of war, including women, children, displaced people, persons with disabilities, older people, and Indigenous Peoples.

Part IV includes chapters on other impacts of war and their documentation. Chapter 12 focuses on physical and mental disorders of active military personnel and veterans—in whom war-related morbidity and mortality has been studied more intensively than in civilians. Chapter 13 describes environmental impacts of war, including contamination of air, water, and land; emission of greenhouse gases, which cause climate change; and other damage to natural and human-made environments. Chapter 14 focuses on determining the health impacts of war with rapid assessments, public health surveillance, and epidemiological studies as well as forensic investigations.

Part V, which consists of Chapter 15, provides a public health perspective on preventing war, promoting peace, and moving toward a world without war.

During the course of war, the issues addressed in this book are intertwined. Reflecting this interconnectedness, some subjects are discussed in multiple chapters. For example, displaced people are discussed in the chapters that address mass displacement, vulnerable populations, and various categories of health impacts. Agent Orange, a carcinogen-containing defoliant that was used extensively by U.S. forces during the Vietnam War, is discussed in the chapters that address cancer, impacts of war on military personnel and veterans, and impacts on the environment. And landmines are discussed in the chapters that address conventional weapons and assaults and injuries.

The front matter includes on pages xvii and xviii a list of 34 wars cited in the text and their timeframes. Given that civil strife has often occurred before the start and after the end of some wars, there is not complete agreement on some of these timeframes.

Finally, the book also features, independent of specific chapters, profiles of individuals who have played—and are playing—vital roles in addressing the health impacts of war. Although individuals are featured, their work has been primarily as members and leaders of groups and organizations, as is typical for work in medical care and public health. And, as the philosopher Søren Kierkegaard said, "Life can only be understood backwards, but it must be lived forwards."[37] So, while the careers of each of the people profiled are described in retrospect, each of them lived life forwards—one step at a time, not necessarily knowing where the next opportunity would eventually take them.

REASONS FOR HOPE

This book describes many horrors of war. Young men killed. Women assaulted. Children separated from their parents. Hospitals bombed. Health workers attacked. Widespread malnutrition. Disease outbreaks. Psychological trauma. Destruction of communities and cultures. Environmental devastation.

But this book also describes many reasons for hope. The settlement of many disputes without violence. Increasing documentation of the horrors of war. Greater public awareness of gender-based violence, mental disorders, and other health impacts of war. Widespread international support to protect civilians during war. Increasing efforts to respect, protect, and fulfill human rights. New insights into the causes of violence. Greater accountability of individuals who violate international humanitarian law. Improved provision of humanitarian aid to victims of war. The success of older treaties in banning antipersonnel landmines and chemical weapons. The promise of newer treaties to control small arms and nuclear weapons. And an increasing number of people and organizations addressing the health impacts of war and working to prevent war and to promote peace.

SUMMARY POINTS

- War creates much morbidity and mortality and many personal tragedies.
- The number of armed conflicts is at a peak level.
- Health professionals can play vital roles in recognizing and preventing the health impacts of war.
- Yet war is addressed relatively infrequently in education, research, and practice in public health.
- Despite the many horrors of war, there are many reasons for hope.

REFERENCES

1. Institute of Medicine, Committee for the Study of Public Health. The Future of Public Health. Washington, DC: National Academy of Sciences, 1988.
2. Stevens A, Lindberg CA (eds.). New Oxford American Dictionary (3rd edition). Oxford: Oxford University Press, 2010, p. 1947.
3. Davis I. "Tracking Armed Conflicts and Peace Processes" in J Batho, C Brown, F Esparraga, et al. (eds.). SIPRI Yearbook 2020: Armaments, Disarmament and International Security. New York: Oxford University Press, 2020, pp. 29-44.
4. Palik J, Rustad SA, Methi F. Conflict Trends: A Global Overview, 1946-2019 (PRIO Paper 2020). Oslo: Peace Research Institute Oslo, 2020. Available at: https://www.prio.org/utility/DownloadFile.ashx?id=2117&type=publicationfile. Accessed on June 1, 2021.

5. Krug EG, Dahlberg LL, Mercy JA, et al. "Collective Violence" in World Report on Violence and Health. Geneva: World Health Organization, 2002, p. 215. Available at: http://www.who.int/violence_injury_prevention/violence/global_campaign/en/chap8.pdf?ua=1. Accessed on April 9, 2021.

6. Galtung J. Violence, peace, and peace research. Journal of Peace Research 1969; 6: 167-191.

7. Hiller PT. "Structural Violence and War: Global Inequalities, Resources, and Climate Change" in WH Wiist, SK White SK (eds.). Preventing War and Promoting Peace: A Guide for Health Professionals. Cambridge, UK: Cambridge University Press, 2017, pp. 90-102.

8. Tirman T. The Death of Others: The Fate of Civilians in America's Wars. New York: Oxford University Press, 2011.

9. Slim H. Killing Civilians: Method, Madness, and Morality in War. New York: Columbia University Press, 2008.

10. Roberts A. Lives and statistics: Are 90% of war victims civilians? Survival 2010; 52: 115-136.

11. Jawad M, Hone T, Vamos EP, et al. Estimating indirect mortality impact of armed conflict in civilian populations: Panel regression analyses of 193 countries, 1990-2017. BMC Medicine 2020; 18: 266. https://doi.org/10.1186/s12916-020-01708-5

12. Department of Peace and Conflict Research, Uppsala University. Uppsala Conflict Data Program: Charts, Graphs, and Maps. Available at: https://ucdp.uu.se/. Accessed on December 24, 2020.

13. Syrian Observatory for Human Rights. Total death toll: Over 606,000 people killed across Syria since the beginning of the "Syrian Revolution," including 495,000 documented by SOHR. Available at: https://www.syriahr.com/en/217360/. Accessed on July 6, 2021.

14. Jabbour S, Leaning J, Nuwayhid I, et al. 10 years of the Syrian conflict: A time to act and not merely to remember (Comment). Lancet 2021; 397: 1245-1248.

15. Jarland J, Nygård HM, Gates S, et al. Conflict Trends: How Should We Understand Patterns of Recurring Conflict? Oslo: Peace Research Institute Oslo, 2020. Available at: https://www.prio.org/utility/DownloadFile.ashx?id=2051&type=publicationfile. Accessed on June 1, 2021.

16. Kreutz J. Conflict trends: How and when armed conflicts end: Introducing the UCDP Conflict Termination dataset. Journal of Peace Research 2010; 47: 243-250.

17. Braithwaite A, Dasandi N, Hudson D. Does poverty cause conflict? Isolating the causal origins of the conflict trap. Conflict Management and Peace Science 2016; 33: 45-66.

18. Pettersson T, Öberg M. Organized violence, 1989–2019. Journal of Peace Research 2020; 57.

19. Fearon JD, Laitin DD. Ethnicity, insurgency, and civil war. American Political Science Review 2003; 97: 75-90.

20. Collier P, Hoeffler A. Greed and grievance in civil war. Oxford Economic Papers 2004; 56: 563-595.

21. von Einsiedel S. Major Recent Trends in Violent Conflict (Occasional Paper 1). United Nations University Centre for Policy Research, 2014. Available at: https://collections.unu.edu/eserv/UNU:6114/MajorRecentTrendsinViolentConflict.pdf. Accessed on December 21, 2020.

22. Gleditsch KS, Ward MD. War and peace in space and time: The role of democratization. International Studies Quarterly 2000; 44: 1–29.

23. Beer FA. The epidemiology of peace and war. International Studies Quarterly 1979; 23: 45–86.

24. Houweling HW, Siccama JG. The epidemiology of war, 1816–1980. Journal of Conflict Resolution 1985; 29: 641-663.

25. Duursma A, Read R. Modelling violence as disease? Exploring the possibilities of epidemiological analysis for peacekeeping data in Darfur. International Peacekeeping 2017; 24: 733-755.

26. Marc A. Conflict and Violence in the 21st Century: Current Trends as Observed in Empirical Research and Statistics. Washington, DC: World Bank Group, 2016.

27. Klare MT, Levy BS, Sidel VW. The public health implications of resource wars. American Journal of Public Health 2011; 101: 1615-1619. doi: 10.2105/AJPH.2011.300267.

28. Mann M. The roots and contradictions of modern militarism. New Left Review 1987; 162: 35-50.

29. Coulter NA. Militarism: A psychosocial disease. Medicine, Conflict and Survival 1992; 8: 7-17.

30. Eisenhower DD. Farewell Address, January 17, 1961. U. S. National Archives & Records Administration. Available at https://www.ourdocuments.gov/. Accessed on June 1, 2021.

31. Smith DT. From the military-industrial complex to the national security state (review essay). Australian Journal of Political Science 2015; 50: 576-590.

32. Johnson H. Why you should care about the military-industrial-media complex. The Miscellany News, April 15, 2021. Available at: https://miscellanynews.org/2021/04/15/opinions/why-you-should-care-about-the-military-industrial-media-complex/. Accessed on June 4, 2021.

33. Levy BS, Sidel VW. Protecting non-combatant civilians during war (commentary). Medicine, Conflict and Survival 2015; 31: 88-91.

34. Geiger HJ, Cook-Deegan RM. The role of physicians in conflicts and humanitarian crises: Case studies from the field missions of Physicians for Human Rights, 1988 to 1993. Journal of the American Medical Association 1993; 270: 616-620.

35. White SK. Public health and prevention of war: The power of transdisciplinary, transnational collaboration. Medicine, Conflict and Survival 2017; 33: 101-109.

36. Hagopian A. Why isn't war properly framed and funded as a public health problem? Medicine, Conflict and Survival 2017; 33: 92-100.

37. Kierkegaard S, Journalen JJ. Søren Kierkegaards Skrifter. Søren Kierkegaard Research Center, Copenhagen 1997; 18: 306.

Profile 1:
Jennifer Leaning, M.D.
Protecting Human Rights

Jennifer Leaning has made many extraordinary contributions as a witness to human rights violations in war-torn countries, as an educator and researcher on the health impacts of war, as an advocate for human rights, as a contributor to public policy, and as an organizational leader. She has researched and written about the protection of civilians, early warning of humanitarian crises, mass displacement, sexual violence, international humanitarian law, and the public health response to war.

Looking back on her career, Dr. Leaning identifies a few key decision points where she consciously disrupted her career path. She took time off from college after her sophomore year and spent 5 months teaching in Dar es Salaam and then 7 months living and teaching in rural Tanzania. A few years later, in the midst of graduate studies in public health and demography, she volunteered for many nights on an obstetrics ward and, as a result of that intense and uplifting experience, she chose to become a physician. Years later, after completing an internal medicine residency, she chose to become an emergency medicine physician— before there was an established career track in emergency medicine.

She also identifies several times when she chose to take on additional major responsibilities. In addition to her clinical practice of emergency medicine, she became director of emergency services and then medical director of a large community health plan. She co-authored a book on the medical implications of nuclear war and, for more than 10 years, edited the journal *Medicine and Global Survival*. In addition to serving in leadership roles with Physicians for Social Responsibility, she helped establish Physicians for Human Rights and actively participated in its field investigations in war zones and elsewhere. And, while engaged in all these activities, she joined the faculty of the Harvard School of Public Health so she could devote more time to teaching and writing. She ultimately left clinical medicine to devote herself full-time to public health and human rights. And then, at a time when many

From Horror to Hope. Barry S. Levy, Oxford University Press. © Oxford University Press 2022.
DOI: 10.1093/oso/9780197558645.003.0002

people would have chosen to retire, she served, for 9 years, as Director of Harvard's FXB Center for Health and Human Rights, while continuing to teach, write, and advocate.

What has enabled Dr. Leaning to be successful in her work? A key skill in being an effective emergency medicine physician is performing triage to simultaneously manage treatment of many individuals while considering how other emergencies might be prevented. Her mastery of this skill has helped her manage many projects over the past four decades while performing research and advocating for preventing war and preventing violations of human rights. Even more important than management skill has been her deep commitment to this work.

But it is the human connections that have most supported her in her work: the connections with colleagues worldwide, with students she has taught and mentored, and with many victims of humanitarian crises whom she has met. She recalls, for example, a conversation she had 17 years ago at the Sudan–Chad border with survivors of mass killing and gender-based violence in Darfur. Although she did not share a common language or many life experiences with them, there was nevertheless a person-to-person connection, and a sense that they appreciated that someone from far away had cared enough to come and learn firsthand about the suffering that they had endured.

She observes: "I have felt a responsibility to bring a moral vision to situations where moral visions have been shattered, to bear witness to the impacts of war on populations, and to help strengthen norms and measures to protect civilians from the consequences of armed conflict."

Dr. Leaning is Senior Research Fellow at, and a former Director of, the FXB Center for Health and Human Rights, Harvard University, and an Associate Professor of Emergency Medicine, Harvard Medical School.

2

The Nature of War

It is forbidden to kill; therefore all murderers are punished unless they kill in
large numbers and to the sound of trumpets.

VOLTAIRE

INTRODUCTION

This chapter describes the nature of recent wars, focusing on attacks on civilians and
civilian infrastructure (including attacks on healthcare), mass displacement, indirect
deaths, and diversion of resources. Assaults on civilians are described in more detail in
Chapters 4, 5, and 6.

The vast majority of recent wars have been intrastate armed conflicts. They have been
fueled by wide availability of guns and automatic weapons, such as in many civil wars in
Africa; ethnic and religious animosity, such as in recent wars in Iraq and Syria; and military
and financial support from other countries, such as in the Yemeni Civil War.

Many recent wars have occurred in low-income countries, which prior to conflict have
had high levels of abject poverty, malnutrition and communicable diseases, and inadequate
health services. Other wars have occurred in middle-income countries, which prior to conflict had better economic conditions and overall health status than low-income countries.
But populations in both low-income countries and middle-income countries suffer from the
devastating health impacts of war.

Civilians suffer high mortality rates during war (Table 2-1). In some recent wars, most
deaths have occurred among civilians—although the exact percentage has been debated.[1,2]
Civilian mortality rates vary widely between wars and between countries engaged in interstate wars. For example, in the Second World War, the approximate proportion of all war-
related deaths that were deaths of civilians was 100% in Czechoslovakia, 93% in Poland, 50%
in the Soviet Union, 50% in Japan, 39% in China, 22% in the United Kingdom, and 14% in
Germany[3]—and less than 3% in the United States.

From Horror to Hope. Barry S. Levy, Oxford University Press. © Oxford University Press 2022.
DOI: 10.1093/oso/9780197558645.003.0003

TABLE 2-1 Selected Estimates of Numbers of Civilian Deaths in Six Wars

War	Civilian Deaths
First World War	6.8 million (~45% of total deaths)[a,b]
Second World War	46 million,[c] including 15 million Soviet civilians[d]
Korean War	2.9 million Korean civilians (34% of all war-related deaths)[d]
Vietnam War	2.1 million Vietnamese civilians[d,e]
Afghanistan War	More than 71,000 civilians (in the Afghanistan and Pakistan war zone)[f]
Iraq War	405,000 excess deaths (more than 60% of excess deaths were directly attributable to violence)[g] (See Chapter 14.)

[a] Hochschild A. To End All Wars: A Story of Loyalty and Rebellion, 1914-1918. New York: Houghton Mifflin Harcourt Publishing Company, 2011.
[b] White M. Source list and detailed death tolls for the primary megadeaths of the twentieth century. Necrometrics. Available at: http://necrometrics.com/20c5m.htm. Accessed on July 6, 2020.
[c] Ferguson N. The War of the World: Twentieth-Century Conflict and the Descent of the West. New York: Penguin Press, 2006.
[d] Garfield RM, Neugut AI. Epidemiologic analysis of warfare: A historical review. Journal of the American Medical Association 1991; 266: 688-692.
[e] Levy BS, Sidel VW. Adverse health consequences of the Vietnam War. Medicine, Conflict and Survival 2015; 31: 162-170. doi: 10.1080/13623699.2015.1090862.
[f] Costs of War: Afghan Civilians. Watson Institute, Brown University. Available at: https://watson.brown.edu/costsofwar/costs/human/civilians/afghan. Accessed on May 18, 2021.
[g] Hagopian A, Flexman AD, Takaro TK, et al. Mortality in Iraq associated with the 2003-2013 war and occupation: Findings from a national cluster sample survey by the University Collaborative Iraq Mortality Study. PLoS Med 2013; 10: e1001533. doi: 10.1371/journal.pmed.1001533.

ATTACKS ON CIVILIANS

During war, civilians are injured and killed by both indiscriminate and targeted attacks. In many wars, civilians live in constant fear of aerial attacks (Figure 2-1). No matter how precisely aerial bombs are aimed at military targets, there frequently are unintended—but predictable—civilian injuries and deaths.[4] Aerial attacks on military targets in populous areas almost always cause civilian casualties. And military forces sometimes aim weapons at civilian targets by mistake. In urban warfare, military forces frequently deploy improvised explosive devices (roadside bombs), with devastating impacts to civilians.

Children have markedly increased death rates in many wars and their aftermath, partly due to indiscriminate attacks. The under-5 child mortality rate in Iraq more than tripled after the Gulf War began in late 1990; in the first 8 months of 1991, there were more than 46,900 excess deaths among young children.[5] During the next 7 years, many additional excess deaths occurred among young children, largely due to imposition by the UN Security Council of trade sanctions, which restricted import of food and medicine.[6] An analysis based on a logistic regression model indicated a minimum of 100,000 and a more likely estimate of 227,000 excess deaths among young children in Iraq from August 1991 through March 1998; about one-fourth of these deaths were mainly associated with the Gulf War, most of which were primarily associated with sanctions (see below).[7]

Military forces have often targeted civilians, especially women, as a planned strategy of war. When husbands and fathers serve in military forces—or are severely injured or killed during war—women become increasingly vulnerable to physical and sexual assaults.

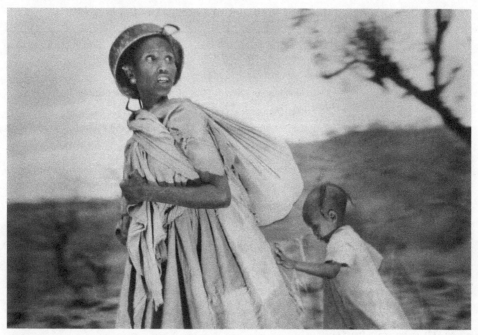

FIGURE 2-1 Woman and her young daughter flee an air attack in Ethiopia in 1985. (Photograph by Sebastião Salgado.)

ATTACKS ON CIVILIAN INFRASTRUCTURE

Military forces have damaged and destroyed homes, workplaces, and vital elements of health-supporting civilian infrastructure, both accidentally and intentionally. These elements of infrastructure have included hospitals and clinics (see below), water treatment plants, farms and food markets, power plants and electrical grids, and transportation and communication networks—with resultant injuries, illnesses, and deaths.

During the Gulf War in Iraq, Coalition military forces bombed water treatment plants and damaged the electric grid, on which the water treatment and supply system was dependent. Backup generators operated for only short periods. The small supply of spare parts was used up and UN economic sanctions for 7 years prohibited or delayed availability of additional spare parts, so much war-related damage was not repaired. Sanctions also severely restricted Iraq's access to technical assistance and water purification chemicals. Eventually, sanctions were lifted, but Iraq recovered only a small fraction of the water service it had before they were imposed. An estimated 90% of Iraqis had access to safe drinking water in 1990, before sanctions were imposed; by 1999, only 41% did (Figure 2-2).[8-11]

In addition to injuring and killing civilians, military attacks damage the economy in other ways. In urban areas, they destroy buildings, roads, electrical grids, and communication systems. In agricultural areas, they destroy farm buildings and irrigation systems, and make farmland unusable with antipersonnel landmines and unexploded ordnance. As a result, less food is grown. Food shortages lead to higher prices, making food less accessible to many people. And malnutrition increases. These conditions often force farmers and their families

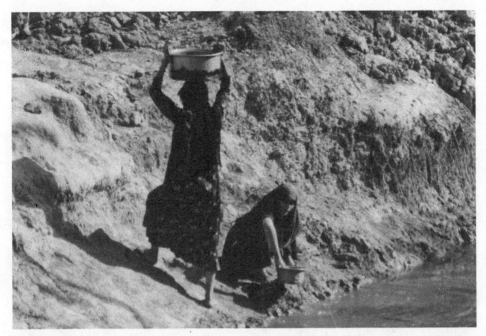

FIGURE 2-2 Two women collecting drinking water from a polluted tributary of the Tigris River near Basra, southern Iraq, August 1991, after the Gulf War. The lack of electricity and wartime damage to the water infrastructure prevented purification and pumping of clean water to most parts of the country. (Photograph by Eric Hoskins.)

to migrate from rural to urban areas—and sometimes to other countries. Unemployment increases, leading to socioeconomic and political instability. (See Chapters 6 and 7.)

Military forces target sociocultural institutions and disrupt the fabric of daily life. This disruption is especially traumatic in cultures where families are interdependent and sociocultural institutions connect people with their values, history, and identity.[12] Persecution of and attacks on leaders of community, academic, and cultural organizations may lead to their being injured, imprisoned, killed, or forced to flee.

War adversely affects the environment. Military vehicles and other equipment powered by fossil fuels emit greenhouse gases, which cause climate change. Military forces contaminate air, water, and land by using weapons that release toxic chemicals, by dumping hazardous materials on land or in water, and by abandoning vehicles and other equipment. (See Chapter 13.)

ATTACKS ON HEALTHCARE FACILITIES AND HEALTH WORKERS

Government forces and armed non-state groups have attacked healthcare facilities and health workers in many ways. They have bombed, shelled, and looted hospitals and clinics. They have assaulted, detained, abducted, tortured, and killed health workers—and patients. And they have obstructed access to care, taken over and occupied healthcare facilities, disrupted public health services, and attacked and blocked humanitarian aid. Despite these clear violations of international humanitarian law, the global community has generally failed to condemn and stop these attacks, and has rarely held perpetrators accountable.[13-15]

In 2019, there were 1,203 reported incidents of violence against or obstruction of healthcare in 20 countries experiencing conflict, including Afghanistan, Burkina Faso, the Democratic Republic of Congo (DRC), Egypt, Libya, Mali, Pakistan, Somalia, and Sudan— almost one-third more than in 2018. In 2019, at least 151 health workers died and 502 were injured in these attacks. Health facilities in at least 19 countries and health transports in at least 14 countries were damaged or destroyed.[16]

Human rights lawyer Leonard Rubenstein, in his book *Perilous Medicine: The Struggle to Protect Health Care from the Violence of War*, presents 12 case studies of health workers who have been attacked while seeking to serve their patients. He reveals how military and political leaders avoid their legal obligations to protect healthcare during war, punish health workers for carrying out their responsibilities to provide care to all people in need, and fail to hold perpetrators accountable. And he describes the lessons that the international community needs to learn in order to protect healthcare workers and civilians during war.[17]

In Afghanistan in 2015, U.S. forces bombed a trauma center hospital operated by Médecins Sans Frontières (MSF, Doctors Without Borders) (Figure 2-3). The attack killed 14 staff members, 24 patients, and four relatives.[18] The destruction of the hospital created a gap in critical healthcare services; in an 18-month period before the bombing, more than 35,000 patients received medical care there, many of them for war-related wounds (Figure 2-4).[19]

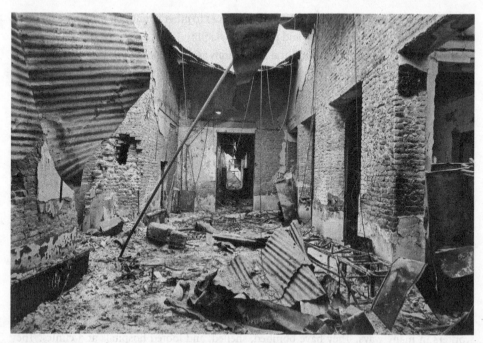

FIGURE 2-3 Iron roofing and rubble litter a corridor in the Médecins Sans Frontières Trauma Center in Kunduz, Afghanistan, after an aerial attack in October 2015. (Photograph by Andrew Quilty. Courtesy of Médecins Sans Frontières.)

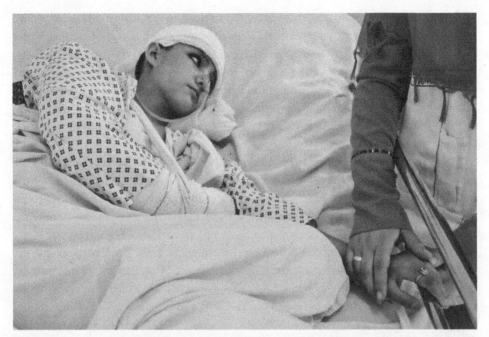

FIGURE 2-4 A 14-year-old girl being treated at the Médecins Sans Frontières Trauma Center in Kunduz, Afghanistan, in May 2015. She had been in her kitchen when a rocket fell on her house and caused the roof to collapse on her. When her family found her body, they thought she was dead. But the villagers realized that she was still breathing and took her to the Trauma Center, where she underwent two operations and was treated in the intensive care unit for 10 days. (Photograph by Matilda Vu. Courtesy of Médecins Sans Frontières.)

In the Yemeni Civil War, since airstrikes began in 2015, many clinics and hospitals have been destroyed. In the first 7 months of the war, 39 hospitals were bombed. Attacks on hospitals, clinics, and ambulances have continued. Blockades of ports of entry have restricted the import of food, essential medicines, vaccines, and healthcare equipment. Healthcare workers have endured major risks to their own safety.[20] Many facilities no longer fully function. In 2018, an estimated 42% of the population lived more than 1 hour by ground travel from the nearest public primary healthcare facility that was at least partially functioning, and almost 40% more than 2 hours from a facility providing comprehensive emergency obstetric and surgical care.[21]

In the Syrian Civil War, Bashar al-Assad government forces have bombed hospitals in an illegal attempt to cut off civilian lifelines and gain military advantage. Since 2012, they have attacked medical facilities in Aleppo, which had been the second largest city in Syria before the war and was a rebel stronghold, often with barrel bombs. The pediatric referral hospital was destroyed in a bomb attack, the largest trauma hospital was closed after three air raids in less than a week, and, by 2016, all hospitals in Aleppo had been damaged. Victims with multiple injuries or severe burns have often been impossible to treat because of damage to healthcare facilities and few remaining specialist physicians. After surgery to treat injuries, serious postoperative infections have often occurred, requiring amputations. And there have been few, if any, rehabilitation services.[22–24]

Syrian government forces have repeatedly targeted health workers. Hundreds have been killed, hundreds more have been incarcerated or tortured, and many have fled. Those who have stayed behind have faced formidable challenges. In Homs, which had been the third largest city in Syria before the civil war, at least 50% left and only three general surgeons remained after 30 months of war. In and around Aleppo in March 2013, only 36 physicians were still practicing, compared with about 5,000 before the start of the war.[25] Most had fled or had been detained or killed. And the absence of healthcare has caused many civilians to flee.[26]

Since the start of the Iraq War in 2003, many health workers have fled the country because they were targeted by militias and gangs—and even by patients and family members. By 2009, 80% of physicians who had been working in emergency hospitals in Iraq had been assaulted by patients or their family members and 35% of them had been directly threatened with a gun.[27]

In addition to health workers, others who have attended to the needs of civilians in the midst of war have been killed and injured. For example, the White Helmets, a volunteer organization operating in parts of opposition-controlled Syria, performed search-and-rescue missions in bombed urban areas, evacuated civilians, and delivered essential services. By early 2018, they had saved more than 100,000 lives. And 252 White Helmet volunteers had died and more than 500 had been injured.[28]

Health workers can be better protected during war by (a) implementing protective mechanisms contained in UN security resolutions to investigate war crimes, to create prosecutable cases, and to establish prosecution by tribunals; (b) applying pressure on parties to the conflict to avoid targeting health workers; (c) collecting and disseminating data on attacks, including data on perpetrators; and (d) strengthening global solidarity to protect health workers during war.[26]

International humanitarian law protects hospitals. In 2011, the UN Security Council passed Resolution 1998 that gave the United Nations authority to publicly identify armed forces and other groups that have attacked hospitals.[29] The United Nations has provided detailed guidance on ending attacks on healthcare during armed conflict.[30]

International organizations can improve assessment of threats to healthcare personnel and facilities by establishing a clearinghouse for information on these threats, creating standard definitions and terminology for reporting attacks, better defining exposed populations, and assessing and publicizing the indirect costs of this violence—such as healthcare workers fleeing, hospitals running out of supplies, and immunization campaigns ending.[31]

MASS DISPLACEMENT

There are three main categories of displaced people: *Refugees* are "people fleeing conflict or persecution"; they "are defined and protected in international law, and must not be expelled or returned to situations where their life and freedom are at risk."[32] *Internally displaced persons* "stay within their own country and remain under the protection of the government, even if that government is the reason for their displacement."[32] *Asylum-seekers* are people "whose request for sanctuary has yet to be processed."[32]

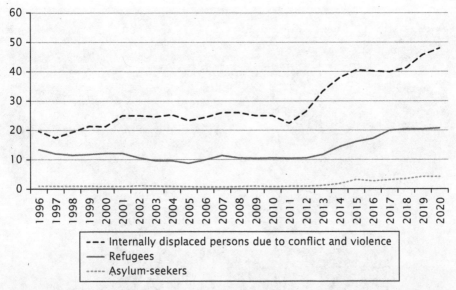

FIGURE 2-5 Millions of internally displaced persons displaced due to conflict and violence, refugees (under UNHCR's mandate), and asylum-seekers, by year, 1996–2020. (*Sources*: UNHCR: The UN Refugee Agency and the Internal Displacement Monitoring Centre. Available at: https://www.unhcr.org/refugee-statistics/. Accessed on January 20, 2022.)

The number of displaced people, most of whom are women and children, has markedly increased since 2012. At the end of 2020, there were 82.4 million people who had been forcibly displaced worldwide: 48.0 million internally displaced persons displaced due to conflict and violence, 20.7 million refugees under UNHCR's mandate, 5.7 million Palestine refugees under UNRWA's mandate, and 4.1 million asylum-seekers. There were also 3.9 million Venezuelans displaced abroad.[33] The numbers of displaced people have markedly increased over the past two decades (Figure 2-5).

The primary causes of displacement are war, civil unrest, persecution, and hunger. In Africa, interstate and intrastate wars, poverty, lack of democratic institutions, and genocides and mass killings have driven much large-scale forced migration (Figure 2-6). The adverse impacts of climate change, especially the effects of heat and drought on agriculture, are displacing many people (Chapter 13).[34]

Before 1990, most refugees had fled from low-income countries, such as Afghanistan, Cambodia, Ethiopia, and Somalia. In the 1990s, many refugees came from middle-income countries, such as Armenia, Georgia, Iraq, Kuwait, and some former Yugoslav republics. Since 2011, there have been major increases in refugees, primarily from war-torn Syria and Yemen—both of which had been middle-income countries.[35] At the end of 2019, most people displaced across borders had come from low- and middle-income countries (LMICs) that had been devastated by intrastate armed conflict, such as in Syria (6.6 million), Afghanistan (2.7 million), and South Sudan (2.2 million).[36]

Most countries to which displaced people have recently migrated have been LMICs, which are often challenged to meet the needs of their own citizens. At the end of 2019, the countries that were hosting the most people displaced across borders

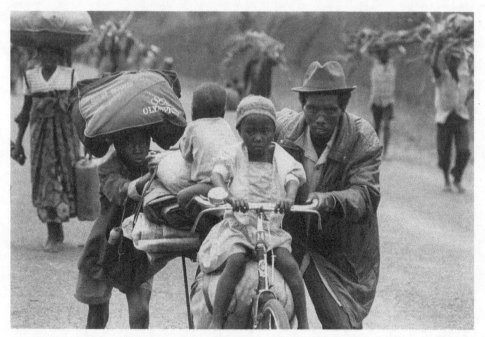

FIGURE 2-6 A family of Rwandan refugees, their bicycle loaded, make their way along the road to the Benaco Camp in the remote Ngara District of Zaire (now the Democratic Republic of the Congo), a day's walk from the river where they crossed from Rwanda in 1994. (© UNICEF/94-0065/Davies.)

were Turkey (3.6 million), Colombia (1.8 million), Pakistan (1.4 million), and Uganda (1.4 million).[36]

Most of the countries with the largest populations of internally displaced persons have been plagued by intrastate conflict. At the end of 2019, the countries that were hosting the largest number of internally displaced persons were Syria (6.5 million), Colombia (5.6 million), the DRC (5.5 million), Yemen (3.6 million), and Afghanistan (3.0 million).[37]

Refugees, who have crossed into other countries, receive assistance from UN agencies, bilateral government aid programs, nongovernmental organizations, and host-country governments; increasingly, they are housed in locations other than refugee camps.[35] People who are internally displaced within their own countries are usually worse off than refugees because they have less security and less access to food, water, shelter, and healthcare than refugees. Internally displaced persons face increased risks of assaults and other injuries, malnutrition, communicable diseases, mental disorders, and other health problems. They are sometimes displaced multiple times or live in protracted displacement. (See Chapter 11.)

Most internally displaced persons are in Africa and the Middle East. In 2020, three countries accounted for more than one-third of those *recently* displaced due to conflict and violence—the DRC with 2.9 million, Syria with 2.4 million, Yemen with 1.7 million. And five other countries (Colombia, Afghanistan, Somalia, Nigeria, and Sudan) each had one million or more recently displaced persons due to conflict and violence.[37]

Internally displaced persons are at especially high risk of dying during war. For example, direct attacks on villages in West Darfur, Sudan, in 2003 displaced many families

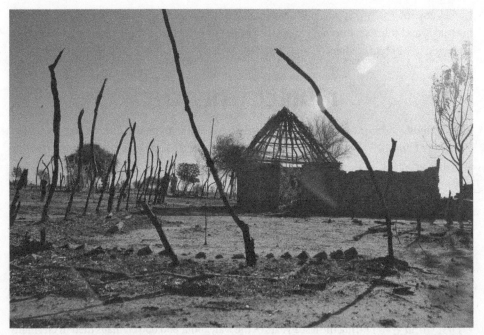

FIGURE 2-7 Remains of village destroyed in 2003 by Janjaweed militia, Darfur, Sudan. (Photograph by Michael Wadleigh [www.gettyimages.org]. Courtesy of Physicians for Human Rights.)

(Figure 2-7). Among the 215,000 internally displaced persons, the daily crude mortality rate was almost 6 per 10,000, with at least two-thirds of deaths caused by violence.[38] The highest death rates are often recorded soon after displaced persons arrive in camps because they have not had adequate food, water, and medical care immediately before and during their migration.

The following situation illustrates the risks that internally displaced persons face:

In 2005 in northern Uganda, after almost two decades of war, about two million people had been internally displaced. In the three districts most affected by violence, almost 90% of the population had relocated to camps. Both the crude mortality rate and the under-5 mortality rate were increased far above emergency thresholds. "Malaria/fever," AIDS, and violence were the most frequently reported causes of death. Persons killed were mostly adult males, but 17% were children under age 15. Between January and July 2005, an estimated 1,168 people were abducted and not returned home, 46% of whom were children. Availability of water was below the minimum standard of 15 liters per person per day.[39]

Children account for about 40% of internally displaced persons.[33] In many countries, internally displaced children lack access to basic services. They are often denied their rights to education, health, protection, and non-discrimination. And they are exposed to many threats and dangers from violence, abuse, and exploitation through child labor and trafficking. Internally displaced girls are at increased risk for sexual assault, abduction, forced marriage, and murder; internally displaced boys are at increased risk for being recruited or abducted to be child soldiers (Chapter 6).[40]

INDIRECT DEATHS

During most wars, more civilians die from the indirect than the direct impacts of war (Chapters 1 and 14). These *indirect deaths* are largely due to damage to civilian infrastructure and displacement, as described above. Health professionals and journalists usually do not recognize or report these deaths as being related to war.

In some wars from which reliable data are available, indirect deaths outnumber direct deaths by more than 15 to 1. The ratio of indirect to direct deaths depends on many factors, including prewar level of development, duration and intensity of combat, access to health services, and effectiveness of humanitarian aid.[41] (Humanitarian aid is discussed in Chapter 11.)

Studies from several wars demonstrate the frequency of indirect deaths among civilians:

- First World War: During the last 2 years of the war, about 800,000 civilians died in Germany due to shortages of medical care, breakdowns of sanitary systems, and war-induced material deprivations. And during the aftermath of the war, more civilians died than during the war, due to nutritional deprivation, crowding, and social disruption—and influenza.
- Angolan and Mozambican civil wars: During these wars, the vast majority of deaths were among civilians. During some years of these wars, for each combat-related death there were up to 14 deaths due to indirect impacts of war.[3]
- Wars in Iraq: During and after three wars in Iraq since 1980, widespread damage to health-care facilities, systems for water treatment and supply, urban infrastructure, and the natural environment caused much morbidity and mortality.[42,43]
- Second Congo War (Civil War in the DRC): During this war, only a small percentage of all deaths were directly caused by violence. Most were due to communicable diseases, malnutrition, pregnancy- and neonatal-related conditions, and other treatable and preventable disorders. The incidence of these diseases increased because of food and water shortages, poor sanitation, disruption of health services, and population displacement. Children were at especially high risk; they constituted 47% of all deaths, although they constituted only 19% of the population. And about 2.1 million of the estimated 5.4 million war-related deaths occurred *after* the formal conclusion of the war.[44,45]
- Darfur Conflict: From 2004 to 2008, there were an estimated 300,000 excess deaths, more than 80% of which were not due to violence. Many were due to diarrheal diseases. Overcrowding, inadequate sanitation, and inadequate health services contributed to the high mortality rate.[46]
- Yemeni Civil War: Attacks on civilian infrastructure have caused much morbidity and mortality. They contributed to a large outbreak of cholera, with 1.2 million cases and more than 3,000 deaths during the first 6 months (Chapter 7).

DIVERSION OF RESOURCES

Maintaining large military forces and fighting wars diverts human and financial resources that could otherwise be used for health and social services, education, and other societal benefits. Global military expenditures were estimated at $1.98 trillion in 2020—the highest annual amount since 1991. This amount was *more than 600 times the $3.07 billion UN budget for 2020.*[47] The $778 billion in U.S. military expenditures was more than 39% of the global total, more expenditures than those of the next 11 countries—China, India, Russia, the United Kingdom, Saudi Arabia, Germany, France, Japan, South Korea, Italy, and Australia—*combined.*[48]

In 1953, U.S. President Dwight D. Eisenhower, who during the Second World War had been Supreme Commander of the Allied Expeditionary Force in Europe, described the consequences of this diversion: "Every gun that is made, every warship launched, every rocket signifies, in the final sense a theft from those who hunger and are not fed, those who are cold and not clothed. This world in arms is not spending money alone. It is spending the sweat of its laborers, the genius of its scientists, the hopes of its children."[49]

The amount of resource diversion varies among countries, as reflected by their ratios of per-capita health expenditures to per-capita military expenditures (Table 2-2). It is noteworthy that, in this analysis, Japan and Germany have, by far, the highest ratios, with Japan spending greater than 11 times and Germany greater than nine times more on health expenditures per capita than military expenditures.

TABLE 2-2 Comparison of Per-Capita Health and Military Expenditures, Selected Countries, 2018

Country	Per-Capita Health Expenditures[a]	Per-Capita Military Expenditures[b]	Ratio of Per-Capita Health to Military Expenditures
Japan	$4,267	$368	11.6
Germany	5,472	597	9.2
Brazil	848	133	6.4
United Kingdom	4,315	752	5.7
United States	10,624	1,983	5.4
France	4,690	952	4.9
South Korea	2,543	835	3.0
China	501	180[c]	2.8[c]
Turkey	390	231	1.7
India	73	49	1.5
Russia	609	425	1.4

[a] The World Bank. Current health expenditure per capita (current US$). Available at: https://data.worldbank.org/indicator/SH.XPD.CHEX.PC.CD. Accessed on June 1, 2021.
[b] Tian N, Fleurant A, Kuimova A, et al. "I. Global developments in military expenditure" in Stockholm International Peace Research Institute. SIPRI Yearbook 2019: Armaments, Disarmament and International Security. Oxford: Oxford University Press, 2019, p. 194; and The World Bank. Population, total. Available at: https://data.worldbank.org/indicator/SP.POP.TOTL. Accessed on June 1, 2021.
[c] Based on estimated military spending for 2018.

Other parameters also reflect diversion of resources for military purposes. For example, the United States ranks first among countries in military expenditures and first in export of conventional weapons, but 35th in life expectancy and 43rd in infant mortality rate.[50,51]

Diversion of resources for a specific war more clearly illustrates the tradeoffs that occur as a result of this diversion. An analysis performed in 2005 found that the first $204 billion allocated by the United States for the Iraq War could have been used to accomplish *all of the following for 3 years*: reduction of world hunger by 50%, provision of a comprehensive global program to address HIV/AIDS, full immunization of all children in "less-developed countries," and meeting all global needs for clean water and sewage treatment.[52]

Countries without military forces do not suffer from this diversion of resources. As of 2018, there were 36 nations and territories that did not have military forces. For some of these countries, international organizations provide for their defense; for others, the national police force acts as the de facto military force.

Costa Rica, which has not had a military since 1948, is an illustrative example. The country has maintained political stability and economic prosperity, even though neighboring countries have been plagued by poverty and violence. By not spending on a military, it has used its resources to improve medical care, education, and its social safety net. The standard of living in Costa Rica is almost double that of other Central American countries, except for Panama, which receives revenues from the Panama Canal.[53] In recent years, Costa Rica has had the third lowest infant mortality rate (8 per 1,000 live births), the third highest adult literacy rate (98%), and the highest life expectancy at birth (80 years) in Central and South America.[54]

SUMMARY POINTS

- Most recent wars have been intrastate conflicts fueled by the availability of guns and automatic weapons, ethnic and religious animosity, and military and financial support from other countries.
- Many wars occur in low-income countries that, prior to armed conflict, were already suffering from abject poverty, high levels of malnutrition and endemic communicable diseases, and inadequate health services.
- In most wars, military forces have attacked civilians and civilian infrastructure, including healthcare, causing much morbidity and mortality as well as mass displacement.
- Indirect deaths account for the vast majority of civilian deaths during war, largely due to damage to the health-supporting infrastructure and to mass displacement.
- War and the preparation for war divert to the military large amounts of human and financial resources.

REFERENCES

1. Aboutanos MB, Baker SP. Wartime civilian injuries: Epidemiology and intervention strategies. Journal of Trauma 1997; 43: 719-726.
2. Roberts A. Lives and statistics: Are 90% of war victims civilians? Survival 2010; 52: 115-136.

3. Garfield RM, Neugut AI. Epidemiologic analysis of warfare: A historical review. Journal of the American Medical Association 1991; 266: 688-692.

4. Crawford NC. Accountability for Killing: Moral Responsibility for Collateral Damage in America's Post-9/11 Wars. New York: Oxford University Press, 2013.

5. Ascherio A, Chase R, Coté T, et al. Effect of the Gulf War on infant and child mortality in Iraq. New England Journal of Medicine 1992; 327: 931-936.

6. Ali MM, Blacker J, Jones G. Annual mortality rates and excess deaths of children under five in Iraq, 1991-98. Population Studies 2003; 57: 217-226.

7. Garfield R. Morbidity and mortality among Iraqi children from 1990 through 1998: Assessing the impact of the Gulf War and economic sanctions. Unpublished paper, 1999. Available at: https://reliefweb.int/sites/reliefweb.int/files/resources/A2E2603E5DC88A4685256825005F211D-garfie17.pdf. Accessed on July 12, 2021.

8. Zolnikov TR. The maladies of water and war: Addressing poor water quality in Iraq. American Journal of Public Health 2013; 103: 980-987. doi: 10.2105/AJPH.2012.301118.

9. Dyer O. Infectious diseases increase in Iraq as public health service deteriorates. British Medical Journal 2004; 329: 940.

10. Center for Economic and Social Rights. The Human Costs of War in Iraq. New York: CESR, 2003.

11. MacQueen G, Nagy T, Santa Barbara J, Raichle C. "Iraq water treatment vulnerabilities": A challenge to public health ethics. Medicine, Conflict and Survival 2004; 20: 109-119.

12. Summerfield D. The social, cultural and political dimensions of contemporary war. Medicine, Conflict and Survival 1997; 13: 3-25.

13. Burnham GM, Lafta R, Doocy S. Doctors leaving 12 tertiary hospitals in Iraq, 2004-2007. Social Science and Medicine 2009; 69: 172-177.

14. Borrie J. Explosive Remnants of War: A Global Survey. London: Landmine Action; 2003, p. 11.

15. Haar RJ, Risco CB, Singh S, et al. Determining the scope of attacks on health in four governorates of Syria in 2016: Results of a field surveillance program. PLoS Medicine 2018; 15: e1002559. doi.org/10.1371/journal.pmed.1002559.

16. Safeguarding Health in Conflict Coalition. Health Workers at Risk: Violence Against Health Care. June 2020. Available at: https://www.safeguardinghealth.org/sites/shcc/files/SHCC2020final.pdf. Accessed on June 26, 2020.

17. Rubenstein L. Perilous Medicine: The Struggle to Protect Health Care from the Violence of War. New York: Columbia University Press, 2021.

18. Shaheen K. Hospitals are now normal targets of war, says Médecins Sans Frontières. The Guardian, June 1, 2006. Available at: https://www.theguardian.com/world/2016/jun/01/hospitals-are-now-normal-targets-of-war-says-medecins-sans-frontieres-adviser. Accessed on April 20, 2020.

19. Hemat H, Shah S, Isaakidis P, et al. Before the bombing: High burden of traumatic injuries in Kunduz Trauma Center, Kunduz, Afghanistan. PLoS One 2017; 12: e0165270. doi: 10.1371/journal.pone.0165270.

20. Mohareb AM, Ivers LC. Disease and famine as weapons of war in Yemen. New England Journal of Medicine 2019; 380: 109-111.

21. Garber K, Fox C, Addalla M, et al. Estimating access to health care in Yemen, a complex humanitarian emergency setting: A descriptive applied geospatial analysis. Lancet Global Health 2020; 8: e1435-e1443.

22. Physicians for Human Rights. Aleppo abandoned: A case study on healthcare in Syria. November 2015. Available at: https://phr.org/wp-content/uploads/2015/11/aleppo-abandoned.pdf. Accessed on April 17, 2020.

23. Dyer O. Hospitals and medical staff are targeted in Syria, as UN report blames regime forces (News). British Medical Journal 2017; 356: 1189. doi: 10.1136/bmj.j1189.

24. Gulland A. Main paediatric centre in Aleppo is destroyed by airstrike (News). British Medical Journal 2016; 353: i2471. doi: 10.1136/bmj.i2471.

25. Assessment Working Group for Northern Syria. Joint Rapid Assessment of Northern Syria—Aleppo City Assessment, March 27, 2013. Available at: https://reliefweb.int/report/syrian-arab-republic/joint-rapid-assessment-northern-syria-aleppo-city-assessment. Accessed on January 30, 2021.

26. Fouad FM, Sparrow A, Tarakji A, et al. Health workers and the weaponisation of health care in Syria: A preliminary inquiry for *The Lancet*-American University of Beirut Commission on Syria. Lancet 2017; 390: 2516-2526.

27. Donaldson RI, Shanovich P, Sheety P, et al. A survey of national physicians working in an active conflict zone: The challenges of emergency medical care in Iraq. Prehospital and Disaster Medicine 2012; 27: 153-161.

28. The White Helmets. Available at: https://www.whitehelmets.org/en/. Accessed on December 10, 2020.

29. United Nations Security Council. Resolution 1998 (2011). Available at: https://digitallibrary.un.org/record/706840?ln=en. Accessed on March 5, 2021.

30. United Nations Office of the Special Representative of the Secretary-General for Children and Armed Conflict. Protect schools + hospitals: Guidance Note on Security Council Resolution 1998. New York: United Nations Secretariat, 2014. Available at: https://childrenandarmedconflict.un.org/publications/AttacksonSchoolsHospitals.pdf. Accessed on April 20, 2020.

31. Jaff D, Singh K, Margolis L. Targeting health care in armed conflicts and emergencies: Is it underestimated? (Commentary). Medicine, Conflict and Survival 2016; 32; 21-29.

32. UNHCR: The UN Refugee Agency. Refugees. Internally Displaced People. Asylum-seekers. Available at: https://www.unhcr.org. Accessed on August 31, 2020.

33. UNHCR: The UN Refugee Agency. Figures at a glance. Available at: https://www.unhcr.org/en-us/figures-at-a-glance.html. Accessed on January 17, 2022.

34. Bayar M, Aral MM. An analysis of large-scale forced migration in Africa. International Journal of Environmental Research and Public Health 2019; 16: 4210. doi: 10.3390/ijerph16214210.

35. Toole M. "Health in Humanitarian Crises" in P Allotey, DD Reidpath (eds.). The Health of Refugees: Public Health Perspectives from Crisis to Settlement. United Kingdom: Oxford University Press, 2019, pp. 54-84.

36. UNHCR: The UN Refugee Agency. Global trends: Forced displacement in 2019. Geneva: UNHCR, 2020. Available at: https://www.unhcr.org/5ee200e37.pdf. Accessed on September 2, 2020.

37. Internal Displacement Monitoring Centre. Global Internal Displacement Database: 2019 Internal Displacement Figures by Country. Available at: https://www.internal-displacement.org/database/displacement-data. Accessed on September 2, 2020.

38. Depoortere E, Checchi F, Broillet F, et al. Violence and mortality in West Darfur, Sudan (2003-04): Epidemiological evidence from four surveys. Lancet 2004; 364: 1315-1320.

39. Ministry of Health, the Republic of Uganda. Health and mortality survey among internally displaced persons in Gulu, Kitgum and Pader districts, northern Uganda. Geneva: World Health Organization, 2005. Available at: https://reliefweb.int/report/uganda/health-and-mortality-survey-among-internally-displaced-persons-gulu-kitgum-and-pader. Accessed on October 29, 2020.

40. United Nations Children's Fund. Lost at Home: The Risks and Challenges for Internally Displaced Children and the Urgent Actions Needed to Protect Them. New York: UNICEF, 2020. Available at: https://www.unicef.org/media/70131/file/Lost-at-home-risks-and-challenges-for-IDP-children-2020.pdf. Accessed on August 26, 2020.

41. "The Many Victims of War: Indirect Conflict Deaths" in Global Burden of Armed Violence 2008, pp. 31-48. Available at: http://www.genevadeclaration.org/fileadmin/docs/GBAV/GBAV08-CH2.pdf. Accessed on July 15, 2020.

42. Levy BS, Sidel VW. Adverse health consequences of the Iraq War. Lancet 2013; 381: 949-958.

43. Lafta RK, Al-Nuaimi MA. War or health: A four-decade armed conflict in Iraq. Medicine, Conflict and Society 2019; 35: 209-226.

44. Coghlan B, Ngoy P, Mulumba F, et al. Mortality in the Democratic Republic of Congo: An Ongoing Crisis. International Rescue Committee. New York: International Rescue Committee; 2007. Available at: https://www.rescue.org/sites/default/files/document/661/2006-7congomortalitysurvey.pdf. Accessed on December 21, 2020.

45. Coghlan B, Brennan RJ, Ngoy P, et al. Mortality in the Democratic Republic of Congo: A nationwide survey. Lancet 2006; 367: 44-51.

46. Degomme O, Guha-Sapir D. Patterns of mortality rates in Darfur conflict. Lancet 2010; 375: 294-300.

47. United Nations. General Assembly approves $3 billion UN budget for 2020. UN News, December 27, 2019. Available at: https://news.un.org/en/story/2019/12/1054431. Accessed on January 10, 2022.

48. da Silva DL, Tian N, Marksteiner A. Trends in World Military Expenditure, 2020 (SIPRI Fact Sheet). SIPRI Military Expenditure Database, Stockholm International Peace Research Institute, April 2021.

49. Eisenhower DD. The Chance for Peace. Address delivered before the American Society of Newspaper Editors, Washington, DC, April 16, 1953. Available at: https://www.eisenhowerlibrary.gov/sites/default/files/file/chance_for_peace.pdf. Accessed on April 24, 2020.

50. Central Intelligence Agency. The World Factbook: Infant Mortality Rate. Available at: https://www.cia.gov/the-world-factbook/field/infant-mortality-rate/country-comparison. Accessed on October 20, 2021.

51. Central Intelligence Agency. The World Factbook: Life Expectancy at Birth. Available at: https://www.cia.gov/the-world-factbook/field/life-expectancy-at-birth/country-comparison. Accessed on October 20, 2021.

52. Bennis P, Leaver E, IPS Iraq Task Force. The Iraq Quagmire: The Mounting Costs of War and the Case for Bringing Home the Troops. Washington, DC: Foreign Policy in Focus, 2005.

53. Trejos A. Why getting rid of Costa Rica's army 70 years ago has been such a success. USA Today, January 5, 2018. Available at: https://www.usatoday.com/story/news/world/2018/01/05/costa-rica-celebrate-70-years-no-army/977107001/. Accessed on December 18, 2020.

54. The World Bank. World Bank Data. Available at: data.worldbank.org/indicator/. Accessed on December 18, 2020.

Profile 2:
Deane Marchbein, M.D.
Providing Medical Care in
War Zones

In 1971, Deane Marchbein was in France, studying French and art history, when Médecins Sans Frontières (MSF, or Doctors Without Borders) was established. Then and for many years afterward, she thought that she might work for MSF someday. And she did.

She became an anesthesiologist and, for 19 years, practiced at Lawrence Community Hospital in Massachusetts, which served a working-class, immigrant community. She had many responsibilities in that position, including performing many types of anesthesiology and serving as director of the intensive care unit. And she recognized that her full-time position there would not enable her to work in other countries for long periods of time. So, in 2005, she changed her work setting to the Cambridge Health Alliance, where her contract enabled her to be away for a 4-month block each year.

For her first MSF assignment, she worked in Côte d'Ivoire (Ivory Coast) as an anesthesiologist and intensive care unit manager at a large community hospital in the midst of a civil war. And, over the next 10 years, Dr. Marchbein worked as part of MSF surgical teams in Nigeria, the Democratic Republic of the Congo (DRC), Libya, South Sudan, Afghanistan, Syria, Haiti, Burundi, and the Central African Republic—often in the midst of armed conflict. Typically, she worked 7 days a week, often with little sleep, and with far fewer available resources than she had in Massachusetts. In Syria, the hospital where she worked had only one operating room and very limited equipment. This contrast was especially striking when she returned from Syria at the time of the Boston Marathon bombing in 2013, as hundreds of healthcare workers and dozens of operating rooms at five nearby trauma centers were available to treat victims.

From Horror to Hope. Barry S. Levy, Oxford University Press. © Oxford University Press 2022.
DOI: 10.1093/oso/9780197558645.003.0004

For the past 4 years, Dr. Marchbein has worked as a project coordinator for MSF, spending 6 to 12 months on a given assignment. In this role, her focus has been on hiring, training, and empowering local health workers, and engaging in community outreach—listening to local people and understanding community priorities.

Some of Dr. Marchbein's most gratifying experiences have involved setting up improved systems for treatment and prevention. After witnessing many preventable maternal deaths in the DRC, she helped to establish a prenatal (antenatal) care unit. And while working in Côte d'Ivoire, she recognized that children with burns were scattered throughout the hospital and were not receiving adequate care. So she set up a six-bed burn unit with limited available supplies, where children received close observation and intensive treatment—and had improved outcomes. Five years later, she was gratified to see that local health workers were continuing to operate the burn unit.

Dr. Marchbein has also brought her expertise and experience to MSF leadership, serving as a member and then President of the board of directors of Médecins Sans Frontières USA and now as an international board member of MSF.

While working in arduous circumstances, her relations with patients and coworkers have kept her energized. She recalls, in Syria, relating to two extensively burned young girls by painting their toenails. She recalls, in Côte d'Ivoire, a boy being treated in the burn unit who, after participating in dance therapy, asked her to dance with him before she left. And she recalls a shy data analyst in Kyrgyzstan, who had managed to complete college on his own after his parents had died, and her helping to support him to prepare for graduate studies in the United States.

What advice does she have for health professionals who may want to do similar work in unstable and potentially dangerous settings? "Develop concrete skills. Make sure you have the fortitude, resilience, and maturity to work in challenging situations. Listen to, train, and empower local health workers. And leave your ego at home."

Dr. Marchbein is a Past President of Médecins Sans Frontières USA and a current member of the international board of MSF.

3

Human Rights, Ethics, and International Humanitarian Law

Peace can only last where human rights are respected, where people are fed,
and where individuals and nations are free.
TENZIN GYATSO, THE 14TH DALAI LAMA

INTRODUCTION

How can civilians be protected during war? Which military practices should be totally
banned? Is cruel punishment or torture of detainees ever justified? What, if anything, consti-
tutes justification for a specific war or war in general? This chapter addresses these and other
questions concerning human rights, ethics, and international humanitarian law as they relate
to war.

HUMAN RIGHTS

Human rights are "norms that aspire to protect people everywhere from severe political,
legal, and social abuses."[1] They include *political and civil rights*, which relate to democracy
and freedom, and *social and economic rights*, which relate to social justice. Human rights
are embodied in international treaties, declarations, and laws, including the United Nations
Charter, the Universal Declaration of Human Rights (UDHR), the International Covenant
on Civil and Political Rights (ICCPR), and the International Covenant on Economic, Social
and Cultural Rights (ICESCR).

The United Nations Charter, which was adopted in 1945, was based on human rights.
Its preamble stated: "We the peoples of the United Nations determined . . . to affirm faith in
fundamental human rights, in the dignity and worth of the human person, in the equal rights
of men and women and of nations large and small." Its purposes included "promoting and
encouraging respect for human rights and for fundamental freedoms for all without distinction as to race, sex, language, or religion."[2]

From Horror to Hope. Barry S. Levy, Oxford University Press. © Oxford University Press 2022.
DOI: 10.1093/oso/9780197558645.003.0005

In 1948, the UN General Assembly adopted the UDHR, which set forth the human rights and fundamental freedoms to which all people are entitled without any discrimination. The United States was among 48 countries that voted in favor of the UDHR. The Declaration proclaims the right to life, liberty, and security of person—essential to the enjoyment of all other rights. It includes other civil and political rights, such as freedom from arbitrary arrest and the right to a fair trial by an independent tribunal. It includes economic, social, and cultural rights, such as the right to equal pay for equal work and the right to a standard of living adequate for health and well-being.[3]

Two additional treaties, which were opened for signature in 1966, built on the UDHR: the ICCPR and the ICESCR. Both covenants prohibit discrimination of any kind regarding race, color, sex, language, religion, political or other opinion, national or social origin, property, birth, or other status. While the UDHR was a declaration of intent, these two additional treaties bind the ratifying parties to comply or suffer consequences. Together, the UDHR, the ICCPR (and its two Optional Protocols), and the ICESCR constitute the International Bill of Human Rights.

The ICCPR attempts to ensure the protection of civil and political rights and to protect basic principles of the rule of law. It requires its parties to respect the civil and political rights of people, including the right to life, freedom of religion, freedom of speech, freedom of assembly, rights to due process and a fair trial, and electoral rights. It includes rights concerning physical integrity, liberty, and security. As of June 2021, the ICCPR had 173 states parties, including the United States; six other countries (states) had signed it but not ratified it. (When a state signs a treaty, it expresses its willingness to continue the treaty-making process and to refrain from acts that would defeat the object and the purpose of the treaty. By ratification, a state "indicates its consent to be bound to a treaty."[4]) The ICCPR binds, under international law, the countries that have ratified it. However, the U.S. government has determined that the ICCPR, which is a non-self-executing treaty that requires legislative implementation before it may be applied by courts, has no legal status in the United States; therefore, in the United States, the ICCPR is generally cited only for its persuasive value and not offered as binding law.

The ICESCR requires that its parties grant economic, social, and cultural rights to people, including:

- Labor rights, such as safe working conditions and the right to form and join trade unions
- The right to education, such as free universal primary education
- The right to health, specifically "the highest attainable standard of physical and mental health"
- The right to an adequate standard of living, with adequate food, clothing, and housing
- Social security, with social insurance.

As of June 2021, the ICESCR had 171 parties; four other countries, including the United States, had signed but not ratified it.

International humanitarian law also includes conventions and treaties that focus on the rights of vulnerable populations, such as women, children, displaced persons, and people with disabilities. These include the UN Convention on the Elimination of All Forms of

Discrimination Against Women, the UN Convention on the Rights of the Child, the UN Convention Relating to the Status of Refugees, and the UN Convention on the Rights of Persons with Disabilities (Chapter 11). In addition, international law includes conventions that address major violations of human rights, such the UN Genocide Convention and the UN Convention against Torture and Other Cruel, Inhuman or Degrading Treatment or Punishment (see later in the chapter).

Despite international law, leaders who have gained power in some countries have ignored or opposed human rights. And in Yemen, Syria, Myanmar, South Sudan, and other countries, military forces have committed atrocities with impunity. These developments have also enabled attacks on healthcare to occur without consequences. None of 25 attacks on hospitals and healthcare workers in 10 countries between 2013 and 2016 led to criminal charges, and most of these attacks have not led to investigations—even though at least 16 may have constituted war crimes.[5] (See Chapter 2.)

PRINCIPLES FOR PROTECTION OF CIVILIANS

This section focuses on justification for war, justified conduct in war, and justice after war.

Justification for War

Can war ever be justified? In limited circumstances, international law provides justification for war. The United Nations Charter addressed this question: "Armed force shall not be used, save in the common interest. . . . All Members shall refrain in their international regulations from the threat or use of force against the territorial integrity or political independence of any state, or in any other manner inconsistent with the Purposes of the United Nations." But the Charter stated that the UN Security Council could authorize use of armed force "to maintain or restore international peace and security" when nonviolent measures were not adequate to address threats to peace, breaches of peace, or acts of aggression. In addition, the Charter specified conditions under which UN member states, individually or collectively, could use armed force in self-defense until the Security Council implemented measures to ensure international peace and security.[2]

Just War Theory, which can be traced to ancient Egypt, Confucian philosophy, a Hindu epic, Aristotle, St. Augustine, and St. Thomas Aquinas, has also addressed this question. It focuses on the justification for war (*jus ad bellum*) and on justified conduct in war (*jus in bello*, see next section). It includes six principles for the justification for war: just cause, legitimate authority (war must be declared by a legitimate authority), right intention (conformity with international law), necessity or last resort, proportionality (anticipated benefits outweigh anticipated harms and destruction), and reasonable probability of success.

Justified Conduct in War

Just War Theory includes three principles for justified conduct in war:

- The *principle of discrimination* (or *distinction*), which concerns the distinction between combatants, who are legitimate targets during war, and noncombatants (civilians), who are not

- The *principle of necessary or minimal force*, which requires combatants to use the minimal amount of force necessary to achieve legitimate military aims and objectives
- The *principle of proportionality*, which addresses the need that anticipated benefits outweigh anticipated costs—that is, the harm caused to civilians and civilian property is not excessive compared to the military advantage anticipated by an attack on a legitimate military objective.

The first international agreements on the protection of civilians during war were developed more than 150 years ago. The First Geneva Convention, which was adopted in 1864, provided that (a) wounded and sick soldiers who were no longer in battle should be humanely treated, (b) all facilities for treating wounded and sick soldiers be immune from capture and destruction, (c) civilians providing aid to wounded and sick soldiers be protected, and (d) the Red Cross symbol be used as a way of identifying people, facilities, and equipment covered by the convention.

The principle of protecting civilians during war was embodied in the Hague Conventions of 1899 and 1907. The 1899 Convention addressed treatment of spies and prisoners of war; prohibition of weapons, arms, and materiel that cause excessive injury; obligation to warn before bombardment; duty to spare hospitals and buildings devoted to religion, arts, and charity; and administration of occupied territory.[6] The 1907 Convention added agreements on the rules of war, collection of debts, rights and obligations of neutral countries, and fines for belligerents who violated regulations.

The League of Nations, which was founded in 1920 with 42 founding members, was the first intergovernmental organization whose main mission was to maintain world peace. Its covenant obligated participating nations to not engage in war and mandated the League of Nations to implement measures to safeguard peace. The League of Nations was successful in helping to bring about nonviolent settlements of some disputes in the 1920s, although there was extensive armed conflict during that decade, including some wars perpetrated by leading countries in the League of Nations. But it was unable to stop aggression by the Axis powers in the 1930s and 1940s. Between 1920 and 1937, an additional 21 countries joined the League of Nations; seven countries left, withdrew, or were expelled by 1946, when it ceased to operate. (The United States never joined the League of Nations.) In 1946, the United Nations was established.[7]

In 1925, a Geneva protocol was adopted that prohibited use in war of asphyxiating, poisonous, or other gases, and of "bacteriological methods of warfare"—an agreement that was the basis for the Biological Weapons Convention five decades later (Chapter 5). In 1929, two additional conventions were adopted: the Second Geneva Convention, which addressed improving the condition of sick, wounded, and shipwrecked members of the armed forces at sea; and the Third Geneva Convention, which addressed treatment of prisoners of war.

In 1949, representatives of 64 countries met in Geneva, where they reviewed, revised, and reaffirmed the three previous Geneva Conventions, the two Hague Conventions, and related documents and adopted the Fourth Geneva Convention, which addressed protection of civilians. In sum, the four Geneva Conventions, which apply only in times of war, were adopted for the purpose of protecting people who had not participated or were no longer participating in war from violence, cruel treatment, torture, humiliation, degrading treatment, and summary execution. In 1977, because wars were increasingly intrastate and asymmetric in nature, two protocols were added as amendments to the Geneva Conventions. They provide additional protection for victims of both international and non-international conflicts.

Because the Geneva Conventions prohibit direct attacks on civilians and indiscriminate attacks in areas where they are present, it is essential to distinguish between civilians and combatants. Combatants include members of military forces; members of guerrilla forces, even those not in uniform; and individuals who take up arms during conflict for reasons other than self-defense.

Civilians include all of the following groups:

- Children (although children have been exploited as child soldiers)
- Older people and sick people
- Soldiers who have been wounded or who have surrendered
- Military personnel clearly identified in civilian roles, such as physicians, nurses, and chaplains
- Individuals whose work sustains a country during war, such as farmers and transportation workers, even though their work supports those who are directly involved in fighting the war
- Citizens of neutral countries, except those performing acts that are incompatible with their neutral status, such as fighting as mercenary soldiers.

Indiscriminate use of conventional weapons, such as in bombing of cities, and use of nuclear weapons are unethical, in part because such use cannot avoid harming civilians.[8] (See Chapters 4, 5, and 6.)

The Geneva Conventions have important implications for military personnel. If a country chooses to wage war in a manner consistent with international humanitarian law, it must instruct its soldiers to avoid injuring civilians whenever possible, train its soldiers in the rules of war, give orders in compliance with the rules of war, and enforce the rules of war and punish anyone who breaches them.[8]

In recent decades, the nature of war has evolved from interstate wars, in which regular armies of two or more countries fight, to intrastate conflicts (including civil wars), which are often fought between the regular army of a country and a rebel group or groups who are not under the control of any country. As has been the case in interstate wars, the principles of Just War Theory have also often been ignored in intrastate wars.[9]

Justice After War

A third broad category of just war principles focuses on the transition of a just war to a just peace, known as *jus post bellum* (justice after war). Its key components are:

- Rights of vindication: The establishment of peace should secure those basic rights whose violation triggered the justified war.

- Proportionality: The settlement of the war should represent measured and reasonable attributes, not revenge.
- Discrimination: Punitive postwar measures should distinguish between leaders, soldiers, and civilians.
- Punishment: People responsible for violations of human rights and international law should be prosecuted.
- Compensation: There should be financial restitution.
- Rehabilitation: Measures should be taken to demilitarize or politically rehabilitate the aggressor country in order to decrease the threat of future conflict.[10,11]

Related Issues

Modern philosophers have analyzed the principles of Just War Theory and found potential inconsistencies and paradoxes, such as the following:

1. If combatants in an unjust war (a war without justification) follow the principles for justified conduct in war, all of their actions during war would be permissible under the principle of *jus in bello*. But the composite of actions by unjust-war combatants would constitute an unjust war—not permissible under the principles of *jus ad bellum*.
2. In this situation, only the political leaders who have instigated the war have done wrong while the combatants bear no responsibility and have not done anything wrong—which could make it easier for governments to start unjust wars.
3. The Just War Theory enables soldiers to believe that they are permitted to kill people who are defending themselves and others from unjust aggression, as long as the victims are wearing uniforms and the killing is done under orders from appropriate authorities.[12]

Political theorist Michael Walzer, in his book *Just and Unjust* Wars,[13] and philosopher Jeff McMahan, in his book *Killing in War*,[14] provide extensive discussion of Just War Theory and its potential inconsistencies and paradoxes.

Another issue concerning just wars involves the distinction between a justifiable *preemptive war*, which is launched on the near-certainty of an imminent attack, and an illegal *preventive war*, which is launched on speculation about what another country might do sometime in the future. A country would be justified to launch a preemptive war if it could justify the war on the basis of self-defense. In contrast, many experts in international law believe that a preventive war, a concept that the United States used to try to justify its invasion and occupation of Iraq in 2003—or it could use to justify an attack on Iran, North Korea, or some other country—is contrary to the principles embodied in the UN Charter.[15]

In his book *Asymmetric Killing*, peace researcher and security policy analyst Neil Renic addresses new ethical issues in the conduct of war that have arisen with the U.S. use of armed drones (unmanned aerial vehicles, or UAVs). Because UAVs are operated from locations far removed from the battlefield, he asserts that this practice challenges existing moral frameworks of war because the UAV operators are not exposed to harm while they kill people thousands of miles away who are suspected of posing security risks to the United States.[16] However, operating UAVs from locations distant from the battlefield does not differ from deploying, from distant locations, cruise missiles or missiles carrying nuclear weapons.

MEDICAL NEUTRALITY

Origins

In 1859, Henry Dunant, a Swiss humanitarian and social activist, organized the Red Cross to provide volunteers to properly care for the sick and wounded during war. In 1863, Francis Lieber, an American jurist and political philosopher, developed a code of laws on armed conflict for the Union army in the Civil War. His code, which became known as the Lieber Code, included directives for generals concerning the release of captured medical personnel and regulations requiring treatment of sick and injured enemy soldiers.

In 1864, the Geneva Conventions established the concept of *medical neutrality*, ensuring that medical personnel are protected during war, and obligating them to care for the sick and wounded, regardless of race, ethnicity, religion, or political affiliation.[17] (Human rights law protects health workers during peacetime.) The term *neutrality* was removed from the Geneva Conventions in 1906 and it was replaced with the obligation *to respect and protect* health facilities and personnel. Although the term *medical neutrality* is still often used, it is a misnomer because both military and civilian health workers cannot be expected to be politically neutral.

Modern-Day Threats

In 2016, the UN Security Council adopted Resolution 2286, reaffirming international humanitarian law and mandating that parties at war respect and protect hospitals and other healthcare facilities, medical and humanitarian personnel, and their transport and equipment.[17] However, unlawful attacks on healthcare professionals and facilities have continued in wars in Syria, Yemen, and elsewhere (Chapter 2). Lack of accountability and the failure to condemn and address attacks like these has led perpetrators to believe that they will not be punished for these attacks.[18]

Mechanisms need to be established to protect healthcare during war and to improve documentation and investigation of attacks on healthcare. Accountability needs to be improved. Academic institutions can help by developing tools to monitor and verify attacks and measures to assess the adverse impact of these attacks on healthcare for affected populations.[19]

GENOCIDE

Origins

The term *genocide* was coined in 1944 by Raphäel Lemkin, a Polish lawyer who organized a campaign to have it recognized as an international crime. In 1946, the UN General Assembly declared that genocide was a crime under international law.[20] Two years later, it adopted the Convention on the Prevention and Punishment of the Crime of Genocide (the Genocide Convention), which entered into force in 1951.[21]

As of June 2021, there were 152 countries, including the United States, that had ratified or acceded to the Genocide Convention. The International Court of Justice has stated that the Convention embodies principles that are recognized as customary international law. Therefore, whether or not a country has ratified the Convention, it is bound, as a matter of law, by the principle that genocide is a crime that is prohibited under international law.[21]

The Convention defined *genocide* as "any of the following [five] acts committed with intent to destroy, in whole or in part, a national, ethnical, racial or religious group, as such:

(a) Killing members of the group;

(b) Causing serious bodily or mental harm to members of the group;

(c) Deliberately inflicting on the group conditions of life calculated to bring about its physical destruction in whole or in part;

(d) Imposing measures intended to prevent births within the group;

(e) Forcibly transferring children of the group to another group."[21]

This definition of genocide has been criticized because it excludes political and social groups from the list of potential victims of genocide. It has also been criticized because it is difficult to establish intent, especially when violence often arises from anonymous—or deliberately obscured—social and economic forces rather than from individuals' decisions, as it often does. American psychologist Ervin Staub and others have offered an alternative definition of genocide: "(T)he attempt to eliminate a whole group of people—a racial, ethnic, religious, or political group—which can involve varied means, ranging from murder to making it impossible for the group to reproduce." He has made a distinction between genocide and mass killing without the aim to eliminate a group, but has noted that mass killing has frequently led to genocide.[22]

States parties' obligations under the Genocide Convention, in addition to not committing genocide, are to prevent genocide, to punish genocide, to enact the necessary legislation to implement the Convention, to try persons charged with genocide in an appropriate court of justice, to grant extradition when genocide charges are involved, and to ensure that effective penalties are given to individuals found guilty of criminal conduct as defined in the Convention. William Schabas, a Canadian specialist in international criminal and human rights law, has suggested that a permanent body be established to monitor the implementation of the Convention and that participating countries issue reports on their compliance with the Convention.[23]

Responsibility to Protect

The *Responsibility to Protect* principle represents the obligation of countries "to protect their own populations from genocide, war crimes, ethnic cleansing and crimes against humanity."[24] It is intended "to narrow the gap between [countries'] pre-existing obligations under international humanitarian and human rights law and the reality faced by populations at risk of genocide, war crimes, ethnic cleansing and crimes against humanity."[24] In 2005, member states of the United Nations affirmed their Responsibility to Protect and agreed to a collective responsibility to assist each other in upholding this commitment. These countries "also declared their preparedness to take timely and decisive action, in accordance with the United Nations Charter and in cooperation with relevant regional organizations, when national authorities manifestly fail to protect their populations."[24]

The Responsibility to Protect principle offers opportunities for UN agencies to assist countries in preventing the listed crimes and violations and in protecting affected populations through early warning, capacity building, and other preventive and protective measures rather than waiting to respond if they should fail to prevent these crimes and violations. Since 2005, the UN Secretary-General has acted on this principle and guided its implementation. UN member states have regularly considered implementing the principle during meetings, and the Responsibility to Protect principle has been often referenced and reaffirmed in relevant UN resolutions.[24]

Military Intervention

Before 2005, there was considerable debate as to whether the United Nations and individual countries were authorized to intervene militarily when a government was perpetrating or permitting genocide or other life-threatening injustice against its own citizens. Nevertheless, in 1971, India militarily intervened in the Bangladesh genocide, and, in 1979, Vietnam militarily intervened in the genocide in Cambodia.

The United Nations has also permitted armed forces and others to intervene in extraordinary humanitarian emergencies. The UN Security Council approved intervention on humanitarian grounds in the civil conflict in Libya. But the United Nations and several high-income countries have been criticized for not intervening in the Rwandan genocide. And the United States and other countries have been criticized for not intervening during a number of genocides, including the Holocaust (Chapter 6).[25]

Short of military invasion and direct attacks on a regime's authority, a variety of coercive measures theoretically could be used to stop genocide. These measures include controlling transportation routes and borders; reinforcing peace operations; enforcing "no-fly zones," safe havens, and arms embargoes; jamming broadcasts and other communications; carrying out precisely targeted strikes; and "demonstrating presence."[26] Another measure that could be implemented is targeting the assets of the elite members of a regime.

Criminal Responsibility for Genocide

In 1993 and 1994, two ad hoc international courts (also known as tribunals) were established by the UN Security Council to try those indicted for genocide, crimes against humanity, and war crimes in the former Yugoslavia and Rwanda. Both of these courts were moderately successful in obtaining prosecutions. Both tribunals clarified the criteria for establishing criminal responsibility for genocide. The Rwanda tribunal stated that genocide included "subjecting a group of people to a subsistence diet, systematic expulsion from homes and the reduction of essential medical services below minimum requirement." The tribunal also ruled that "rape and sexual violence constitute genocide . . . as long as they were committed with the specific intent to destroy, in whole or in part, a particular group, targeted as such." The Yugoslav tribunal ruled that genocidal intent can be manifest in the persecution of small groups of people as well as large ones.

In 1998, the Rome Statute of the International Criminal Court (ICC) was adopted by 120 countries and entered into force in 2002. The Rome Statute gave the ICC jurisdiction for the crime of genocide, crimes against humanity, and war crimes.[27] The United States opposed establishing the ICC and refused to accept its jurisdiction when it was established. The opposition by the United States reflects its emphasis on sovereignty and also accounts for its refusal to ratify the ICESCR and United Nations conventions concerning the rights of children, people with disabilities, and other matters—although the United States *did* ratify the Convention Against Torture (see below).

TORTURE

International Law

Torture and other forms of cruel, inhuman, or degrading treatment or punishment are extreme violations of human rights (Chapter 6). In 1984, the UN General Assembly adopted the Convention against Torture and Other Cruel, Inhuman, or Degrading Treatment or Punishment (the Convention Against Torture), which entered into force in 1987. As of June 2021, the Convention had 171 states parties, including the United States; five other countries had signed but not ratified it. The Convention defined *torture* as "any act by which severe pain or suffering, whether physical or mental, is intentionally inflicted on a person," for such purposes as obtaining information or a confession, punishment for an act committed or suspected of having been committed, intimidation or coercion, or discrimination, "when such pain or suffering is inflicted by or at the instigation of or with the consent or acquiescence of a public official or other person acting in a public capacity."

The Convention stated that each party to it must "take effective legislative, administrative, judicial or other measures to prevent acts of torture in any territory under its jurisdiction." It did not allow for any exceptions.[28] Preventing torture depends on making countries and individuals accountable by implementing civil, criminal, and administrative laws and regulations.[29]

The Convention Against Torture compels states parties to investigate all allegations of torture, to bring to justice the perpetrators, and to provide a remedy for tortured victims. Because the United States ratified it, the Convention applies to all U.S. actions, both inside and outside the country—including government actions in all prisons and jails and in all police departments and other state and local law-enforcement agencies. It also applies to private contractors who perform government functions.

The Committee Against Torture, comprising 10 independent experts, monitors implementation of the Convention. Countries that have ratified the Convention must report to the Committee every 4 years. Domestic human-rights organizations and other nongovernmental organizations (NGOs) are encouraged to participate whenever the Committee considers a country's compliance with the Convention. The Committee relies partly on information provided by NGOs in assessing the validity and completeness of information submitted by the government in its report.

Participation in Torture by Health Professionals

In violation of their ethical and legal obligations, physicians and other health professionals have sometimes participated in torture. Health professionals and lawyers working together after 9/11 played a critical role in designing, justifying, and carrying out the U.S. state-sponsored torture program in the CIA "Black Sites" and U.S. military detention centers, including in Iraq, Afghanistan, and Guantanamo Bay, Cuba. Analysts have compared this role by health professionals to the roles of Nazi physicians used by the Third Reich. In both situations, health professionals discarded their ethical obligation to prevent harm to people and instead became agents of the state. In 2009, the Obama administration released memoranda that further detailed the critical role of medical personnel in the CIA torture program. It likely would have been difficult for the United States to carry out the torture program without the collusion of health professionals and lawyers, who looked to the approval of the Department of Justice to approve torture. In 2014, the Executive Summary of the U.S. Senate Select Committee on Intelligence Report on Torture provided a detailed account of the critical role that medical professionals, working with lawyers, served to implement the torture program.[30]

Forensic medicine, which deals with applying medical knowledge to establish facts in civil or criminal legal cases, can be a constraint against torture by confirming information regarding the use of torture and by making those responsible accountable. Military forces generally do not perform forensic investigations. Alleged perpetrators of lethal torture often go unprosecuted.[31]

However, Physicians for Human Rights and some other organizations have performed forensic investigations of alleged cases of torture. These investigations have included examinations of torture survivors and bodies of deceased persons, systematic interviews of witnesses, and other methods.[32-34] The Istanbul Protocol, published by the United Nations, is a manual to guide investigation and documentation of torture and other cruel, inhuman, or degrading treatment or punishment.[33] An updated edition is scheduled for publication in 2022. (See Profile 3 and the section on Forensic Investigations in Chapter 14.)

Several national and international organizations of healthcare providers have established rules concerning human rights violations and healthcare in specific types of situations. The Code of Medical Ethics of the American Medical Association states: "Physicians must oppose and must not participate in torture for any reason."[35] The American Public Health Association, in a policy statement, has condemned the cooperation of health professionals in the physical and medical abuse and torture of military prisoners and detainees.[36] And the Declaration of Tokyo of the World Medical Association strictly forbids physicians to use medical knowledge in the service of torture or to allow the continuation of torture.[37]

ENFORCED DISAPPEARANCE

An *enforced disappearance*, also known as a forced disappearance, has been defined as

> the arrest, detention, abduction or any other form of deprivation of liberty by agents of the State or by persons or groups of persons acting with the authorization, support

or acquiescence of the State, followed by a refusal to acknowledge the deprivation of liberty or by concealment of the fate or whereabouts of the disappeared persons, which places such a person outside the protection of the law.

In 2020, the Working Group on Enforced or Involuntary Disappearances of the United Nations Commission on Human Rights reported 58,606 cases of enforced or involuntary disappearances since 1980, affecting 109 countries, many of which were engaged in intrastate conflicts. The countries with the largest numbers of missing persons were Iraq (16,571) and Sri Lanka (12,708), followed by Argentina, Algeria, Guatemala, Peru, El Salvador, Colombia, and Pakistan.[38]

In 2006, the United Nations adopted the Declaration on the Protection of All Persons from Enforced Disappearance, and later adopted a convention on this subject. The Declaration stated: "Any act of enforced disappearance is an offence to human dignity. It is condemned as a denial of the purposes of the Charter of the United Nations and as a grave and flagrant violation of the human rights and fundamental freedoms" stated in the UDHR and various international conventions and treaties.[39]

MORAL AND ETHICAL DILEMMAS

Health professionals and humanitarian relief workers as well as the organizations for which they work are often faced with *moral dilemmas*—"situations in which each possible course of action breaches some otherwise binding moral principles."[40] These dilemmas arise when moral principles conflict, forcing a choice between two seemingly necessary actions. In addition, they can be faced with tough choices, such as choosing between speaking out against human rights abuses or continuing to manage a humanitarian relief program in silence.[41]

An army that captures enemy soldiers or others is responsible for providing them with impartial medical care. Healthcare workers must protect the health of captured persons and provide treatment with the same standards as they do in treating others. They must not do any of the following:

- Participate in torture—or be complicit in, incite to, or attempt to commit torture—or other cruel, inhuman, or degrading treatment or punishment
- Assist in interrogating captured persons in a manner that may adversely affect their physical or mental health
- Participate in any procedure for restraining a captured person unless such a procedure is necessary for the protection of the physical or mental health or the safety of captured persons and their guardians
- Participate in or cooperate with torture or cruel, inhuman, or degrading treatment or punishment.

They must limit their professional relationships with captured persons to evaluating, protecting, and improving the physical and mental health of captured persons. And they must report all violations of human rights to appropriate authorities.[42,43]

Military physicians face "dual-loyalty" dilemmas from the urgent needs and demands of war, the necessity to conserve troop strength, and the moral requirements of treating enemy civilians and prisoners of war. They face an additional potential conflict between traditional medical ethics, in which physicians' primary loyalties are directed to the sick and the wounded, and the ethics of the U.S. military, which mandates obedience to orders, loyalty to fellow soldiers and one's country, and honor and integrity.[44,45] In addition, they sometimes have been restricted from providing care for civilians (including those of the adversary) and punished for treating enemy soldiers and not giving preferential access to treatment for personnel in their own military units.

Military physicians also face dilemmas concerning confidentiality and other issues: Is knowledge of a soldier's HIV infection or drug abuse to be reported for "the good of the service" when it may result in discharge of the soldier? Should soldiers receive, against their wishes, vaccinations and/or medications not approved by the U.S. Food and Drug Administration? Should physicians participate in research involving chemical, biological, or nuclear warfare?[44,45]

In some situations, punitive actions have been taken against healthcare workers because of their provision of healthcare. In violation of international human rights law and international humanitarian law, healthcare workers have been harassed, arrested, and prosecuted for providing healthcare to those in need. In some countries, laws that criminalize support for "terrorists" and others who oppose the national government are applied to healthcare providers in an inappropriate manner, designating healthcare as a prohibited form of support to the "enemy" and designating as criminals individuals who provide healthcare. In some countries, general laws have been implemented to punish healthcare workers, stating reasons unrelated to the provision of healthcare (such as spreading false news or assembling illegally)—although the actual reasons for punishing them is their provision of healthcare to people opposing the national government. And in some situations, healthcare workers have faced suspension or other administrative sanctions, intimidation, or harassment for fulfilling their responsibility of providing healthcare.[46] (See Chapter 2.)

ETHICAL ISSUES IN RESEARCH

There are many ethical issues concerning research performed on war-affected populations. Ethical issues include obtaining informed consent, ensuring anonymity and confidentiality of data, ensuring accountability of researchers, and protecting subjects from exploitation, abuse, and other harms.[47,48] Researchers, funding agencies, institutional review boards, international relief organizations, and journal editors need to be responsible for inadequacies in adherence to these standards—and for improving ethical conduct of research in these settings.[49]

Ethical lapses in research on war-affected populations occur frequently. For example, a scoping review of research performed on refugees and war-affected populations in the Arab world found that only 48% of research publications reported institutional approval and only 54% reported informed consent/assent from research participants.[49] Another study found that during the armed conflict in Darfur, only 13% of research projects obtained institutional approval and only 43% obtained informed consent from participants. These findings may be due, in part, to exemptions from ethical review, assumptions that ethical review had been granted, and pre-approval of research protocols.[50] However, these findings should lead to improved oversight of research on populations affected by war.

CONSCIENTIOUS OBJECTION TO MILITARY SERVICE

A *conscientious objector* is a person who claims the right to refuse to perform military service based on freedom of thought, conscience, or religion. Conscientious objection to military service is based on the right to freedom of thought, conscience, and religion as stated in the UDHR and the ICCPR. Article 18 of the UDHR states: "Everyone has a right to freedom of thought, conscience and religion; this right includes freedom to change his religion or belief, and freedom, either alone or in community with others and in public or private, to manifest his religion or belief in teaching, practice, worship and observance."[3,51] Article 18 of the ICCPR contains similar wording.

The United States legally recognizes conscientious objection only for religious and moral reasons. It provides noncombatant service in the military or civilian service as alternatives.[52] During the Vietnam War, 170,000 applicants received conscientious objections deferments, and as many as 300,000 other applicants were denied deferment.

Over the course of U.S. history, many conscientious objectors have been imprisoned or punished in other ways. Journalist Chris Lombardi, in her book *I Ain't Marching Anymore*, provides a detailed account of soldier dissent from 1754 to 2020.[53]

SUMMARY POINTS

- Human rights relate to democracy, freedom, and social justice.
- Just war principles address justification for war, justified conduct in war, and justice after war.
- In times of war, the Geneva Conventions protect people who have not participated or are no longer participating in war.
- International humanitarian law addresses genocide, torture, and enforced disappearance and supports medical neutrality during war.
- The Responsibility to Protect principle obligates countries to protect their populations from genocide, war crimes, and crimes against humanity.

REFERENCES

1. Nickel J. "Human rights" in EN Zalta, U Nodelman, C Allen, et al. (eds.). Stanford Encyclopedia of Philosophy (revised 2019). Available at: https://plato.stanford.edu/entries/rights-human/. Accessed on December 26, 2020.

2. United Nations. United Nations Charter (full text). Available at: https://www.un.org/en/sections/un-charter/un-charter-full-text/. Accessed July 14, 2020.
3. United Nations. Universal Declaration of Human Rights. Available at: https://www.un.org/en/universal-declaration-human-rights/. Accessed on July 14, 2020.
4. United Nations. What is the difference between signing, ratification and accession of UN treaties? Dag Hammarskjöld Library. Available at: https://ask.un.org/faq/14594. Accessed on March 29, 2021.
5. Lohman D. Retreat from human rights and adverse consequences for health. Journal of the American Medical Association 2018; 319: 861–862.
6. Convention (II) with Respect to the Laws and Customs of War on Land and Its Annex: Regulations Concerning the Laws and Customs of War on Land. The Hague, July 29, 1899. Available at: https://ihl-databases.icrc.org/ihl/INTRO/150?OpenDocument. Accessed on July 14, 2020.
7. Covenant of the League of Nations. Available at: http://avalon.law.yale.edu/20th_century/leagcov.asp. Accessed on July 14, 2020.
8. British Broadcasting Company. In an Ethical War, Whom Can You fight? Available at: http://www.bbc.co.uk/ethics/war/just/whom_1.shtml. Accessed on June 10, 2020.
9. McMahan J. Rethinking the "Just War," Part I. New York Times, November 11, 2012. Available at: https://opinionator.blogs.nytimes.com/2012/11/11/rethinking-the-just-war-part-1/. Accessed on July 11, 2020.
10. Orend B. *Jus Post Bellum*: The perspective of a just-war theorist. Leiden Journal of International Law 2007; 20: 571-591.
11. Bass GJ. Jus post bellum. Philosophy & Public Affairs 2004; 32: 384-412.
12. McMahan J. Rethinking the "Just War," Part II. New York Times, November 12, 2012. Available at: https://opinionator.blogs.nytimes.com/2012/11/12/rethinking-the-just-war-part-2/. Accessed on July 11, 2020.
13. Walzer M. Just and Unjust Wars: A Moral Argument with Historical Illustrations (5th edition). New York: Basic Books, 2015.
14. McMahan J. Killing in War. Oxford: Oxford University Press, 2009.
15. Weiss P. "International law" in BS Levy, VW Sidel (eds.). War and Public Health (2nd edition). New York: Oxford University Press, 2008, pp. 357–368.
16. Renic NC. Asymmetric Killing: Risk Avoidance, Just War, and the Warrior Ethos. Oxford: Oxford University Press, 2020.
17. Gross ML. Bioethics and Armed Conflict: Moral Dilemmas of Medicine and War. Cambridge, MA: MIT Press, 2006.
18. Crawford NC. Accountability for Killing: Moral Responsibility for Collateral Damage in America's Post-9/11 Wars. New York: Oxford University Press, 2013.
19. Taylor GP, Castro I, Rebergen C, et al. Protecting health care in armed conflict: Action towards accountability (correspondence). Lancet 2018; 391: 1477-1478.
20. United Nations General Assembly Resolution 1946. 96 (I): The Crime of Genocide. December 11, 1946. Available at: http://www.armenian-genocide.org/Affirmation.227/current_category.6/affirmation_detail.html. Accessed on July 14, 2020.
21. Office of the High Commissioner, United Nations Human Rights. Convention on the Prevention and Punishment of the Crime of Genocide, December 9, 1948. Available at: https://www.ohchr.org/en/professionalinterest/pages/crimeofgenocide.aspx. Accessed on June 30, 2021.
22. Staub E. Building a peaceful society: Origins, prevention, and reconciliation after genocide and other group violence. American Psychologist 2013; 68: 576-589.
23. Schabas W. War Crimes and Human Rights: Essays on the Death Penalty, Justice and Accountability. London: Cameron May, 2008.
24. United Nations Office on Genocide Prevention and the Responsibility to Protect. Responsibility to Protect. Available at: https://www.un.org/en/genocideprevention/about-responsibility-to-protect.shtml. Accessed on February 25, 2021.
25. Power S. "A Problem from Hell": America and the Age of Genocide. New York: Basic Books, 2002.
26. Waxman MC. Intervention to Stop Genocide and Mass Atrocities: International Norms and U.S. Policy (Council Special Report No. 49). Washington, DC: Council on Foreign Relations, 2009.

Available at: https://www.cfr.org/report/intervention-stop-genocide-and-mass-atrocities. Accessed on December 11, 2020.

27. Totten S, Bartrop PR. The United Nations and genocide: Prevention, intervention, and prosecution. Human Rights Review 2004; 5: 8-31.

28. Office of the High Commissioner, United Nations Human Rights. Convention against Torture and Other Cruel, Inhuman or Degrading Treatment or Punishment. Available at: https://www.ohchr.org/en/professionalinterest/pages/cat.aspx. Accessed on December 21, 2020.

29. Rubenstein LS, Iacopino V. "Preventing Torture" in BS Levy (ed.). Social Injustice and Public Health (3rd edition). New York: Oxford University Press, 2019, p. 567.

30. Crosby SS, Benavidez G. From Nuremberg to Guantanamo Bay: Uses of physicians in the War on Terror. American Journal of Public Health 2018; 108: 36-41.

31. Miles SH. Medical investigations of homicides of prisoners of war in Iraq and Afghanistan. Medscape General Medicine 2005; 7: 4.

32. Physicians for Human Rights. Torture. Available at: https://phr.org/issues/torture/. Accessed on May 14, 2021.

33. Office of the United Nations High Commissioner for Human Rights. Istanbul Protocol: Manual on the Effective Investigation and Documentation of Torture and other Cruel, Inhuman or Degrading Treatment or Punishment. New York and Geneva: United Nations, 2004. Available at: https://www.ohchr.org/documents/publications/training8rev1en.pdf. Accessed on May 14, 2021.

34. Iacopino V, Frank MW, Bauer HM, et al. A population-based assessment of human rights abuses committed against ethnic Albanian refugees from Kosovo. American Journal of Public Health 2001; 91: 2013-2018.

35. American Medical Association. Torture: Code of Medical Ethics Opinion 9.7.5. Available at: https://www.ama-assn.org/delivering-care/ethics/torture. Accessed on January 16, 2021.

36. American Public Health Association. Condemning the Cooperation of Health Professional Personnel in Physical and Mental Abuse and Torture of Military Prisoners and Detainees (Policy Number 20051), December 14, 2005. Available at: https://www.apha.org/policies-and-advocacy/public-health-policy-statements/policy-database/2014/07/30/12/59/condemning-health-prof-personnel-in-physical-mental-abuse-torture-of-military-prisoners-detainees. Accessed on January 16, 2021.

37. World Medical Association. WMA Declaration of Tokyo—Guidelines for Physicians Concerning Torture and Other Cruel, Inhuman or Degrading Treatment or Punishment in Relation to Detention and Imprisonment, Tokyo, 1975; Revised Taipei, 2016. Available at: https://www.wma.net/policies-post/wma-declaration-of-tokyo-guidelines-for-physicians-concerning-torture-and-other-cruel-inhuman-or-degrading-treatment-or-punishment-in-relation-to-detention-and-imprisonment/. Accessed on January 23, 2021.

38. Human Rights Council, United Nations General Assembly. Enforced or Involuntary Disappearances: Report of the Working Group on Enforced or Involuntary Disappearances. August 7, 2020. Available at: https://undocs.org/A/HRC/45/13. Accessed on December 14, 2020.

39. Office of the High Commissioner, United Nations Human Rights. Declaration on the Protection of all Persons from Enforced Disappearance. Adopted by General Assembly Resolution 47/133, December 18, 1992. Available at: https://www.ohchr.org/en/professionalinterest/pages/enforceddisappearance.aspx. Accessed on December 14, 2020.

40. Blackburn S. The Oxford Dictionary of Philosophy. Oxford: Oxford University Press, 1994. Available at: https://www.oxfordreference.com/view/10.1093/acref/9780199541430.001.0001/acref-9780199541430-e-2073. Accessed on December 29, 2020.

41. Slim H. Doing the right thing: Relief agencies, moral dilemmas and moral responsibility in political emergencies and war. Disasters 1997; 21: 244-257.

42. Simpson RG, Wilson D, Tuck JJ. Medical management of captured persons. Journal of the Royal Army of Medical Corps 2014; 160: 4-8.

43. London L, Rubenstein LS, Baldwin-Ragaven L, van Es A. Dual loyalty among military health professionals: Human rights and ethics in times of armed conflict. Cambridge Quarterly of Healthcare Ethics 2006; 15: 381-391.

44. Sidel VW, Levy BS. "Physician-Soldier: A Moral Dilemma?" in TE Beam, LR Sparacino (eds.). Military Medical Ethics: Volume 1 (Textbooks of Military Medicine). Falls Church, VA: Office of the Surgeon General, United States Army; Washington, DC: Borden Institute, Walter Reed Army Medical Center; and Bethesda, MD: Uniformed Services University of the Health Sciences, 2003, pp. 293–312.

45. Pellegrino ED. Societal duty and moral complicity: The physician's dilemma of divided loyalty. International Journal of Law and Psychiatry 1993; 16: 371-391.

46. Buissonniere M, Woznick S, Rubenstein L. The Criminalization of Healthcare. Safeguarding Health in Conflict, the Center for Public Health and Human Rights at the Johns Hopkins Bloomberg School of Public Health, and the University of Essex, June 2018. Available at: https://www1.essex.ac.uk/hrc/documents/54198-criminalization-of-healthcare-web.pdf. Accessed on March 5, 2021.

47. Wood EJ. The ethical challenges of field research in conflict zones. Qualitative Sociology 2006; 29: 373-386.

48. Boyden J. Conducting research with war-affected and displaced children: Ethics and methods. Cultural Survival Quarterly Magazine, June 2000. Available at: https://www.culturalsurvival.org/publications/cultural-survival-quarterly/conducting-research-war-affected-and-displaced-children. Accessed on July 10, 2021.

49. Makhoul J, Chehab RF, Shaito Z, Sibai AM. A scoping review of reporting "Ethical Research Practices" in research conducted among refugees and war-affected populations in the Arab world. BMC Medical Ethics 2018; 19: 36. doi: 10.1186/s12910-018-0277-2.

50. Hussein G, Elmusharaf K. Mention of ethical review and informed consent in the reports of research undertaken during the armed conflict in Darfur (2004–2012): A systematic review. BMC Medical Ethics 2019; 20: 40. doi: 10.1186/s12910-019-0377-7.

51. Office of the High Commissioner, United Nations Human Rights. Conscientious Objection to Military Service. New York and Geneva: United Nations, 2012.

52. Selective Service System. Conscientious Objectors. Available at: https://www.sss.gov/conscientious-objectors/. Accessed on July 14, 2020.

53. Lombardi C. I Ain't Marching Anymore: Dissenters, Deserters, and Objectors to America's Wars. New York: New Press, 2020.

Profile 3:
Vincent Iacopino, M.D., Ph.D.
Investigating Torture

When Vincent Iacopino spent 2 months during his final year in medical school working at a refugee camp in Thailand, he did not anticipate what a profound impact that experience would have on his future career. He liked being engaged in international humanitarian assistance for refugees. He enjoyed the challenges of problem-solving with limited resources. And he saw that this work made a profound contribution to people's lives.

After completing 1 year of a residency in internal medicine, he took a year off and returned to Thailand, where he was chief physician at a refugee camp in a war zone on the Thai-Cambodian border. There was no electricity or running water. There was much violence inside the camp, and intense armed conflict just outside the camp. Mortar shells landed in the camp. To address the refugees' medical needs, he trained nurses, medics, and others to provide 90% of the medical care.

Dr. Iacopino returned to the United States to complete his internal medicine residency. He then participated in a 2-year clinical scholars program, during which he studied suffering in torture survivors and others. He learned about torture, including documenting and preventing it.

For the next 6 years, he served as medical director of Survivors International, which documented physical and psychological evidence of torture and provided courtroom testimony on behalf of torture victims who were seeking asylum in the United States.

Then, he began performing forensic investigations for Physicians for Human Rights in Thailand and India, where there was intense violence in Kashmir and Punjab. These forensic investigations involved taking histories from and performing examinations on victims of torture and other human rights violations, and visiting sites and interviewing witnesses where the alleged abuses had been committed. During this period, he developed and taught

From Horror to Hope. Barry S. Levy, Oxford University Press. © Oxford University Press 2022.
DOI: 10.1093/oso/9780197558645.003.0006

a course on health and human rights for public health students at the University of California at Berkeley.

By then, Dr. Iacopino had recognized that documentation and accountability are necessary for preventing torture. He saw the need for developing rigorous methodologies for forensic investigations and for writing publications on torture in leading medical journals. And he also saw the need to train, mentor, and guide other health professionals in documenting torture and other human rights violations.

Working with 75 other torture experts from 15 countries, he led the development of an 80-page UN document, known as the Istanbul Protocol, which has been used in many countries to guide medico-legal investigation and documentation of torture and ill-treatment. (Dr. Iacopino and more than 180 colleagues from 51 countries have completed an update of the Istanbul Protocol, which is scheduled for release in 2022.)

Recognizing that long-term, multisectoral programs at the national level are needed to prevent torture, Dr. Iacopino and his colleagues initiated programs to implement the Istanbul Protocol in Mexico, Kyrgyzstan, Tajikistan, and Kazakhstan. These programs involved awareness-raising and assessment; capacity building, such as by training lawyers, prosecutors, and judges on documentation of torture; policy reform, such as by changing laws as well as judicial and administrative rules and practices; and establishing national plans for torture prevention, accountability, and redress.

When asked what has motivated and supported him for more than 30 years in doing this work, Dr. Iacopino replies: "Directly participating in work to address inhumanity. Problem-solving on a large scale. Being part of a group of committed professionals. And the support of my family."

Dr. Iacopino is a member of the Advisory Council of Physicians for Human Rights and an Adjunct Professor of Medicine at the University of Minnesota Medical School.

PART II

Types of Weapons

4

Conventional Weapons

The very existence of armaments and great armies psychologically accustoms us to accept the philosophy of militarism. They inevitably increase fear and hate in the world.
    NORMAN THOMAS

I know not with what weapons World War III will be fought, but World War IV will be fought with sticks and stones.
    ALBERT EINSTEIN

INTRODUCTION

Conventional weapons include small arms, light weapons, and heavy weapons. They also include bombs, other explosives, and incendiaries. These weapons are described as "conventional" to distinguish them from *weapons of mass destruction*—chemical, biological, and nuclear weapons (Chapter 5). However, some conventional weapons, such as multiple launch rocket systems, cause mass destruction. And it can be argued that antipersonnel landmines and many other conventional weapons, in the aggregate, are weapons of mass destruction, although they kill only a few people at a time.

Categories and examples of conventional weapons are shown in Table 4-1. *Small arms* are weapons designed for use by individuals. *Light weapons* are designed for use by groups of two or three people.

Small arms are the primary weapons used in intrastate wars. They are inexpensive, sturdy, low-tech, and easy to carry, maintain, and use. Small arms typically stay in circulation for decades, as reflected in the large market for secondhand small arms. When an intrastate conflict ends, small arms have sometimes been turned in by military forces and then destroyed (Figure 4-1). But often, small arms end up in the hands of civilians or enter the black market and emerge in other war zones—or in a war in the same country years later.

From Horror to Hope. Barry S. Levy, Oxford University Press. © Oxford University Press 2022.
DOI: 10.1093/oso/9780197558645.003.0007

TABLE 4-1 Categories and Examples of Conventional Weapons

Small Arms	Light Weapons	Heavy Weapons
Revolvers	Heavy machine guns	Battle tanks
Self-loading pistols	Grenade launchers	Armored combat vehicles
Rifles	Portable anti-tank and anti-aircraft guns	Large-caliber artillery
Carbines	Recoilless rifles	Combat aircraft
Submachine guns	Portable anti-tank missile and	Attack helicopters
Assault rifles	rocket launchers	Armed drones (unmanned aerial vehicles)
Light machine guns	Portable anti-aircraft missile launchers	Missiles
	Mortars of less than 100 mm caliber	Warships

Widespread availability of small arms and light weapons can create sociopolitical insta-bility—and armed conflict. A vicious cycle may occur in which small arms and light weapons create instability, which leads to increased availability of these weapons, which creates more instability. And sociopolitical instability, in combination with poverty and inadequate health services, adversely affects the health of populations.[1]

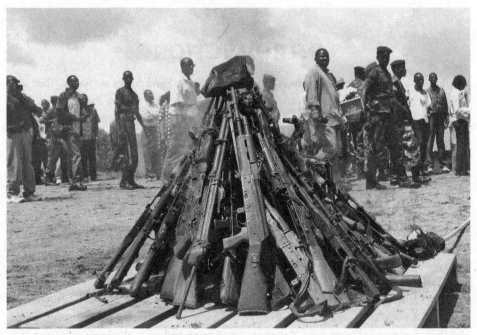

FIGURE 4-1 Stack of guns during demobilization of the Burundian military in 2004. While demobiliza-tion is commendable, open burning of these weapons creates risks to human health and the environ-ment. (UN/Martine Perret.)

THE INTERNATIONAL ARMS TRADE

Overview

The international arms trade makes conventional weapons available directly to armies, militias, and insurgent groups, and indirectly to civilians. In 2017, the total value of the international arms trade was estimated to be at least $95 billion—not including domestic sales of small arms. During the 2015–2019 period, the volume of the international arms trade in major conventional weapons increased by 5.5% over the previous 5-year period, to reach its highest level since the end of the Cold War. In 2019, the five largest arms-exporting countries were the United States ($10.7 billion), Russia ($4.7 billion), France ($3.4 billion), China ($1.4 billion), and Germany ($1.2 billion).[2] The five largest recipients of major conventional weapons were Saudi Arabia ($3.7 billion), India ($3.0 billion), Qatar ($2.3 billion), South Korea ($1.5 billion), and Australia ($1.4 billion).[3]

The Arms Trade Treaty

In 2013, the UN General Assembly overwhelmingly approved the Arms Trade Treaty (ATT), which entered into force in 2014. The treaty, which was designed to promote accountability and transparency of arms transfers, links sales of conventional weapons to human rights records of purchasing countries. It requires all states parties to:

- Adopt basic regulations and approval processes for the flow of weapons across international borders
- Establish common international standards that must be met before arms exports are authorized
- Annually report imports and exports
- Establish and maintain a transparent national control system regulating the transfer of conventional arms
- Assess the potential that the arms exported would "contribute to or undermine peace and security" or could be used to commit or facilitate serious violations of international humanitarian or human rights law, acts of terrorism, or transnational organized crime
- Consider measures to mitigate the risk of these violations; and, if there remains an "overriding risk" of "negative consequences," to "not authorize the export."[4]

The treaty also prohibits arms transfer authorizations to states if the transfer would violate arms embargoes or other relevant international obligations, or if it is known that the arms would be used for genocide, crimes against humanity, grave breaches of the 1949 Geneva Conventions, attacks against civilians or "civilian objects," or other war crimes.[4]

As of June 2021, the treaty had been signed by 130 countries and ratified by 110. The United States has signed, but not ratified, the treaty. The treaty only regulates *international* arms transfers, and it affirms "the sovereign right of any State to regulate and control conventional arms" within its own territory.[5]

The ATT has some significant limitations. It does not restrict the types or amounts of arms that may be bought, sold, or possessed by countries. It does not impact a country's domestic gun-control laws or other policies concerning ownership of arms. It does not address conventional weapons that are transferred as aid, loans, leases, or gifts. And it has no enforcement power—although it creates a set of standards that can facilitate efforts to shame violators and possibly hold them accountable.[6]

Illicit Transfers

The illicit transfer of arms—those that are produced, transferred, held, or used in violation of national or international law—contributes to their availability and accessibility. Illicit transfer also contributes to sociopolitical instability, political repression, human rights violations, crime, and armed conflict. In Africa, sophisticated organizations and networks arrange illicit flows of small arms and light weapons (and their ammunition) across national borders, mainly by land. These weapons originate from national stockpiles, previous wars, and other countries, including Middle Eastern and Eastern European nations that violated arms embargoes.[7]

ANTIPERSONNEL LANDMINES AND OTHER EXPLOSIVE REMNANTS OF WAR

Overview

Explosive remnants of war, which include antipersonnel landmines, unexploded ordnance (UXO), and abandoned explosive ordnance (AXO), injure and kill civilians, especially in rural areas of war-torn countries. Explosive remnants of war can deter people from seeing a physician, sending their children to school, and using land for farming or other purposes.

Antipersonnel landmines have been planted during wars to prevent travel by opposing military forces and to prevent land from being inhabited or used for agriculture or other purposes. Inexpensive and simple to produce, landmines can be activated by pressure, tripwire, or remote detonation. They may be thrown, dropped from aircraft, mounted on trees or stakes, or buried in the ground.[8]

At least 82 countries have been adversely affected by explosive remnants of war, which often persist for years after war had ended. Millions of landmines are still deployed in about 58 countries, including Cambodia, Mozambique, and Angola. UXO poses additional safety hazards. In some war-torn countries, residents have collected UXO charges and reused them to bomb underwater areas to "harvest" fish—a hazardous activity that destroys fragile ecosystems.[8] Putting themselves at great risk, residents also collect casings and sell them as scrap metal. Landmines and UXO adversely affect childhood education, economic productivity, and agriculture and food security.[9,10]

Studies have documented many civilian injuries and deaths caused by landmines and UXO in numerous countries (Table 4-2), sometimes long after armed conflict has ended. Many victims suffer arm or leg amputations and some lose one or both eyes (Figure 4-2). Many die before they can receive medical care. Displaced persons and children are at increased risk of being injured or killed by landmines. Common activities of child victims when they were injured or killed have been playing, tending animals, and tampering with

TABLE 4-2 Selected Studies on Civilian Deaths and Injuries from Landmines and Unexploded Ordnance

Country (Timeframe)/Number of Victims	Other Information
Iraq, Kurdistan Region (1970–2003)[a] 12,863 deaths and injuries	Males, children, and older people were at higher risk. Landmine training and awareness programs did not reduce the landmine mortality rate. The rate of incidents declined over time.
Vietnam, nine districts of one province (1975–2009)[b] 2,620 killed 4,410 injured 1.1% of provincial population	Highest rates were among low-income families and ethnic minorities living in mountainous areas. Most common activities leading to injuries and deaths were farming, collecting scrap metal, and herding cattle.
Iran (1980–1988)[c] 78 injured children Mean age at time of injury: 8.2 years (range 2–15 years)	80% of injuries caused by landmines and 20% by UXO. 63% of incidents injured 2 or more people. Most prevalent injuries were amputations (in 53%) and hearing loss (in 30%).
Chechnya (1994–2005)[d] 3,021 victims (25% children)	Case-fatality rate was 23%. Among children, 14% suffered lower-limb amputations and 12% suffered upper-limb amputations. Injury rates among civilians from landmines and UXO were 10 times higher than those reported from Afghanistan, Angola, and Cambodia.
Laos (approximately 1975–1996)[e] 870 UXO death and injury victims (46% under age 15)	Case-fatality rate ranged between 30% and 70% among districts. Most injuries involved multiple fragments, which usually required complex surgery and medical management.
Chad and Thailand (2000 and 2001)[f] Chad: 339 death and injury victims Thailand: 346 death and injury victims	Landmine risk associated with community size, closeness to another community with victims, proximity of UXO or anti-tank mines, placement of landmines in previous 2 years, and water or pasture blockage by landmines or UXO.
Turkey (2001–2008)[g] 23 injured children (20 from landmines and 3 from UXO); mean age = 13	Most children lost a hand, a leg, and/or an eye.
Afghanistan (2002–2006)[h] 5,471 victims (92% civilians, 47% children)	Case-fatality rate was 17%. Among surviving victims, 28% who had received mine awareness training reported that the area where in the incident occurred was marked; 2% of those who did not receive such training reported that it was marked.
Cambodia (2003–2006)[i] 356 victims (26% children)	Among child victims, 5.3% died, 21% became blind, and 23% had permanent damage to upper limbs. 62% of child victims were injured by UXO, 72% of adult victims by landmines.

[a] Heshmati A, Khayyat NT. Analysis of landmine fatalities and injuries in the Kurdistan Region. Journal of Interpersonal Violence 2015; 30: 2591-2615.
[b] Phung TK, Viet L, Husum H. The legacy of war: An epidemiological study of cluster weapon and land mine accidents in Quang Tri Province, Vietnam. Southeast Asian Journal of Tropical Medicine and Public Health 2012; 43: 1035-1041.
[c] Mousavi B, Soroush MR, Masoumi M, et al. Epidemiological study of child casualties of landmines and unexploded ordnances: A national study from Iran. Prehospital and Disaster Medicine 2015; 30: 472-477. doi: 10.1017/S1049023X15005105.
[d] Bilukha OO, Brennan M, Anderson M, et al. Seen but not heard: Injuries and deaths from landmines and unexploded ordnance in Chechnya, 1994-2005. Prehospital and Disaster Medicine 2007; 22: 507-512.
[e] Morikawa M, Taylor S, Persons M. Deaths and injuries due to unexploded ordnance (UXO) in northern Lao PDR (Laos). Injury 1998; 29: 301-304.
[f] Moulton LH, Benini AA. Community-level risk factors for numbers of landmine victims in Chad and Thailand. Journal of Epidemiology and Community Health 2003; 57: 956-959.
[g] Can M, Yildirimcan H, Ozkalipci O, et al. Landmine associated injuries in children in Turkey. Journal of Forensic and Legal Medicine 2009; 16: 464-468.
[h] Bilukha OO, Brennan M, Anderson M. The lasting legacy of war: Epidemiology of injuries from landmines and unexploded ordnance in Afghanistan, 2002-2006. Prehospital and Disaster Medicine 2008; 23: 493-499.
[i] Bendinelli C. Effects of land mines and unexploded ordnance on the pediatric population and comparison with adults in rural Cambodia. World Journal of Surgery 2009; 33: 1070-1074.

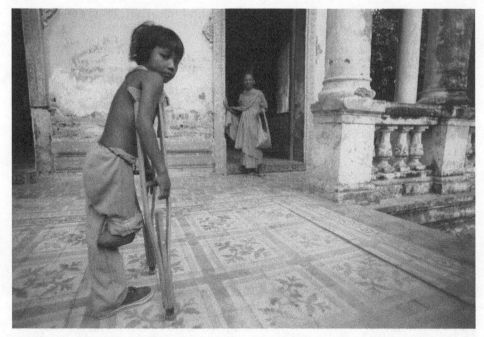

FIGURE 4-2 A disabled boy maimed by a landmine stands in 1992 in a courtyard of a UNICEF-assisted rehabilitation center located in the Wat Tan Temple in Phnom Penh, Cambodia. (© UNICEF/UNI53638/ Lemoyne.)

explosive devices. Common activities of adult victims when they were injured or killed have been traveling and performing activities of economic necessity, such as farming and herding cattle, and collecting scrap metal.[9,10]

Prevention of Injuries and Deaths

Areas contaminated with landmines and UXO need to be cleared to prevent further injuries and deaths. Because UXO is more visible than landmines and because UXO-contaminated areas are cheaper to clear than minefields, UXO injuries are highly preventable and UXO clearance and risk education deserve priority attention.[11] So does education about landmines in areas where they are present, recognizing that various activities, such as working outdoors and walking distances to obtain water, may put people at risk of coming into contact with landmines or UXO (Figure 4-3).[12] Healthcare workers in countries where landmines or UXO are deployed can educate their patients and ask them to report the presence of these devices. They can support community efforts to recognize and report these devices. And health workers in all countries can advocate for more effective policies and programs to address landmines and UXO.

The Mine Ban Treaty

The Convention on the Prohibition of the Use, Stockpiling, Production and Transfer of Anti-Personnel Mines and on Their Destruction—also known as the "Ottawa Convention" and the "Mine Ban Treaty"—was adopted in 1997 and entered into force in 1999. It prohibits the

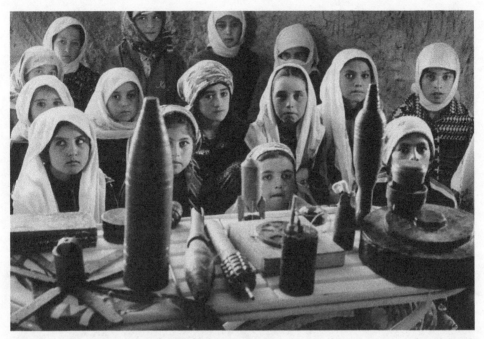

FIGURE 4-3 Tajik refugees in a class on landmines and unexploded ordnance in Mazar-i-Sharif, Afghanistan, in1996. (Photograph by Sebastião Salgado.)

use, development, production, acquisition, retention, stockpiling, or transferring of anti-personnel landmines.[13]

The Mine Ban Treaty resulted primarily from the advocacy work of the International Campaign to Ban Landmines (ICBL, a coalition of Handicap International, Human Rights Watch, Medico International, the Mines Advisory Group, Physicians for Human Rights, and the Vietnam Veterans of America Foundation), the International Committee of the Red Cross, and a small group of countries. (See Profile 4.) The development of the treaty was unusual in that it arose from a coalition of nongovernmental organizations rather than the initiative of the United States or other world powers. The ICBL used education and shaming campaigns to bring antipersonnel landmines onto the global agenda. It also successfully appealed to universal norms that acknowledge the protection of civilians, the sanctity of children, and the fragility of the environment. In doing so, the ICBL engaged in the process outside traditional mechanisms for developing international humanitarian law.[14,15]

Within 4 years of joining the Mine Ban Treaty, each state party was expected to destroy all antipersonnel landmines it possessed, except for landmines retained for training deminers. States parties have destroyed over 50 million stockpiled landmines. Within 10 years of joining the treaty, each state party committed to clear all mined areas within its territory. (Since 1999, a total of 28 states parties have removed all landmines in areas where they were deployed.) States parties have also committed to conducting mine risk education, ensuring that civilians are excluded from mined areas, and providing assistance for the care and rehabilitation of mine victims and their social and economic reintegration.

As of June 2021, there were 164 states parties to the Mine Ban Treaty. Although the United States has not signed the Mine Ban Treaty, the Obama administration said that it would abide by the treaty except on the Korean Peninsula. In 2020, the Trump administration rescinded the Obama administration policy. As of early July 2021, the Biden administration had not reinstituted it. Few of the other 32 countries that have not joined the treaty produce or use antipersonnel landmines.[16,17]

Although most countries do not produce landmines, approximately 36 stockpile them. In 2018, the countries that stockpiled the most landmines were Russia (more than 26 million), Pakistan (6 million), India (4 to 5 million), China (less than 5 million), and the United States (3 million).[18]

Clearance of landmines and UXO in postwar countries usually continues for many years after war has ended. Mine clearance personnel face risks of serious injury or death. Between 1991 and 2000, there were 92 traumatic injuries in 73 mine clearance personnel working in seven countries; their case-fatality rate was 15%. Of all victims, 44% suffered severe injuries of the arm or face and 30% required amputations of arms or legs.[19]

CLUSTER MUNITIONS

Overview

Cluster munitions (also known as *cluster bombs*) are canisters containing tens to thousands of sub-munitions ("bomblets") that are delivered by aircraft, rocket, or artillery, and are designed to separate and spread when canisters break open in midair. Although cluster bombs can cover vast areas, they are difficult to target and guide precisely and sub-munitions are widely dispersed. Unexploded sub-munitions (*duds*), which represent UXO, pose major threats to civilians during war and its aftermath. Duds can lay dormant for decades until they are discovered by children, who are attracted to their small size and bright colors, or by farmers plowing their land. In Afghanistan in 2001, the failure (dud) rate of U.S. cluster munitions was estimated at 17%. Mine clearance personnel have reported failure rates between 5% and 30%. When many cluster munitions are used, even a 1% failure rate results in many explosive remnants.[20]

Cluster munitions were first used during the Second World War by Germany and the Soviet Union. The most extensive deployment of cluster munitions occurred during the Vietnam War, when the United States dropped at least 300 million sub-munitions over Vietnam, Cambodia, and Laos. During the wars in Afghanistan and Iraq, the U.S.-led coalition used cluster munitions widely. In 2006, Israel used cluster munitions in southern Lebanon. An increasing number of countries possess cluster munitions. Some of these countries have a history of attacking their own civilians. Non-state armed groups use cluster munitions; for example, Hezbollah used them against Israel in 2006.[20] Millions of people in at least 30 countries live in areas with unexploded cluster munitions.

Injuries and Deaths

In 2018, there were 149 cluster-munition injuries and deaths reported worldwide—a substantial decrease from 971 injuries and deaths in 2016. In 2018, injuries and deaths from cluster munition remnants were recorded in Afghanistan, Iraq, Laos, Lebanon, South Sudan, Syria, Ukraine, Yemen, and the Nagorno Karabakh area in the South Caucasus region. Many injuries and deaths have gone unrecorded or have lacked sufficient documentation, especially in Southeast Asia, Afghanistan, and Iraq.[21]

The World Health Organization reported in 2018 that cluster munitions had been used in civilian areas in Syria and Yemen. In Yemen, cluster munitions had been used in 18 attacks between 2015 and early 2017, leading to 21 civilian deaths and 74 injured victims. Most cluster munitions used in Syria since 2012 and in Yemen since 2015 were manufactured in Brazil, Russia, the United Kingdom, and the United States.[22] Since mid-2012, there have been at least 674 cluster munition attacks in Syria. From mid-2018 to mid-2019, cluster munitions continued to be used by Syrian government forces with support from Russia.[21]

Unexploded sub-munitions have caused at least 55,000 casualties. In recent years, more than 98% of recorded casualties from cluster munitions have been among civilians. Poor and uneducated men, who are often the main sources of income for their households, suffer most injuries and deaths caused by cluster munitions. If they are injured or killed, their families may suffer for years afterward. In some countries, children account for about 60% of victims.[22] In Kosovo, Laos, Vietnam, Afghanistan, and Lebanon, injuries and deaths from cluster munitions increased as people returned home as war subsided or ended.[20] Cluster munition injuries cause amputations and other body disfigurations, loss of function, chronic pain, and posttraumatic stress disorder and other psychosocial problems.[23]

U.S. military forces last used cluster munitions in large quantities during the Gulf War, where there were high failure rates and little evidence that cluster munitions deterred Iraqi forces. Cleanup efforts in Kuwait and Iraq to find and destroy landmines and cluster munitions continued at least through February 2020. Between 1993 and early 2020, the United States spent $3.4 billion to demine and eradicate UXO in the Middle East and Southeast Asia, and spent more to clean up UXO on former military practice ranges in Hawaii and Puerto Rico. Sections of military bombing and artillery ranges where cluster weapons had been used are considered so hazardous that only bomb disposal personnel may enter. And cleanup of military practice ranges presents challenges, such as air pollution from burning hazardous materials.[17]

During the Second Lebanon War (between Israel and Lebanon), which lasted 34 days, Israel dropped approximately four million sub-munitions in south Lebanon, mainly in rural villages, making much farmland inaccessible. One-fourth remain unexploded. Between 2006 and 2011, there were at least 51 people killed and 356 injured, of whom 83 required amputations. Among the victims, 122 (30%) were children, 10 of whom died. Among those injured, 85% developed functional disabilities.[23] A study found that 19% of victims developed infections with various bacterial and fungal organisms.[24] A 10-year longitudinal study in Lebanon of adult civilian victims of sub-munition blasts found that they had a high long-term prevalence of PTSD, which was associated with severe functional impairment, and a very high rate of job instability.[25]

Convention on Cluster Munitions

The Convention on Cluster Munitions (CCM) bans the use, stockpiling, production, and transfer of most cluster munitions—except for bombs that self-destruct or self-deactivate.

It also requires that states parties destroy their stockpiles within 8 years, clear contaminated land within 10 years, and provide assistance to victims. The CCM was opened for signature in 2008 and entered into force in 2010. As of June 2021, it had 110 states parties; an additional 13 countries had signed but not ratified the Convention; and the United States had not signed the Convention—nor had Russia or Syria.[26]

In 2008, President George W. Bush issued a policy declaring that the United States would remove all but a few of the cluster munitions in its active stockpile by the end of 2018. However, the Department of Defense in late 2017 indefinitely delayed the implementation of this policy and issued a new policy that permits the U.S. military to use the cluster munitions that it possesses and facilitates acquisition of cluster munitions from sources in other countries to replenish its stocks.

The CCM, based on the principle of discrimination (or distinction), states that "the parties to a conflict shall at all times distinguish between the civilian population and combatants and between civilian objects and military objectives and accordingly direct their operations against military objectives only."[26] The CCM bans standard cluster munitions because they are indiscriminate weapons that fail to permit those who employ them from distinguishing between combatants and civilians. A weapon can fail to discriminate between combatants and civilians spatially or temporally. Due to the high dud rates of their sub-munitions, cluster bombs fail to discriminate temporally.[27]

From the adoption of the CCM in 2008 until 2019, almost 1.5 million cluster munitions and more than 178 million sub-munitions were destroyed by 35 states parties, representing 99% destruction of declared stocks of these weapons (Figure 4-4). Although states parties

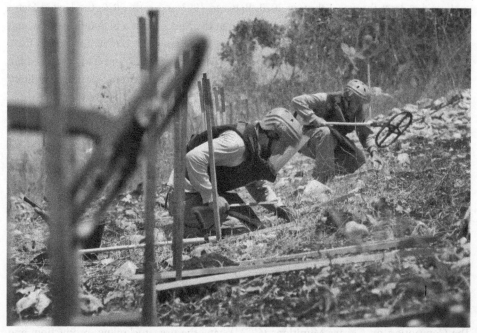

FIGURE 4-4 A team from the Mines Advisory Group clear unexploded cluster munitions in farmland in southern Lebanon in 2010. (Sipa via AP Images.)

had committed to improving assistance for cluster munition victims, by 2019 funding for community-based work of local organizations had decreased, thereby hampering access to rehabilitation and economic activities. As of 2019, a total of 16 countries outside the CCM continued to produce cluster munitions or had not committed to cease production in the future, and 13 states parties to the CCM, almost all in Europe, were retaining live cluster munitions or sub-munitions for training and research.[21]

Overall, however, the CCM seems to be working well. No state party has violated the prohibition on using cluster munitions. With the glaring exception of Syria, which has not joined the CCM, the stigma against cluster munitions appears to be strong, even with almost all of the countries that have not signed it, according to Human Rights Watch.[28]

AUTONOMOUS WEAPONS SYSTEMS

Overview

Autonomous weapons systems (AWS), which use sensors and computer algorithms to independently identify targets and use onboard weapon systems to destroy them without meaningful human control, present new ethical, legal, and other challenges.[29] Representing a major paradigm shift in weaponry, AWS are designed to be used without communication systems or human control, and to respond to an evolving environment.[30]

AWS, because they are precise weapons, could theoretically have benefits during war, such as by reducing civilian injuries and deaths and reducing the number of soldiers needed on a battlefield. In addition, they react more quickly than humans, do not develop fatigue or "war weariness," and do not get emotional when fellow soldiers are seriously injured or killed during combat. But a growing number of countries, defense experts, humanitarian and nongovernmental organizations, and others oppose AWS because:

- AWS might lead to widespread killing.
- AWS represent increased risks of accidental escalation of conflicts.
- Military forces using AWS might lose all control over them.
- AWS could proliferate; even non-state actors could acquire and use them.
- It is fundamentally immoral to give machines, operating without direct human control, the ability to determine who lives and who dies during war.[30]

Some military officials believe that handing the capability of selecting military targets and executing attacks over to a machine undermines command-and-control frameworks and renders the participation of humans redundant.[31]

Challenges and Concerns

Human Rights Watch has argued that machines cannot judge whether their actions create a justifiable proportionate risk to civilians. It has also argued that AWS would make wars more likely because they might make tragic mistakes and it would not be clear who should be held responsible. In addition to moral issues, there is much concern about the unpredictability in computer-based thinking, which diverges from human logic in ways that might cause civilian casualties. Another concern is that AWS components are being developed without restrictions by technology companies, rather than by defense contractors or the U.S. military.[32]

Any new weapon system needs to be able to distinguish between combatants and civilians and operate in accordance with the *principle of proportionality*—the risk of unintended damage to civilians and civilian infrastructure should be proportionate to the anticipated military benefit of attacking the target. Many analysts believe that AWS could never meet these requirements.[33-35]

Another challenge is determining responsibility and accountability for the use of these weapons and their consequences, especially when their use violates moral or legal standards. Who will be judged to be responsible for the actions of AWS? Existing legal norms will likely be inadequate to properly attribute criminal responsibility to anyone. A major barrier for determining accountability for harm caused by AWS is the inherent uncertainty associated with their behavior. It would be inappropriate to blame military personnel who initiated use of AWS in a specific incident for any harm to civilians. But should one blame those who designed and developed AWS and the government and military officials who authorized their use? One option will be developing international laws and legal doctrines to address these issues. Another would be to criminalize the use of AWS in armed conflict.[36]

The Campaign to Stop Killer Robots, a global civil-society coalition coordinated by Human Rights Watch, is attempting to preemptively ban AWS and retain meaningful human control over the use of force. The campaign has proposed an international treaty that would apply to all weapons systems that select and engage targets based on sensor processing, rather than human inputs. The proposed treaty would have three categories of obligations:

1. "A general obligation that requires maintaining meaningful control over the use of force"
2. "Prohibitions that ban the development, production, and use of weapons systems that autonomously select and engage and, by their nature, pose fundamental moral or legal problems; these prohibitions cover weapons that always operate without meaningful human control and those that rely on data, such as weight, heat, or sound, to select human targets."
3. "Specific positive obligations that aim to ensure that meaningful human control is maintained in the use of all other systems that select and engage targets."[37]

Such a treaty would build on precedents of previous treaties, such as the Chemical Weapons Convention, the Mine Ban Treaty, the Convention on Cluster Munitions, and the Treaty on the Prohibition of Nuclear Weapons, which prohibit use, development, production, acquisition, stockpiling, retention, transfer, testing, and threat of use of specific weapons—and prohibit use of these weapons under any circumstances in times of war or peace, including operations by law enforcement entities.[37]

As of early 2021, the U.S. military remained ambivalent about the use of AWS. However, the U.S. Navy was experimenting with vessels that could travel long distances independently, hunting for enemy submarines or ships that could attack U.S. forces. The U.S. Army was experimenting with autonomous systems to identify targets and automatically aim tank guns. And the U.S. Air Force was developing AWS that could accompany combat aircraft or proceed on their own.[32]

CYBER WARFARE

Overview

Cyber warfare refers to the use of digital attacks by one country to disrupt the vital computer systems of another by attacking with computer viruses or by hacking into computer systems. Its potential goals include causing chaos and confusion, damage and destruction, and/or death. In future wars, hackers could use cyber warfare to attack an adversary's infrastructure while military troops attack with conventional weapons.

Computer systems may be targeted because they are integral to managing civilian infrastructure, such as airports, power grids, the Internet, and systems for communication, transportation, food distribution, water supply, and finance. A country attacked by cyber warfare could experience gridlock and chaos. Attackers could both physically destroy critical civilian infrastructure and carry out massive manipulation of data.

Cyber attacks could also be used for other military purposes, such as performing reconnaissance, gathering intelligence information, and disabling weapon systems and military communication systems.[38] They could threaten the integrity of systems that control the launch of weapons, including nuclear weapons—either by preventing them from functioning or by preventing them from being accurately targeted. They might increase the possibility that nuclear weapons could be launched accidentally.

Cyber attacks by national governments or military forces against other countries occur frequently. It is likely that the United States, Russia, China, and other major world powers have targeted and/or infiltrated each other's critical infrastructure. Several years ago, Israel and the United States developed sophisticated malware to destroy centrifuges in Iran that were being used to refine fissile material that could be used in nuclear weapons. China has carried out an espionage campaign against governments and corporations to try to steal records, intellectual property, and consumer information.[38] In May 2021, a major fuel pipeline in the United States was shut down by a ransomware attack.[39]

Challenges and Concerns

Under international law, countries are allowed to use force to defend themselves against an armed attack. Therefore, if a country were hit by a significant cyber attack, it might have the right to strike back with military force. Cyber warfare, however, is not adequately addressed in existing international law.[40]

State-based hacking and physical warfare have been converging for two decades. The first reporting of a cyber attack that led to a physical attack occurred in 2019 when the Israel Defense Force targeted and partially destroyed a building in Gaza that it claimed was associated with an ongoing cyber attack on Israel by Hamas.[38] This physical attack was a crucial turning point in the evolution of hybrid warfare (a combination of cyber warfare and physical warfare), setting a dangerous precedent that offensive hackers are fair game for physical retaliation. More incidents of violent physical retaliation against hackers are inevitable.

The first reported physical attack that led to a cyber attack also occurred in 2019, after Iran used a surface-to-air missile to down an unmanned U.S. surveillance drone that was flying over the Strait of Hormuz. In response, the United States launched a cyber attack against computer systems in Iran that controlled missile and rocket launches.[41]

While many people believe that legal restrictions should apply to cyber warfare, the international community has yet to agree on how international humanitarian law applies or could be applied to this new form of conflict. Two key principles of international humanitarian law are *distinction* (during war, parties must distinguish between combatants and civilians and also between military objectives and civilian objects) and *neutrality* (during a specific war, some countries abstain from participating). Violations of distinction and neutrality might occur more frequently in cyber warfare than in conventional warfare.[42]

MILITARIZATION OF OUTER SPACE

Militarization of space, which involves placement of technological military equipment into outer space, has been taking place for decades. Military forces rely on outer space for purposes such as surveillance of opposing military forces in order to defend against ground invasion or a missile attack—a potential deterrent against aggression. *Space warfare*—combat that targets objects in space—could occur with satellites attacking each other or ground-based missiles attacking satellites.

At the same time, individual countries and the global community greatly rely on outer space for many peaceful purposes: cellphone, satellite-television, radio, and other communications; global positioning systems (GPS), air traffic control, and other transportation-related uses; weather forecasting; observation and analyses of environmental resources and the consequences of climate change; surveillance of disasters; and partial verification of international treaties.[43]

The international community has for more than five decades regulated the use of outer space, including defining and regulating the weaponization of outer space.[43] The provisions of the UN Outer Space Treaty, first signed in 1967, include the following:

- Outer space shall be free for exploration, use, and benefit by all countries.
- Activities in outer space shall be carried out in accordance with international law.
- No nuclear weapons or other weapons of mass destruction shall be placed in orbit around the Earth or placed on any celestial body.
- Responsibility and liability shall be placed for damage caused by an object launched or by its components on the Earth.
- Countries shall be responsible for national space activities, including those carried out by both governments and nongovernmental organizations.
- Countries shall be liable for damage caused by their outer space objects.
- Countries shall avoid harmful contamination of outer space and celestial bodies.[44]

An ominous development was the creation, by the U.S. Congress in 2019, of the U.S. Space Force as an independent military service within the U.S. Air Force.[45] Its establishment received widespread criticism and received little initial support from the leadership of the

U.S. military.[46,47] As of June 2021, it was not clear what the long-term implications of the U.S. Space Force would be.

SUMMARY POINTS

- Small arms and light weapons are the primary weapons that have been used in intrastate wars.
- The international arms trade increases availability of conventional weapons in many countries.
- Antipersonnel landmines and unexploded ordnance have accounted for much injury and death among civilians.
- Effectiveness of treaties concerning conventional weapons partially depends on mechanisms for enforcement, including identifying violators and holding them accountable.
- Autonomous weapons systems, cyber warfare, and militarization of outer space represent new challenges in preventing armed conflict.

REFERENCES

1. Bowsher G, Bogue P, Patel P, et al. Small and light arms violence reduction as a public health measure: The case of Libya. Conflict and Health 2018; 12: 29. doi: 10.1186/s13031-018-0162-0.
2. Wezeman ST, Kuimova A, da Silva DL, et al. "Developments Among the Suppliers of Major Arms, 2015-19" in J Batho, C Brown, F Esparraga, et al. (eds.). SIPRI Yearbook 2020: Armaments, Disarmament and International Security. New York: Oxford University Press, 2020, pp. 275-289.
3. Wezeman ST, Kuimova A, da Silva DL, et al. "Developments Among the Recipients of Major Arms, 2015-19" in J Batho, C Brown, F Esparraga, et al. (eds.). SIPRI Yearbook 2020: Armaments, Disarmament and International Security. New York: Oxford University Press, 2020, pp. 290-306.
4. Arms Control Association. The Arms Trade Treaty at a Glance, updated August 2017. Available at: https://www.armscontrol.org/factsheets/arms_trade_treaty. Accessed on March 22, 2021.
5. Stohl R. Tell the truth about the arms treaty (Op-ed). New York Times, April 11, 2013. Available at: https://www.nytimes.com/2013/04/12/opinion/tell-the-truth-about-the-arms-trade-treaty.html. Accessed on August 13, 2020.
6. MacFarquhar N. U.N treaty is first aimed at regulating global arms sales. New York Times, April 2, 2013. Available at: https://www.nytimes.com/2013/04/03/world/arms-trade-treaty-approved-at-un.html. Accessed on August 13, 2020.
7. African Union, Small Arms Survey. Weapons Compass: Mapping Illicit Small Arms Flows in Africa. Geneva: Small Arms Survey, Graduate Institute of International and Developmental Studies, 2019.
8. Kett ME, Mannion SJ. Managing the health effects of the explosive remnants of war. Journal of the Royal Society for the Promotion of Health 2004; 124: 262-267.
9. Frost A, Boyle P, Autier P, et al. The effect of explosive remnants of war on global public health: A systematic mixed-studies review using narrative synthesis. Lancet Public Health 2017; 2: e286-e296.
10. Borrie J. Explosive Remnants of War: A Global Survey. London: Landmine Action, 2003. Available at: https://unidir.org/files/medias/pdfs/erw-a-global-survey-eng-0-69.pdf. Accessed on August 17, 2020.
11. Bilukha OO, Brennan M, Anderson M. The lasting legacy of war: Epidemiology of injuries from landmines and unexploded ordnance in Afghanistan, 2002-2006. Prehospital and Disaster Medicine 2008; 23: 493-499.
12. Boyd AT, Becknell K, Russell S, et al. Risk factors for unsafe behaviors toward grenades among rural populations affected by explosive devices in Colombia. Conflict and Health 2018; 12: 4. doi: 10.1186/s13031-018-0141-5.

13. Convention on the Prohibition of the Use, Stockpiling, Production and Transfer of Anti-Personnel Mines and on their Destruction, September 18, 1997. Available at: https://www.apminebanconvention.org/overview-and-convention-text/. Accessed on August 16, 2020.

14. Rutherford KR. Disarming States: The International Movement to Ban Landmines. Santa Barbara, CA: Praeger Security International, 2011.

15. Wexler L. The international deployment of shame, second-best responses, and norm entrepreneurship: The Campaign to Ban Landmines and the Landmine Ban Treaty. Arizona Journal of International and Comparative Law 2003; 20: 561-606.

16. Arms Control Association. The Ottawa Convention at a Glance. Available at: https://www.armscontrol.org/factsheets/ottawa. Accessed on June 1, 2021.

17. Ismay J, Gibbons-Neff T. 160 nations ban these weapons: The U.S. now embraces them. New York Times, February 7, 2020. Available at: https://www.nytimes.com/2020/02/07/us/trump-land-mines-cluster-munitions.html. Accessed on August 13, 2020.

18. International Campaign to Ban Landmines. Available at: http://www.icbl.org. Accessed on January 9, 2021.

19. Brown R, Chaloner E, Mannion S, Cheatle T. 10-year experience of injuries sustained during clearance of anti-personnel mines. The Lancet 2001; 358: 2048-2049.

20. Parikh SM. Cluster munitions: A threat to health and human rights. Medicine, Conflict & Survival 2010; 26: 101-107.

21. Landmine & Cluster Munition Monitor. Cluster Munition Monitor 2019. Available at: http://the-monitor.org/en-gb/reports/2019/Cluster-Munition-Monitor-2019. Accessed on August 13, 2020.

22. Fares J, Fares Y. Cluster munitions: Military use and civilian health hazards. Bulletin of the World Health Organization 2018; 96: 584-585.

23. Fares Y, Fares J. Anatomical and neuropsychological effects of cluster munitions. Neurological Sciences 2013; 34: 2095-2100.

24. Fares Y, El-Zaatari M, Fares J, et al. Trauma-related infections due to cluster munitions. Journal of Infection and Public Health 2013; 6: 482-486.

25. Fares J, Gebeily S, Saad M, et al. Post-traumatic stress disorder in adult victims of cluster munitions in Lebanon: A 10-year longitudinal study. BMJ Open 2017; 7: e017214. doi: 10.1136/bmjopen-2017-017214.

26. Convention on Cluster Munitions. Available at: www.clusterconvention.org. Accessed on June 1, 2021.

27. Cavanaugh TA. Temporal indiscriminateness: The case of cluster bombs. Science and Engineering Ethics 2010; 16: 135–145.

28. Human Rights Watch. Cluster Munitions: Ban Treaty Is Working: Glaring Exception Is Syria Where Attacks Continue. August 29, 2019. Available at: https://www.hrw.org/news/2019/08/29/cluster-munitions-ban-treaty-working. Accessed on November 5, 2020.

29. Sayler KM. Defense Primer: U.S. Policy on Lethal Autonomous Weapons Systems. Infocus, Congressional Research Service. Updated September 1, 2020. Available at: https://fas.org/sgp/crs/natsec/IF11150.pdf. Accessed on March 3, 2021.

30. Future of Life Institute. Lethal Autonomous Weapons Systems. Available at: https://futureoflife.org/lethal-autonomous-weapons-systems/. Accessed on March 3, 2021.

31. Roff HM. The strategic robot problem: Lethal autonomous weapons in war. Journal of Military Ethics 2014; 13: 211-227.

32. Fryer-Biggs Z. Can computer algorithms learn to fight wars ethically? Washington Post Magazine, February 17, 2021. Available at: https://www.washingtonpost.com/magazine/2021/02/17/pentagon-funds-killer-robots-but-ethics-are-under-debate/?arc404=true. Accessed on March 3, 2021.

33. Etzioni A, Etzioni O. Pros and cons of autonomous weapons systems. Military Review 2017; May-June: 72-81.

34. Bieri M, Dickow M. Lethal Autonomous Weapons Systems: Future Challenges (CSS Analyses in Security Policy [No. 164]). Center for Security Studies, November 2014. Available at: https://css.ethz.ch/content/dam/ethz/special-interest/gess/cis/center-for-securities-studies/pdfs/CSSAnalyse164-EN.pdf. Accessed on March 3, 2021.

35. Meier MW. Lethal autonomous weapons systems (LAWS): Conducting a comprehensive weapons review. Temple International and Comparative Law Journal 2016; 30: 119-132. Available at: https://sites.temple.edu/ticlj/files/2017/02/30.1.Meier-TICLJ.pdf. Accessed on March 3, 2021.

36. Bhuta N, Beck S, Geiß R, et al. (eds.). Autonomous Weapons Systems: Law, Ethics, Policy. Cambridge, UK: Cambridge University Press, 2016.

37. Docherty B. New Weapons, Proven Precedents: Elements of and Models for a Treaty on Killer Robots. Human Rights Watch. October 20, 2020. Available at: https://www.hrw.org/report/2020/10/20/new-weapons-proven-precedent/elements-and-models-treaty-killer-robots. Accessed on March 3, 2021.

38. Newman LH. What Israel's strike on Hamas hackers means for cyberwar. WIRED, May 6, 2019. Available at: https://www.wired.com/story/israel-hamas-cyberattack-air-strike-cyberwar/. Accessed on September 28, 2020.

39. Plumer B. Pipeline hack points to growing cybersecurity risk for energy system. New York Times, May 13, 2021. Available at: https://www.nytimes.com/2021/05/13/climate/pipeline-ransomware-hack-energy-grid.html. Accessed on May 14, 2021.

40. Ranger S. What is cyberwar?: Everything you need to know about the frightening future of digital conflict. ZDNet, December 4, 2018. Available at: https://www.zdnet.com/article/cyberwar-a-guide-to-the-frightening-future-of-online-conflict/. Accessed on September 28, 2020.

41. Sussman B. Cyber war versus traditional war: The difference is fading. SecureWorld, December 27, 2019. Available at: https://www.secureworldexpo.com/industry-news/cyber-war-vs-traditional-war. Accessed on September 28, 2020.

42. Kelsey JTG. Hacking into international humanitarian law: The principles of distinction and neutrality in the age of cyber warfare. Michigan Law Review 2008; 106: 1427. Available at: https://repository.law.umich.edu/cgi/viewcontent.cgi?article=1381&context=mlr. Accessed on September 28, 2020.

43. DeFrieze DC. Defining and regulating the weaponization of space. Joint Force Quarterly 2014; 74: 110-115.

44. United Nations Office for Outer Space Affairs. Treaty on Principles Governing the Activities of Space and the Exploration and Use of Outer Space, Including the Moon and Other Celestial Bodies. Available at: https://www.unoosa.org/oosa/en/ourwork/spacelaw/treaties/introouterspacetreaty.html. Accessed on September 26, 2020.

45. Garamone J. Trump signs law establishing U.S. Space Force. DOD News, December 20, 2019. Available at: https://www.defense.gov/Explore/News/Article/Article/2046035/trump-signs-law-establishing-us-space-force/. Accessed on December 28, 2020.

46. Farley R. Space Force: Ahead of its time, or dreadfully premature? Policy Analysis No. 904. Cato Institute, Washington, DC, December 1, 2020. Available at: https://www.cato.org/publications/policy-analysis/space-force-ahead-its-time-or-dreadfully-premature. Accessed on December 28, 2020.

47. Morales C. The newest guardians of the galaxy are run by the U.S. military. New York Times, December 19, 2020. Available at: https://www.nytimes.com/2020/12/19/us/space-force-guardians-mike-pence.html. Accessed on January 4, 2021.

Profile 4:
James C. Cobey, M.D., M.P.H.
Documenting Impacts of Landmines

By the time Jim Cobey began his orthopedic surgery practice in the mid-1970s, he had more public health and preventive medicine experience than most physicians have during their entire careers.

As a college student in the 1960s, Jim volunteered on a pediatric nutrition and re-hydration project for refugees in the Gaza Strip. As a medical student, he spent a summer in Nigeria studying the effectiveness of a nurse practitioner in improving childhood nutrition. And he spent another summer in Haiti, where he learned from his then girlfriend—now wife of more than 50 years—that, from a public health nurse's perspective, setting up a water purification system would be more beneficial for children's health than his repeatedly treating cases of diarrheal illnesses.

Jim studied both medicine and public health in medical school, and he received both an M.D. and an M.P.H. degree when he graduated. For 2 years in the U.S. Army, he served as Chief of Preventive Medicine at Fort Lewis in Washington State, where he ensured that soldiers received appropriate vaccinations—and that children in all schools in the surrounding county received measles immunizations. And later, during the last 3 months of his orthopedic surgery residency, he treated tuberculosis and polio patients in Hong Kong.

Fast forward to 1979. More than 100,000 Cambodians crossed the border into Thailand after the genocidal Khmer Rouge regime collapsed, and many others were stranded on the border. Dr. Cobey left his U.S.-based orthopedic surgery practice to serve for 3 months as medical coordinator at a camp on the border as a volunteer for the International Committee of the Red Cross (ICRC). There he performed surgery with minimal resources, including on

From Horror to Hope. Barry S. Levy, Oxford University Press. © Oxford University Press 2022.
DOI: 10.1093/oso/9780197558645.003.0008

people with horrific landmine injuries. A few years later, he returned and again observed the impact of landmines on this population.

In 1991, with two colleagues from Physicians for Human Rights (PHR), Dr. Cobey conducted an epidemiological study on the impact of landmines among Cambodians. After reviewing records at a dozen hospitals inside Cambodia, they found that one out of every 236 Cambodians, many of them children, had landmine injuries—not including those killed by landmines. Their work led to the landmark report "Land Mines in Cambodia: A Coward's War," published jointly by PHR and Human Rights Watch and presented to leaders in the U.S. government and at the United Nations.

Over the next few years, Dr. Cobey helped to translate the study's findings into policy that would have profound impacts on preventing landmine injuries. He helped establish the International Campaign to Ban Landmines (ICBL), which led to the Mine Ban Treaty, for which the ICBL was awarded the Nobel Peace Prize in 1997.

His work on landmines did not stop there. He has worked with other ICBL members and the World Health Organization to develop standardized tools to measure the impact of landmine injuries in many countries and to help them improve capacity to provide medical care and rehabilitation for landmine victims.

Dr. Cobey has continued his U.S.-based practice as an orthopedic surgeon, specializing in major trauma, spine reconstruction, and total joint replacement. He has written numerous journal articles, taught medical students and residents, and served as an instructor on disaster relief for ICRC. He has directed Health Volunteers Overseas, which sends healthcare professionals to practice and train local counterparts in low- and middle-income countries, while using locally available technology. He has trained orthopedic surgeons in many of these countries. And he helped establish the G4 Alliance for Surgical, Obstetric, Trauma, and Anesthesia Care, which aims to improve surgical care for two-thirds of the world's population.

Dr. Cobey is an orthopedic surgeon in Washington, DC, a Professor of Orthopedics at Georgetown University School of Medicine, and a Senior Associate at the Johns Hopkins Bloomberg School of Public Health.

5

Chemical, Biological, and Nuclear Weapons

A nuclear war cannot be won and must never be fought. The only value in . . . possessing nuclear weapons is to make sure they will never be used. But then, would it not be better to do away with them entirely?
RONALD REAGAN

The nuclear arms race is like two sworn enemies standing waist deep in gasoline, one with three matches, the other with five.
CARL SAGAN

INTRODUCTION

Chemical, biological, and nuclear weapons are considered *weapons of mass destruction*. Although the vast majority of nations have agreed to international bans on chemical and biological weapons, they could still be used by government military forces or non-state actors to cause illness, disability, and death.

Nuclear weapons, which are held by the United States, Russia, and seven other countries, pose immensely greater risks than chemical and biological weapons. They threaten the survival of the human species. Even a limited nuclear war—triggered by miscalculation or accident—could cause millions of deaths and many more severe injuries. Huge amounts of soot spewed into the atmosphere from a nuclear war could result in dramatic decreases in ambient temperature, which would cause catastrophic damage to agriculture, widespread famine, and hundreds of millions of deaths.

CHEMICAL WEAPONS

Until recently, chemical weapons posed a significant threat to combatants and civilians. One of the great successes in arms control has been the almost total elimination of chemical

From Horror to Hope. Barry S. Levy, Oxford University Press. © Oxford University Press 2022.
DOI: 10.1093/oso/9780197558645.003.0009

weapons. This section provides an overview of chemical weapons and when and where they have been used as well as information on their control.

Overview and Use

Chemical weapons are toxicants that have been designed to kill or disable people. Because they are relatively easy to produce and deploy but difficult to detect, they can have devastating effects. Chemical weapons have been used to kill or disable military personnel and civilians—sometimes by their own government. Chemical weapons have contaminated food and water and adversely affected ecosystems, where they can persist for long periods of time.[1] After the Second World War, the United States, Canada, Russia, Japan, and other countries dumped hundreds of thousands of tons of chemical weapons at sea (Chapter 13).[2]

Major categories of chemical weapons are:

- Asphyxiants, including (a) simple asphyxiants, such as carbon dioxide, which can cause oxygen deficiency in confined or closed spaces; and (b) chemical asphyxiants, such as carbon monoxide and cyanides, which interfere with cellular respiration and/or oxygen transport, causing tissue hypoxia
- Cholinesterase inhibitors, including the nerve agents sarin and VX, which inhibit acetylcholinesterase and thereby cause cholinergic overstimulation
- Respiratory tract irritants (choking agents), including chlorine and lacrimogenic agents ("tear gas"), which can cause severe injuries to the skin and eyes and permanent disabilities[3]
- Vesicants and skin caustics (blister agents), including sulfur mustard, arsenical vesicants (such as lewisite), and halogenated oximes. Mustard gas and arsenic are human carcinogens.[4]

Although infrequent, attacks with chemical weapons still occur—and have occurred dozens of times during the past decade in Syria. Separate from their use in armed conflict, police forces have used lacrimogenic agents for crowd control, accounting for injuries among civilians, including major head injury and vision loss.[3]

Chemical weapons have been used in war since about 1000 B.C.E., when China used arsenical smoke as a weapon. During the Peloponnesian War (460 to 445 B.C.E.), Sparta deployed noxious smoke and flame against urban populations. During the First World War, chemical weapons were first used on a large scale (Figure 5-1). Among the chemical agents deployed were mustard gas, chlorine, phosgene, and lewisite. Use of chemical weapons endangered not only soldiers but also first responders, physicians, and nurses who were treating affected soldiers as well as workers who manufactured chemical weapons.[5]

> [I watched] figures running wildly in confusion over the fields. Greenish-gray clouds swept down upon them, turning yellow as they traveled over the country blasting everything they touched and shriveling up the vegetation. . . . Then there staggered into our midst French soldiers, blinded, coughing, chests heaving, faces an ugly purple color, lips speechless with agony, and behind them in gas soaked trenches, we learned that they left hundreds of dead and dying comrades.[6]
>
> *A British soldier, describing the scene at Ypres, Belgium,*
> *after the use of mustard gas there by German forces*

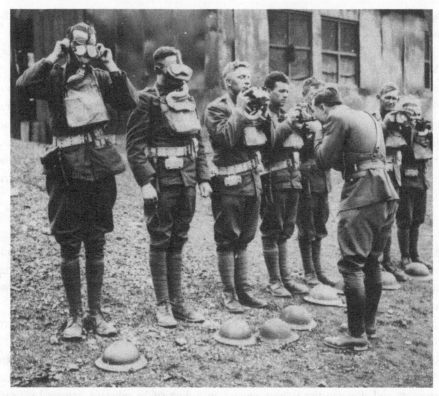

FIGURE 5-1 U.S. soldiers in France learning to use gas masks before deployment in the First World War. (Library of Congress, Negative LC-USZ 62-92733.)

By November 1918, chemical weapons had adversely affected approximately 1.3 million soldiers and caused about 90,000 deaths. The use of these weapons also caused much stress, anxiety, and panic.[1]

Between 1940 and 1945, Germany used Zyklon B (a form of hydrogen cyanide) to kill millions of people in concentration camps during the Holocaust. Between 1919 and 1988, military forces used chemical weapons in wars in Russia, Morocco, Abyssinia, Manchuria, Yemen, Vietnam, Iraq, and Iran.[4] In the Iraq–Iran War, Iraq used chemical weapons, mainly mustard gas and nerve agents, against Iranian troops, causing at least 122 deaths.[7] In 1988, Iraq used chemical agents against Kurdish rebels in Halabja and surrounding villages in northern Iraq.

In 1994, a Japanese cult, Aum Shinrikyo, used sarin in an attack on an apartment complex, causing seven deaths and 300 other injuries. In 1995, it used sarin in attacks in the Tokyo subway system, causing 12 deaths and seriously affecting 1,500 others.[8]

Since 2012, Syrian President Bashar al-Assad has used chemical weapons, likely sarin and chlorine gas, during the Syrian Civil War dozens of times, killing hundreds of civilians.[9–11] Chemical weapons were also used during the past decade by the Islamic State (ISIS) (Figure 5-2).

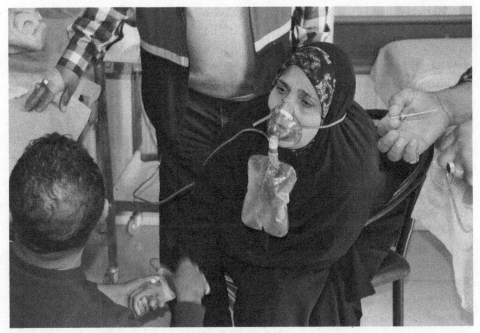

FIGURE 5-2 A woman exposed to a chemical attack by ISIS is treated at a hospital in Taza, near Kirkuk, northern Iraq, in 2016. (AP Photo.)

Chemical Weapons Convention

In 1925, the Geneva Protocol designated chemical weapons as illegitimate weapons of war. The Biological and Toxin Weapons Convention (see page 82), which entered into force in 1975, reinforced the prohibition on use of these weapons. The Chemical Weapons Convention (CWC), which entered into force in 1997, prohibits the development, production, acquisition, stockpiling, transfer, and use (or preparation for use) of chemical weapons. It also mandates that states parties cannot assist, encourage, or induce other countries to engage in prohibited activities.

The CWC requires states parties to declare their chemical weapons stockpiles and production facilities, relevant chemical industry facilities, and other weapons-related information. And it requires states parties to destroy their chemical weapons, facilities that produce them, and chemical weapons it has abandoned in other participating countries. As of June 2021, a total of 193 countries, including the United States, had ratified the CWC, one nation had signed but not ratified it, and three countries had neither signed nor ratified it.[12]

The Organization for the Prohibition of Chemical Weapons (OPCW), with about 500 employees and based in The Hague, implements the CWC. It receives states parties' declarations that describe activities or material related to chemical weapons, and then, in order to ensure compliance, it inspects and monitors relevant states parties' facilities and reviews their activities. The Scientific Advisory Board of the OPCW has provided recommendations on pre- and post-exposure treatments as well as decontaminants and adsorbing materials.[13]

Several states parties have completely destroyed their declared stockpiles of chemical weapons. In 2013, Syria joined the CWC under international pressure and allowed for the removal and destruction of its declared stockpile of nerve agents, mustard agents, precursor chemicals, and associated equipment, but the OPCW and the United Nations report that Syria still has undeclared chemical weapons. As of June 2021, the United States had destroyed 2,067 tons from its stockpile of chemical weapons and estimated that it would destroy the rest by September 2023.[14,15]

A major issue is how to prevent environmental contamination when destroying chemical weapons, as well as antipersonnel landmines and some other weapons. In the past, the primary practices were "open-burn" and "open-detonation" methods, which were inexpensive but harmful to the environment. New technologies have been developed, primarily for chemical weapons, including "closed burn" and "closed detonation," which contain emissions.

A small number of countries continue to develop chemical weapons using modern technology.[16] A recently recognized concern is the category of highly dangerous organophosphorus chemical warfare agents known as novichoks, which bind to acetylcholinesterase.[17,18] Several times, Russia President Vladimir Putin has ordered the use of military-grade novichok nerve agents to poison political adversaries, including Sergei Skripal in England in 2018 and Alexei Navalny in Russia in 2020.

BIOLOGICAL WEAPONS

Overview and Use

Biological weapons contain living organisms (usually microorganisms) or their toxic products. Although these weapons target people, they can also be used to target animals or plants—and thereby reduce human food supplies. People fear these agents because they are invisible, are easy to disseminate, could spread easily from person to person, and could cause serious illnesses.

Over the past 2,600 years, there have been relatively few reports of the use of biological weapons. These reports have included poisoning wells with human bodies, hurling plague victims into cities, mixing wine with blood of leprosy patients, and firing saliva from rabid dogs toward enemies.[19] A critical review of the history of biological warfare found that many reports could not be verified.[20] However, a number of planned or accidental exposures to biological agents have occurred, including the following:

- In the mid-1700s, during the French and Indian War, a British commander sent smallpox-infected blankets to Native Americans.
- During the First World War, the German military developed a program to spread animal diseases, such as anthrax and glanders, to humans.
- In 1942, the British government contaminated Gruinard Island, off the coast of Scotland, with anthrax spores during a test of these biological agents on sheep.
- In 1979, a Soviet military research facility near Sverdlovsk accidentally released anthrax spores, which caused between 68 and 105 fatal cases of anthrax.[21,22]

- In 1984 in Oregon, more than 750 people developed salmonella gastroenteritis after members of a religious commune deliberately contaminated restaurant food.[23]
- In 2001, a still-unidentified person or persons—possibly a worker or workers in a U.S. biodefense laboratory—disseminated anthrax spores through the U.S. Postal Service, exposing thousands of people and causing 23 cases of anthrax, five of which were fatal.[24]

Between the two world wars, Japan developed a biological weapons program, which included exposing prisoners to the organisms that cause smallpox, plague, and anthrax. Japan conducted experiments on prisoners and also dropped plague-infected fleas and infected food and clothing from planes into China, causing thousands of deaths. During the Second World War, Germany performed research on prisoners with biological agents, but did not use them. Fearing Germany's use of biological weapons, the United States increased its research on these agents. After the war, the U.S. government granted immunity to the leaders of Japan's biological weapons program in exchange for knowledge gained through its experiments.[25]

The United States ultimately developed a large biological weapons infrastructure with laboratories, test facilities, and production plants (Figure 5-3). It weaponized existing

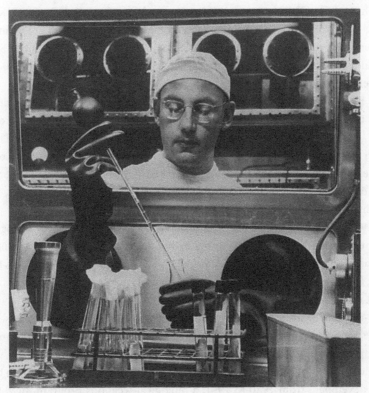

FIGURE 5-3 A technician works in a laboratory at Fort Detrick in Frederick, MD, in the late 1960s under the offensive biological weapons program that the U.S. Army operated there from 1943 to 1969. (AP Photo/Department of Defense.)

strains of bacteria and developed new strains that were resistant to antibiotics.[21] And it conducted in the United States 239 top-secret, open-air disseminations of alleged non-pathogenic bacteria to test the efficiency of dispersal. During the 1960s, the Soviet Union also developed an extensive offensive biological weapons program, which it expanded in 1972 (see below).[26]

Biological Weapons Convention

By 1970, the United States had stockpiles of at least 10 biological and toxin weapons. But the Nixon administration realized that it was in the strategic interest of the United States to develop and support an international convention to ban these weapons, given the large U.S. stockpile of nuclear weapons. Together with the Soviet Union and other nations, the United States negotiated the Convention on the Prohibition of the Development, Production and Stockpiling of Bacteriological and Toxin Weapons and on their Destruction (also known as the Biological Weapons Convention, the Biological and Toxin Weapons Convention, the BWC, and the BTWC), which was signed in 1972 and entered into force in 1975.[27]

The BWC bans the development, production or acquisition, stockpiling, retention, transfer, or assistance with acquiring biological and toxin weapons. (It does not ban the *use* of biological and toxin weapons, but it reaffirms the 1925 Geneva Protocol, which prohibits such use.) The BWC requires states parties to destroy—or to divert for peaceful purposes—agents, toxins, weapons, equipment, and means of delivery that are banned under the Convention.[27] As of June 2021, a total of 183 countries, including the United States, had signed and ratified the BWC; four countries had signed but not ratified it; and 10 countries had neither signed nor ratified it.

The BWC does not have any mechanism for ensuring verification or compliance. It mandates that states parties consult with one another and cooperate to address compliance concerns. It allows states parties to submit complaints to the UN Security Council if they believe other member states are violating the Convention. Although the Security Council can investigate complaints, this power has never been used.[28] Implementation of the BWC has been less than satisfactory. States parties have not consistently submitted reports, and there has been inadequate financial support for the Convention.[29]

In 1972, the Soviet Union began to massively expand its bioweapons program—the same year that it signed the BWC. At one point, the Soviet program employed 60,000 workers at more than 100 facilities. It stockpiled, for possible use against the United States and allied countries, hundreds of tons of the microorganisms that cause anthrax and dozens of tons of those that cause plague and smallpox. It mounted smallpox virus on missiles. It developed antibiotic-resistant forms of the organisms that cause plague and anthrax. It mass-produced the viruses that cause hemorrhagic fever. The program continued for almost two decades, until the dissolution of the Soviet Union in 1991.[26]

In violation of its obligations as a signatory (although not a state party) to the BWC, Iraq also developed, from 1980 to 1991, a biological weapons program, in violation of its having signed (but not ratified) the BWC. This program was uncovered after the Gulf War, at which time Iraq discontinued the program and ratified the Convention.[28]

However, in 2002 and 2003, the George W. Bush administration inaccurately stated that Iraq continued to possess biological weapons and used this allegation to justify the U.S. invasion of Iraq.

The BWC does not ban *biodefense* programs, which aim to protect against biological weapons attacks. During the 1980s, the Reagan administration initiated the Biological Research Defense Program, which was criticized for research that had the potential to increase capabilities for offensive use of biological weapons. Since the anthrax attack in 2001, the U.S. government has spent tens of billions of dollars on preparedness against bioterrorism, including more biodefense research. Some biodefense research laboratories are located in or near densely populated areas, concentrations of livestock, and areas vulnerable to flooding, where an accidental leak or a terrorist attack could have disastrous consequences. Frequent safety incidents at biodefense laboratories have been reported; for example, in 2015, there were more than 230 safety incidents reported at these laboratories, hundreds of workers in these laboratories were monitored for possible hazardous exposures, and a few laboratories had their permits suspended because of violations that raised "significant concerns for imminent danger."[30] The COVID-19 pandemic has increased public awareness about the potential dangers of the release of microorganisms from laboratories and exposing people in adjacent communities and beyond.

Categories of Biological Agents

The Centers for Disease Control and Prevention (CDC) has identified three categories of biological agents that could be used during war or terrorist attacks:

- Category A consists of biological agents that can be easily disseminated or transmitted from person to person, result in high mortality rates, might have a major public health impact, might cause public panic and social disruption, and require special action for public health preparedness.
- Category B consists of biological agents that are moderately easy to disseminate, result in moderate morbidity rates and low mortality rates, and require enhanced diagnostic capacity and enhanced disease surveillance.
- Category C consists of emerging pathogens that could be engineered for mass dissemination because of availability, ease of production and dissemination, and potential for high morbidity and mortality rates and major health impact.[31]

These agents and the diseases that they cause are listed in Box 5-1. More information is available from the CDC, including at: https://emergency.cdc.gov/agent/agentlist-category.asp.

Potential new dangers could arise from genetic technologies that enable development of genetically altered organisms not known to exist in nature. These organisms could be used as biological weapons that could travel far and remain infectious, become resistant to antibiotic treatment, and rapidly infect a population, causing much illness and death.

BOX 5-1 Categories of Diseases and the Biological Agents That Cause Them

Category A

    Anthrax (*Bacillus anthracis*)

    Botulism (*Clostridium botulinum toxin*)

    Plague (*Yersinia pestis*)

    Smallpox (variola major)

    Tularemia (*Francisella tularensis*)

    Viral hemorrhagic fevers (filoviruses, such as Ebola and Marburg; and arena-viruses, such as Lassa and Machupo)

Category B

    Brucellosis (*Brucella* species)

    Epsilon toxin of *Clostridium perfringens*

    Food safety threats (such as salmonella species, *Escherichia coli* O157:H7, and shigella)

    Glanders (*Burkholderias mallei*)

    Melioidosis (*Burkholderia pseudomallei*)

    Psittacosis (*Chlamydia psittaci*)

    Q fever (*Coxiella burnetii*)

    Ricin toxin from *Ricinus communis* (castor beans)

    Staphylococcal enterotoxin B

    Typhus fever (*Rickettsia prowazeki*)

    Viral encephalitis (alphaviruses, such as Eastern equine encephalitis, Venezuelan equine encephalitis, and Western equine encephalitis)

    Water safety threats (such as *Vibrio cholerae* and *Cryptosporidium parvum*)

Category C

    Emerging infectious disease, such as those caused by Nipah virus and hantavirus

(Source: Centers for Disease Control and Prevention. Available at: https://emergency.cdc.gov/agent/agentlist-category.asp. Accessed on June 1, 2021.)

NUCLEAR WEAPONS

Overview and Use

Nuclear weapons release vast amounts of energy by fission and/or fusion. They generate huge explosive forces, create extraordinarily high temperatures, and emit ionizing radiation. Nuclear weapons cause immediate deaths due to blast and thermal injuries. And they cause acute radiation syndrome,[32] many types of cancer, and other diseases related to radiation exposure. The detonation by the United States of "atomic bombs" over Hiroshima and

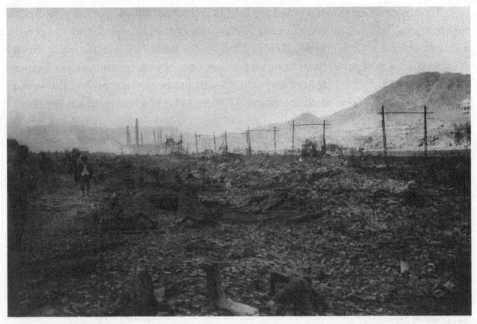

FIGURE 5-4 View of Nagasaki after detonation of an atomic bomb in August 1945. (Yosuke Yamahata/ 1945.08.10/Nagasaki.)

Nagasaki, Japan, in August 1945, at the end of the Second World War, caused by the end of 1945 more than 200,000 deaths—due to heat, blast force, and ionizing radiation—and ultimately tens of thousands of cases of malignant and nonmalignant diseases (Figure 5-4). Since then, thermonuclear weapons (hydrogen bombs) with explosive force much greater than those detonated in 1945 have been developed. The most powerful hydrogen bomb, which was tested by the Soviet Union in 1961, had more than 3,000 times the explosive force of the bombs exploded in Japan.

Survivors of the atomic bomb explosions at Hiroshima and Nagasaki have been extensively studied with prospective cohort studies, which have demonstrated increased rates of cancer and other diseases. (Results of these studies are described in Chapter 10.) Long-term studies of the psychological effects of the Hiroshima and Nagasaki bombings have also been performed, such as a study of survivors 52 years after the Nagasaki bombing, which found that they had severe apathy, disordered relationships, and anhedonia (inability to feel pleasure).[33]

Nuclear Weapons Production and Testing

Production of nuclear weapons has created extensive radioactive and toxic waste, which has contaminated the environment. Nuclear weapons industry sites in the United States, such as former sites of plutonium production in Washington and Tennessee, have been highly contaminated. During 50 years of operation, the Hanford site in Washington produced 500 million gallons of highly radioactive and chemically toxic waste, some of which was released into the environment, extensively contaminating soil and groundwater.[34]

Throughout the development and production cycle of nuclear weapons, adverse health, environmental, and socioeconomic impacts have disproportionately affected Indigenous, minority, and other vulnerable populations.[35] Indigenous lands have been the major sources of materials for nuclear weapons and the primary sites of atmospheric nuclear weapons testing worldwide. In the United States, Native Americans performed much of the work in uranium mines with little or no protection (Chapter 11).[36] Workers in Africa also mined much uranium for nuclear weapons.[37]

More than 2,000 nuclear weapons tests, extensive research, and large-scale production of nuclear weapons has led to contamination of air, water, and soil, causing human disease and damage to ecosystems. Many military personnel deployed for atmospheric tests of nuclear weapons received large doses of radiation.

Native Americans, Marshallese people, and other Indigenous Peoples have been disproportionately affected by the testing of nuclear weapons and disposal of radioactive material.[38] The United States tested nuclear weapons on or near the Bikini and Enewetak atolls in the Pacific Ocean between 1946 and 1958, vaporizing islands that had been homeland for Marshallese people for generations and releasing about 6.3 billion curies of radioactive iodine into the atmosphere—42 times greater than the amount emitted from the Nevada Test Site (Figure 5-5).[39]

An issue of concern is that operation of nuclear reactors can provide materials and technical expertise for possible development of nuclear weapons. At the end of 2019, there were 443 nuclear reactors operating in 30 countries, and 54 more reactors were under construction.[40]

Yet another issue of concern is the waste from the production of nuclear weapons. The United States has more than 40,000 nuclear weapons waste sites. Cleanup costs for these wastes have been estimated at $41.1 billion.[41] (See Chapter 13.)

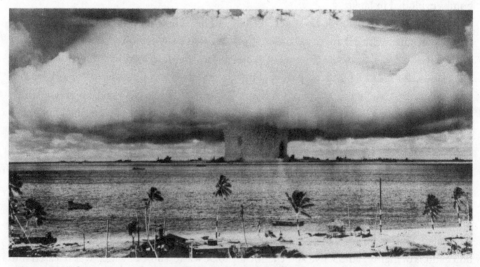

FIGURE 5-5 U.S. atomic bomb test at Bikini Atoll in the Pacific in 1946. (Library of Congress, Negative LC-USZ62-66049.)

Costs of Maintaining and Modernizing Nuclear Weapons

The huge cost of maintaining and modernizing nuclear weapons arsenals diverts human and financial resources away from public health, education, and other activities that benefit society. Between 1945 and 1996, the United States spent $5.5 trillion on nuclear weapons and related programs, a cost that was, during that period, greater than all other categories of U.S. government spending, except for Social Security and non-nuclear national defense.[42] Over the next decade, modernization, maintenance, and storage of nuclear weapons will cost the United States $494 billion.[43] Over the next 30 years, the United States plans to spend an estimated $1.2 trillion to upgrade and modernize its nuclear weapons and delivery systems.[44]

Risks of Nuclear War

The total number of nuclear weapons reached a peak of more than 64,000 in the mid-1980s.[45] There has been a major decrease since then. As of January 2021, nine countries possessed a total of more than 13,000 nuclear warheads: Russia (6,255), the United States (5,550), China (350), France (290), the United Kingdom (225), Pakistan (165), India (156), Israel (90), and North Korea (40 to 50, an uncertain figure). Russia and the United States possessed 90% of them; 1,625 (26%) of the nuclear warheads possessed by Russia were deployed, and 1,800 (32%) of those possessed by the United States were deployed.[46]

Current concerns include:

- Proliferation of nuclear weapons
- An accidental launch of nuclear weapons[47]
- A terrorist attack with nuclear weapons by non-state actors
- The possibility that hostile governments or non-state actors could launch a cyber attack, which could lead to the accidental launch of nuclear weapons (Chapter 4)
- Inadequate security for tons of highly enriched uranium and plutonium, posing risks of nuclear theft and diversion of these materials into nuclear weapons programs.[48]

The nuclear strategy of both the United States and Russia has been based on *mutually assured destruction*. Neither country could "win" a nuclear war. Each country has perceived that its huge arsenals of nuclear weapons, on bombers, land-based missiles, and submarine-based missiles, prevent a "first-strike" attack by the other country. Arsenals of nuclear weapons have been used to deter a nuclear attack. But are more than 3,400 nuclear warheads deployed by the United States and Russia necessary for deterrence?

Some nuclear-weapon states, including the United States, reserve the right of "first use" of nuclear weapons—that is, they do not rule out the possibility of their using nuclear weapons to counter either an aggressive threat or the use of conventional weapons against them. However, first use of nuclear weapons could very quickly escalate into a large-scale nuclear war.[49]

Even a "limited" nuclear war, such as between India and Pakistan, could create dramatic decreases in ambient temperature, with widespread crop failures and famine affecting huge numbers of people. If only 250 of the nuclear weapons in the combined arsenals of India and Pakistan were used against each other, fatalities could reach 50 to 125 million people and nuclear-ignited fires could release 16 to 36 teragrams (Tg) of black carbon (soot), which would rise up to the stratosphere and, within weeks, spread globally. Surface sunlight would decline by 25% to 35%, reducing surface temperature by 2° to 5°C and decreasing precipitation by 15% to 30%. Recovery could take more than 10 years. Mass starvation could occur, with many more collateral fatalities. On a much larger scale, a major nuclear war between the United States and Russia could kill many more people and would send 150 Tg of soot into the stratosphere, decreasing temperatures worldwide by an average of 8°C (14.4°F). Agriculture would come to a halt. Ecosystems would be destroyed. Worldwide, most people would starve to death. And the human species could become extinct.[50,51] (See Profile 5.)

Daniel Ellsberg, an activist and former U.S. military analyst, stated in his book *The Doomsday Machine: Confessions of a Nuclear War Planner*: "The arsenals and plans of the two superpowers represent not only an insuperable obstacle to an effective global anti-proliferation campaign: they are themselves a clear and present existential danger to the human species, and most others."[52]

International Control Measures

International control of nuclear weapons has relied on treaties to reduce arsenals, ban nuclear weapon tests, control fissile material, and prevent proliferation of nuclear weapons to countries that do not possess them. Several international treaties pertaining to the possession, proliferation, testing, and other aspects of nuclear weapons are briefly described in Table 5-1.

TABLE 5-1 Major Nuclear Weapons Treaties

Treaty (Year)	Description
Partial Test Ban Treaty (PTBT) (1963)	Prohibits explosive tests of nuclear weapons in the atmosphere, under water, and in outer space
Treaty on the Non-Proliferation of Nuclear Weapons (the Nuclear Non-Proliferation Treaty, or NPT) (1968)	Prohibits nuclear-weapon states from transferring nuclear weapons to any recipient and prohibits them from assisting, encouraging, or inducing any non–nuclear-weapon state to acquire nuclear weapons.
	Prohibits acquisition of nuclear weapons by non-nuclear-weapon states. Commits nuclear-weapon states to pursue nuclear and general disarmament.
Strategic Arms Limitation Talks (SALT I) (1969–1972)	Produced both the Anti-Ballistic Missile Treaty (see below) and an interim agreement between the U.S. and Soviet Union on measures to limit strategic offensive arms, in which both pledged to not construct new intercontinental ballistic missile silos, to not increase the size of existing silos significantly, and to cap the number of launch tubes for submarine-launched ballistic missiles and submarines carrying these missiles
Anti-Ballistic Missile Treaty (ABM Treaty) (1972)	Limited anti-ballistic missile systems used in defending areas against ballistic missile–delivered nuclear weapons

(continued)

TABLE 5·1 Continued

Treaty (Year)	Description
Strategic Arms Limitation Talks II (SALT II) (Signed in 1979, but never entered into force)	Would have called for numerical limits on missiles, bans on certain missiles, definitions of limited systems, and verification
Strategic Arms Reduction Treaty I (START I) (1994)	Required U.S. and Russian reductions of strategic nuclear weapons
Strategic Arms Reduction Treaty II (START II) (Signed in 1993, but never entered into force)	Obligated the U.S. and Russia to reduce their arms to specific limits and to eliminate all heavy intercontinental ballistic missiles
Intermediate-Range Nuclear Forces (INF) Treaty (1988)	Required the U.S. and Soviet Union to verifiably eliminate all ground-launched ballistic and cruise missiles with ranges between 311 and 3,416 miles
Comprehensive Nuclear-Test-Ban Treaty (CTBT) (1996)	Prohibits test explosions of nuclear weapons, but not computer simulations or explosions involving nuclear material that do not produce nuclear criticality (subcritical tests), and establishes an international monitoring system to detect and deter clandestine nuclear test explosions. Signed by 185 states and ratified by 170, but will not enter into force until 8 states (China, Egypt, India, Israel, Iran, North Korea, Pakistan, and the United States) ratify it. (As of June 2021, no state was actively engaged in explosive testing of nuclear weapons.)
Strategic Offensive Reductions Treaty (SORT or Moscow Treaty) (2002)	U.S. and Russia reduced their strategic arsenals to 1,700 to 2,200 warheads each. Permanent arsenal reductions are not required. Warheads need not be destroyed. Either side may quickly withdraw. Treaty expires when arsenal limits are reached.
New START (2010)	Caps U.S. and Russia to 1,550 deployed strategic nuclear warheads and 700 deployed strategic delivery systems, and requires regular reporting and on-site monitoring.
Treaty on the Prohibition of Nuclear Weapons (TPNW) (Opened for signature in 2017, entered into force in 2021)	Bans nuclear weapons, including their possession. Makes it illegal for states parties to develop, test, produce, acquire, possess, store, transfer, transport, plan to use (or threaten to use), or use nuclear weapons. Would require nuclear-weapon states that are states parties (none of them is a state party at present) to destroy their nuclear weapons and terminate their nuclear-weapons programs. Mandates that states parties assist victims of nuclear-weapons testing and use. Requires that areas contaminated by nuclear weapons be environmentally remediated.

The most recent nuclear weapons-related agreement is the Treaty on the Prohibition of Nuclear Weapons (TPNW), which was adopted at the UN General Assembly in 2017 by more than 120 countries and entered into force in 2021. It bans the development, testing, production, acquisition, possession, storage, transfer, transport, plan or threaten to use, and use of nuclear weapons. The treaty also obligates states parties to provide environmental remediation and victim assistance to those affected by the testing or use of nuclear weapons.[53] As of June 2021, the TPNW had 86 signatories and 54 states parties. The United States and the other eight nuclear-weapon states have not signed the TPNW.[54]

Some countries that possess nuclear weapons argue that the TPNW risks undermining the system of preexisting safeguards to prevent the spread of nuclear weapons and risks aggravating tensions between countries with and those without nuclear weapons. Proponents argue that the TPNW supports and reinforces important norms and institutions for nonproliferation and disarmament, including the 1968 Treaty on the Non-Proliferation of Nuclear Weapons (NPT) and the 1996 Comprehensive Nuclear-Test-Ban Treaty (CTBT).

The NPT obligates non-nuclear-weapon states to never acquire nuclear weapons and obligates all states parties, including the five states parties that are nuclear-weapon states and permanent members of the UN Security Council (China, France, Russia, the United Kingdom, and the United States), to "pursue negotiations in good faith on effective measures relating to cessation of the nuclear arms race at an early date and to nuclear disarmament, and on a treaty on general and complete disarmament under strict and effective international control."[55] (The other four nuclear-weapon states—India, Israel, North Korea, and Pakistan—are not yet states parties to the NPT.)

Developing the popular will necessary for the elimination of nuclear weapons worldwide will depend on the actions of civil society organizations, including organizations of health professionals.[56,57] For example, in 2020, the American Public Health Association adopted a policy urging the United States and other nuclear-weapon states to sign and ratify the TPNW and to pursue measures to end the nuclear arms race.[58] Other organizations of health professionals, such as the International Physicians for the Prevention of Nuclear War and Physicians for Social Responsibility, its U.S. affiliate, have for decades informed the public and policymakers about the projected impact of a nuclear war and have promoted the abolition of nuclear weapons.[59,60]

The president of the United States and the leaders of some of the other eight nuclear-weapon states have had unchecked power to launch a nuclear weapons attack. William Perry, a former U.S. Secretary of Defense who has worked to promote nuclear disarmament and to prevent nuclear war, has recommended that (a) the president share the decision to use nuclear weapons with a select group of U.S. senators and congressional representatives, (b) the United States declare that it will never start a nuclear war and would use nuclear weapons only in retaliation, and (c) the United States retire its land-based ballistic missiles, which are not needed for deterrence because of the deployment of submarine-based nuclear weapons.[61]

A national grassroots campaign, Back from the Brink: The Call to Prevent Nuclear War, outlines a plan for the United States to lead a global effort to prevent nuclear war by:

- Renouncing the option of using nuclear weapons first
- Ending the sole, unchecked authority of any U.S. president to launch a nuclear attack
- Taking U.S. nuclear weapons off hair-trigger alert
- Canceling the plan to replace its entire nuclear arsenal with enhanced weapons
- Actively pursuing a verifiable agreement among nuclear-armed states to eliminate their nuclear arsenals.

As of June 2021, members of the campaign included more than 350 nongovernmental and professional organizations as well as 53 municipalities and seven states and counties in the

United States. The campaign provides advocacy tools, including an organizing guide and organizing materials, a sample resolution, and an endorsement request.[62]

Accidental Detonation

Despite safeguards, accidental detonation remains a possibility. There have been several false alarms since the late 1970s, when the United States and Russia (and the Soviet Union) have come close to launching nuclear missiles in response to a perceived immediate attack from the other side:

- On November 9, 1979, computers at the Pentagon provided a preliminary warning of a massive Soviet nuclear strike aimed at the U.S. command system and nuclear forces. It was later determined that a realistic training tape had been inadvertently inserted into the computer running the U.S. early warning programs.
- On June 3, 1980, U.S. command posts received a warning that the Soviet Union had launched a nuclear attack. Although there were internal inconsistencies in the number of Soviet missiles perceived, a threat assessment was performed to evaluate the possibility that the attack was real. Later investigations showed that a single computer chip failure had caused random numbers of attacking missiles to be displayed.
- On September 26, 1983, the new Soviet early warning satellite system caused a false alarm when it perceived five missiles launched by the United States. In retrospect, this was probably caused by light reflected from clouds or snowbanks. This incident did not start a nuclear war, perhaps because the Soviet command did not want to start a war based on data from a new system. However, had the system falsely reported hundreds of missiles heading to the Soviet Union, it might have mistakenly launched its missiles.
- On January 25, 1995, Boris Yeltsin, then president of Russia, had only a few minutes to decide whether to launch Russian nuclear-armed missiles against the United States in response to what, on radar, looked like a U.S. air attack with multiple re-entry vehicles. It turned out to be a rocket launched by a team of Norwegian and U.S. scientists who were studying the aurora borealis ("the Northern lights").[63]

Today, false alarms may be more likely because nuclear weapons and warning systems could be vulnerable to cyber attacks (Chapter 4).

Other Concerns

There have been other incidents that provoked widespread concern. On August 29, 2007, six cruise missiles, each loaded with a nuclear warhead, were mistakenly loaded onto a U.S. Air Force B-52 bomber in North Dakota and transported to Louisiana without using mandatory security precautions for nuclear weapons.[64] In January 2014, it was reported that 92 officers at Malmstrom Air Force Base in Montana—about half of the nuclear launch crew there—had been suspended in a cheating scandal; the Air Force acknowledged a "systemic problem" in the culture of the team that is entrusted to launch intercontinental ballistic missiles.[65]

Other situations have occurred when nuclear-armed delivery systems have narrowly failed to detonate. For example, in 1961, a B-52 loaded with nuclear weapons crashed in

Goldsboro, North Carolina, and in 1980, a nuclear-tipped Titan missile exploded in Damascus, Arkansas. Journalist Eric Schlosser, in his book *Command and Control: Nuclear Weapons, the Damascus Accident, and the Illusion of Safety*, describes that accident in detail and provides a 70-year account about the nuclear age, documenting "the mixture of human fallibility and technological complexity that can lead to disaster."[66]

Proliferation of nuclear weapons remains a serious threat. During the past two decades, North Korea has obtained nuclear technology and fissile materials, and has developed and tested nuclear weapons. Given the widespread knowledge about nuclear technology and the potential availability of fissile material, non-state actors might be able to acquire—or construct—and detonate nuclear weapons. Highly enriched uranium (HEU), the fissile material that is used in nuclear weapons, is distributed globally; it has been used to power nuclear reactors used for research, make medical isotopes, and fuel aircraft carriers and submarines. Converting to low-enriched uranium would eliminate the possibility of HEU being stolen or otherwise diverted to produce nuclear weapons.

Another potential threat is a conventional weapon to which radioactive materials (such as cesium-137 or cobalt-60) have been added—also known as a *radiological weapon* or a *dirty bomb*. There is a concern that some radioactive materials could be stolen or illegally obtained from medical research and healthcare facilities and industries that use them. If such a device were to be deployed, it would have immediate effects, both in terms of explosive damage and potentially radiation-induced illness in individuals who inhaled or ingested radioactive materials. And it likely would have longer-term impacts by making people unnecessarily avoid the contaminated area, even after it was remediated and determined to be safe.[67,68]

Another major concern is the huge diversion of financial resources to maintain and modernize the U.S. nuclear weapons arsenal, estimated to be about $1.2 trillion over the next 30 years—an inherent contradiction with U.S. nonproliferation policy. As the nuclear weapons budget of the U.S. Department of Energy increases, there have been substantial cuts proposed in the budgets of programs to dismantle and prevent proliferation of nuclear weapons—and in programs to reduce poverty and to protect human rights. To most Americans, all these concerns are unfortunately out of sight and out of mind.

Putting the threats of nuclear weapons in context, Eric Schlosser concluded *Command and Control* with the following:

> America's nuclear weapons are among the safest, the most advanced, the most secure against unauthorized use that have ever been built. And yet the United States has narrowly avoided a long series of nuclear disasters. Other countries, with less hard-earned experience in the field, may not be as fortunate. . . . [Nuclear weapons] also pose a grave threat to any country that possesses them.
>
> Right now thousands of missiles are hidden away, literally out of sight, topped with warheads and ready to go, awaiting the right electrical signal. They are a collective death wish, barely suppressed. Every one of them is an accident waiting to happen, a potential act of mass murder. They are out there, waiting, soulless and mechanical, sustained by our denial—and they work.[66]

TOWARD A WORLD WITHOUT CHEMICAL, BIOLOGICAL, AND NUCLEAR WEAPONS

Countries have traditionally attempted to reduce threats posed by chemical, biological, and nuclear weapons by promoting peace in conjunction with efforts in arms control and disarmament. Measures concerning nuclear weapons have included:

- Unilateral responses, such as South Africa's decision in 1993 to abandon its program to develop nuclear weapons and the decisions of Belarus, Kazakhstan, and Ukraine to turn over the former Soviet Union nuclear weapons that they possessed
- Bilateral (and reciprocal) responses, such as the United States and the Soviet Union cooperating to reduce their nuclear arsenals and missile capabilities during the Cold War and deciding in the late 1980s to reciprocally eliminate their chemical weapons stockpiles
- Responses by more than two countries, such as the effort by the United States, Russia, the United Kingdom, China, France, and Germany, which resulted in the Joint Comprehensive Plan of Action (the "Iran nuclear deal") in 2015
- Regional responses, such as treaties that established nuclear-weapon–free zones in Latin America and the Caribbean, Africa, the South Pacific, Central Asia, and Southeast Asia—with a combined population of more than 2.6 billion people
- Global responses, such as development and implementation of the CWC, the BWC, the NPT, and other international conventions as well as the Global Partnership that helped some republics of the former Soviet Union to eliminate their chemical and biological agents and to secure and reduce their stockpiles of nuclear weapons.

These traditional responses have had limitations, including lack of universal participation by countries in specific conventions and treaties, the potential for countries to withdraw from these agreements, inadequate systems for inspections and verification, countries not complying with their treaty obligations (including annual reports and declarations), and inadequate measures to enforce treaties.[69]

As the Weapons of Mass Destruction Commission stated in its final report: "Weapons of mass destruction cannot be uninvented. But they can be outlawed, as biological and chemical weapons already have been, and their use made unthinkable." The report recommended measures to decrease the danger of nuclear weapon arsenals by ensuring no first use by countries and no access by non-state actors, preventing proliferation of new weapon systems and new countries possessing these weapons, and outlawing all weapons of mass destruction.[69]

SUMMARY POINTS

- International conventions have restricted development, testing, and potential use of chemical, biological, and nuclear weapons.
- Chemical and biological weapons have been used infrequently, but nevertheless represent continuing threats.

- Approximately 13,000 nuclear weapons possessed by nine countries represent a grave threat.
- Current nuclear threats include accidental launch, potential theft of nuclear materials by non-state actors, and miscalculation that could lead to a nuclear war.
- A nuclear war would have catastrophic consequences worldwide that could threaten the survival of humankind.

REFERENCES

1. Ekzayez A, Flecknoe MD, Lillywhite L, et al. Chemical weapons and public health: Assessing impact and responses. Journal of Public Health 2020; 42: e334-e342. doi: 10.1093/pubmed/fdz/145.
2. Greenberg MI, Sexton KJ, Vearrier D. Sea-dumped chemical weapons: Environmental risk, occupational hazard. Clinical Toxicology 2016; 54: 79-91.
3. Haar RJ, Iacopino V, Ranadive N, et al. Health impacts of chemical irritants used for crowd control: A systematic review of the injuries and deaths caused by tear gas and pepper spray. BMC Public Health 2017; 17: 831. doi: 10.1186/s12889-017-4814-6.
4. Lee EC, Bleek PC, Kales SN. "Chemical weapons" in BS Levy, VW Sidel (eds.). Terrorism and Public Health (2nd edition). New York: Oxford University Press, 2012, pp. 183-202.
5. Fitzgerald GJ. Chemical warfare and medical response during World War I. American Journal of Public Health 2008; 98: 611-625. doi: 10.2105/AJPH.2007.11930.
6. Watkins OS. "Methodist Report," cited in A Fries, CJ West. Chemical Warfare. New York: McGraw Hill, 1921.
7. Salamati P, Razavi SM, Shokraneh F, et al. Mortality and injuries among Iranians in Iraq-Iran war: A systematic review. Archives of Iranian Medicine 2013; 15: 542-550.
8. Bismuth C, Borron SW, Baud FJ, Barriot P. Chemical weapons: Documented use and compounds on the horizon. Toxicology Letters 2004; 149: 11-18.
9. Arms Control Association. Timeline of Syrian chemical weapons activity, 2012–2020. Available at: https://www.armscontrol.org/factsheets/Timeline-of-Syrian-Chemical-Weapons-Activity. Accessed on June 4, 2020.
10. Gladstone R. U.S. says Syria has used chemical weapons at least 50 times during war. New York Times, April 13, 2018. Available at: https://www.nytimes.com/2018/04/13/world/middleeast/un-syria-haley-chemical-weapons.html. Accessed on August 25, 2020.
11. Hubbard B. Syria used chemical weapons 3 times in one week, watchdog says. New York Times, April 8, 2020. Available at: https://www.nytimes.com/2020/04/08/world/middleeast/syria-assad-chemical-weapons.html. Accessed on August 25, 2020.
12. Chemical Weapons Convention. Available at: https://www.opcw.org/chemical-weapons-convention. Accessed on June 1, 2021.
13. Timperley CM, Abdollahi M, Al-Amri AS, et al. Advice on assistance and protection from the Scientific Advisory Board of the Organisation for the Prohibition of Chemical Weapons: Part 2. On preventing and treating health effects from acute, prolonged, and repeated nerve agent exposure, and the identification of medical countermeasures able to reduce or eliminate the longer term health effects of nerve agents. Toxicology 2019; 413: 13-23.
14. Arms Control Association. Fact Sheets & Briefs: Chemical Weapons Convention. Available at: www.armscontrol.org/factsheets/cwcglance. Accessed on April 13, 2021.
15. Program Executive Office, Assembled Chemical Weapons Alternatives. Available at: https://www.peoacwa.army.mil/. Accessed on June 1, 2021.
16. Pitschmann V. Overall view of chemical and biochemical weapons. Toxins 2014; 6: 1761-1784.
17. Kloske M, Witkiewicz A. Novichoks: The A group of organophosphorus chemical warfare agents. Chemosphere 2019; 221: 672-682.

18. Franca TCC, Kitagawa DAS, Cavalcante SF, et al. Novichoks: The dangerous fourth generation of chemical weapons. International Journal of Molecular Sciences 2019; 20: 1222. doi: 10.3390/ijms20051222.
19. Barras V, Greub G. History of biological warfare and bioterrorism. Clinical Microbiology and Infection 2014; 20: 497-502.
20. Carus WS. The history of biological weapons use: What we know and what we don't. Health Security 2015; 13: 219-255.
21. Miller J, Engelberg S, Broad W. Germs: Biological Weapons and America's Secret War. New York: Simon and Schuster, 2001.
22. Guillemin J. Anthrax: The Investigation of a Deadly Outbreak. Berkeley: University of California Press, 1999.
23. Török TJ, Tauxe RV, Wise RP, et al. A large community outbreak of salmonellosis caused by intentional contamination of restaurant salad bars. Journal of the American Medical Association 1997; 278: 389-395.
24. Brachman PS. "The Anthrax Epidemic of 2001" in BS Levy, VW Sidel (eds.). Terrorism and Public Health: A Balanced Approach to Strengthening Systems and Protecting People (2nd edition). New York: Oxford University Press, 2012, pp. 80-95.
25. Ilchmann K, Reville J. Chemical and biological weapons in the "new wars." Science and Engineering Ethics 2014; 20: 753-767.
26. Alibek K with Handelman S. Biohazard: The Chilling True Story of the Largest Covert Biological Weapons Program in the World—Told from Inside by the Man Who Ran It. New York: Random House, 1999.
27. Convention on the Prohibition of the Development, Production and Stockpiling of Bacteriological (Biological) and Toxin Weapons and on Their Destruction. Available at: https://ihl-databases.icrc.org/applic/ihl/ihl.nsf/INTRO/450. Accessed on November 16, 2021.
28. Arms Control Association. Fact Sheets & Briefs: Biological Weapons Convention. Available at: www.armscontrol.org/factsheets/BWC. Accessed on August 21, 2020.
29. Millett K. Financial woes spell trouble for the Biological Weapons Convention. Health Security 2017; 15: 320-322.
30. Young A. Hundreds of safety incidents with bioterror germs reported by secretive labs. USA Today, June 30, 2016. Available at: https://www.usatoday.com/story/news/2016/06/30/lab-safety-transparency-report/86577070/. Accessed on April 13, 2021.
31. Centers for Disease Control and Prevention. Emergency preparedness and response: Bioterrorism Agents/Diseases. Available at: https://emergency.cdc.gov/agent/agentlist-category.asp. Accessed on April 3, 2019.
32. DiCarlo AL, Maher C, Hick JL, et al. Radiation injury after a nuclear detonation: Medical consequences and the need for scarce resources allocation. Disaster Medicine and Public Health Preparedness 2011; 5(Suppl 1): S32-S44.
33. Ohta Y, Mine M, Wakasugi M, et al. Psychological effect of the Nagasaki atomic bombing on survivors after half a century. Psychiatry and Clinical Neurosciences 2000; 54: 97-103.
34. Crowley KD, Ahearne JF. Managing the environmental legacy of the U.S. nuclear-weapons production. American Scientist 2002; 90: 514-523.
35. Gould RM, Sutton PM. "Nuclear Weapons and Social Injustice" in BS Levy (ed.). Social Injustice and Public Health (3rd edition). New York: Oxford University Press, 2019, pp. 339-341.
36. Brugge D, Goble R. The history of uranium mining and the Navajo people. American Journal of Public Health 2002; 92: 1410-1419.
37. Hecht G. An elemental force: Uranium production in Africa, and what it means to be nuclear. Bulletin of the Atomic Scientists 2012; 68: 22-33.
38. U.S. Government Accountability Office. Uranium Contamination: Overall Scope, Time Frame, and Costs Information is Needed for Contamination Cleanup on the Navajo Reservation, May 2014. Available at: https://www.gao.gov/assets/670/662964.pdf. Accessed on November 27, 2020.
39. Johnston BR, Barker HM. Consequential Damage of Nuclear War: The Rongelap Report. New York: Routledge, 2008.
40. Gospodarcyk MM, Fisher MN. IAEA releases 2019 data on nuclear power plants operating experience. International Atomic Energy Agency. Available at: https://www.iaea.org/newscenter/news/iaea-releases-2019-data-on-nuclear-power-plants-operating-experience. Accessed on June 2, 2021.

41. Groeger L, Grochowski Jones R. Bombs in your backyard. Propublica, November 30, 2017. Available at: https://projects.propublica.org/bombs/. Accessed on November 27, 2020.

42. Schwartz SI. Atomic Audit: The Costs and Consequences of U.S. Nuclear Weapons Since 1940. Washington, DC: Brookings Institution Press, 1998, pp. 4–5.

43. Congressional Budget Office. Projected Costs of U.S. Nuclear Forces, 2019 to 2028, January 2019. Available at: https://www.cbo.gov/system/files/2019-01/54914-NuclearForces.pdf. Accessed on April 23, 2021.

44. Congressional Budget Office. Approaches for Managing the Costs of U.S. Nuclear Forces, 2017 to 2046. October 2017. Available at: https://www.cbo.gov/system/files/115th-congress-2017-2018/reports/53211-nuclearforces.pdf. Accessed on April 23, 2021.

45. Kristensen HM, Norrish RS. Global nuclear weapons inventories, 1945–2013. Bulletin of the Atomic Scientists 2013; 69: 75-81. doi: 10.1177/0096340213501363.

46. Kristensen HM, Korda M. World Nuclear Forces, January 2021. SIPRI Yearbook 2021: Armaments, Disarmament and International Security. Oxford: Oxford University Press on behalf of the Stockholm International Peace Research Institute, 2021, p. 334.

47. Forrow L, Blair BG, Helfand I, et al. Accidental nuclear war—A post-Cold War assessment. New England Journal of Medicine 1998; 338: 1326-1331.

48. Pomper MA, Tarini G. Nuclear Terrorism—Threat or Not? Nuclear Weapons and Related Security Issues. AIP Conference Proceedings 1898, 050001. Available at: https://doi.org/10.1063/1.5009230. Accessed on November 27, 2020.

49. Murray RK. Nuclear weapons and the law. Medicine, Conflict and Survival 1999; 15: 126-137.

50. Toon OB, Bardeen CG, Robock A, et al. Rapidly expanding nuclear arsenals in Pakistan and India portend regional and global catastrophe. Science Advances 2019; 5: eaay5478.

51. Baum S. The risk of nuclear winter. Federation of American Scientists, May 29, 2015. Available at: https://fas.org/pir-pubs/risk-nuclear-winter/. Accessed on June 4, 2020.

52. Ellsberg D. The Doomsday Machine: Confessions of a Nuclear War Planner. New York: Bloomsbury USA, 2017, p. 20.

53. Arms Control Association. The Treaty on the Prohibition of Nuclear Weapons at a Glance. Available at: https://www.armscontrol.org/factsheets/nuclearprohibition. Accessed on March 22, 2021.

54. ICAN. Treaty on the Prohibition of Nuclear Weapons: Signature and ratification status. Available at: https://www.icanw.org/signature_and_ratification_status. Accessed on June 1, 2021.

55. Arms Control Association. The Nuclear Nonproliferation Treaty at a Glance. Available at: https://www.armscontrol.org/factsheets/nptfact. Accessed on March 22, 2021.

56. Egeland K, Hugo TG, Løvold M, Nystuen G. The nuclear weapons ban treaty and the non-proliferation regime. Medicine, Conflict and Survival 2018; 34: 74-94.

57. Paxton B. 2017 saw 122 countries—but none of the nuclear-weapons states—support the treaty for the prohibition of nuclear weapons. Why is nuclear disarmament so difficult and what should be the next steps for those aiming for prohibition? Medicine, Conflict and Survival 2019; 35: 336-343.

58. American Public Health Association. Towards a Nuclear Weapons-Free World (Policy Statement). Adopted by the American Public Health Association Governing Council, October 2020. Available at: https://www.apha.org/policies-and-advocacy/public-health-policy-statements/policy-database/2021/01/13/toward-a-world-free-of-nuclear-weapons. Accessed on November 16, 2021.

59. The medical consequences of thermonuclear war: Special articles. New England Journal of Medicine 1962; 266: 1126-1155.

60. International Physicians for the Prevention of Nuclear War. Abolition of nuclear weapons: Campaign material and research. Available at: https://www.ippnw.org/resources-abolition-nuclear-weapons.html. Accessed on August 25, 2020.

61. Perry WJ, Collins TZ. Who can we trust with the nuclear button? No one. New York Times, June 22, 2020. Available at: https://www.nytimes.com/2020/06/22/opinion/nuclear-weapons-trump.html?action=click&module=Opinion&pgtype=Homepage. Accessed on June 23, 2020.

62. Back from the Brink: The Call to Prevent Nuclear War. Available at: https://preventnuclearwar.org/. Accessed on June 2, 2021.

63. Forden G. False alarms in the Nuclear Age. NOVA, Public Broadcasting System, November 6, 2001. Available at: https://www.pbs.org/wgbh/nova/article/nuclear-false-alarms/. Accessed on August 25, 2020.
64. Associated Press. Flight of nuclear warheads over U.S. is under inquiry. New York Times, September 6, 2007. Available at: https://www.nytimes.com/2007/09/06/us/06bomber.html. Accessed on August 25, 2020.
65. Cooper H. 92 Air Force officers suspended for cheating on their missile exam. New York Times, January 30, 2014. Available at: https://www.nytimes.com/2014/01/31/us/politics/92-air-force-officers-suspended-for-cheating-on-their-missile-exam.html. Accessed on August 25, 2020.
66. Schlosser E. Command and Control: Nuclear Weapons, the Damascus Accident, and the Illusion of Safety. New York: Penguin Books, 2013.
67. Prockop LD. Weapons of mass destruction: Overview of the CBRNEs (Chemical, Biological, Radiological, Nuclear, and Explosive). Journal of the Neurological Sciences 2006; 249: 50-54.
68. Tan CM, Barnett DJ, Stolz AJ, Links JM. Radiological incident preparedness: Planning at the local level. Disaster Medicine and Public Health Preparedness 2011; 5: S151-S158.
69. Weapons of Mass Destruction Commission. Weapons of Terror: Freeing the World of Nuclear, Biological, and Chemical Arms (Final Report). Stockholm, Sweden, June 1, 2006.

Profile 5:
Ira Helfand, M.D.
Preventing Nuclear War

Each week for almost 40 years, Ira Helfand, an internist based in western Massachusetts, has worked treating patients with medical emergencies. And he has also spent much time helping to prevent the most terrifying global emergency: nuclear war.

In 1977, Dr. Helfand was inspired by a book that raised his awareness about threats posed by nuclear power, and soon afterward he learned that nuclear weapons posed even greater threats. Along with physicians Helen Caldicott and Eric Chivian, he resurrected Physicians for Social Responsibility (PSR), which had been founded in the early 1960s by a number of physicians, including Victor Sidel, Jack Geiger, and Bernard Lown, who wrote seminal articles about the devastating effects that nuclear weapon attacks would have on U.S. cities.

Dr. Chivian organized a conference on the dangers of nuclear war, which received widespread media attention. Afterward, Dr. Helfand presented the main message from that conference—the imminent threat of catastrophic nuclear war—to many audiences, starting with his father's Rotary Club in Milford, Massachusetts. And he has been presenting that message frequently ever since to many audiences worldwide.

From the 1950s through the 1980s, there was much public concern about the threat of nuclear war between the Soviet Union and the United States. But after the Soviet Union dissolved in 1991, many people no longer recognized that threat—although it remained as large as, if not larger than, it had been during the Cold War.

In 2006, Dr. Helfand read a paper about the "nuclear autumn" that would occur after even a relatively small nuclear war. He estimated that as many as one billion people could starve to death from the global famine that would ensue. And he facilitated agricultural research, which ultimately validated his concern.

From 2012 through 2021, Dr. Helfand served as Co-President of the International Physicians for the Prevention of Nuclear War (IPPNW, of which PSR is the U.S. affiliate),

From Horror to Hope. Barry S. Levy, Oxford University Press. © Oxford University Press 2022.
DOI: 10.1093/oso/9780197558645.003.0010

which had received the 1985 Nobel Prize for Peace. In his role as Co-President, he made numerous presentations to organizations of health professionals and peace activists, to government policymakers and nongovernmental organizations, to faith communities and student organizations, and other groups. He presented to Nobel laureates. And he presented to a meeting of the United Nations General Assembly—to 196 national delegates, including those of the nine nuclear-weapon states. Although he is no longer IPPNW Co-President, he continues to make an average of five presentations a month.

In his presentations, Dr. Helfand reviews the consequences of a relatively small nuclear war between India and Pakistan (as described in Chapter 5). He then describes a large nuclear war between the United States and Russia, which could destroy all major cities in both countries. Each of the largest cities might be targeted with 10 to 20 nuclear weapons, each having 10 to 50 times the explosive force of the Hiroshima bomb. In each large metropolitan area, a firestorm with a 30-mile diameter would result, killing every living organism. Perhaps half a billion people would die in the first half-hour and many more afterward. Worldwide temperatures would drop to the coldest level in 18,000 years. The resultant famine could lead to the extinction of the human species.

He then observes, "We humans created these weapons. We can disassemble them. The only thing missing is the political will. We can literally save the world."

Dr. Helfand concludes: "We, as a global society, failed to fully recognize the dangers of climate change. We failed to fully recognize the dangers of COVID-19. And we are failing to fully recognize the dangers of nuclear weapons. Time is running out."

Dr. Helfand is a Former Co-President of the International Physicians for the Prevention of Nuclear War (IPPNW) and a Co-Founder and Past President of Physicians for Social Responsibility, the U.S. affiliate of IPPNW.

PART III

Health Impacts
on Civilians

6

Assaults and Injuries

When the rich wage war, it's the poor who die.
Jean-Paul Sartre

INTRODUCTION

During war, civilians are injured and killed by both indiscriminate and targeted attacks. This chapter primarily addresses these attacks and what can be done to reduce their health consequences and to prevent them from occurring.

INDISCRIMINATE ATTACKS ON CIVILIANS

Civilians have long suffered from indiscriminate attacks during war. But the intensity of these attacks markedly increased when aerial bombing began about 100 years ago. Even though targeting of bombs has become more precise in recent decades, bombs and other explosive weapons continue to injure and kill many civilians.

During the First World War, aerial bombing attacks killed almost 2,000 civilians. Despite moral outrage, these attacks continued, with widespread civilian injuries and deaths. For example, in 1932, Japan bombed a worker district in Shanghai, China. In 1936, Italy bombed Addis Ababa, the capital of Ethiopia. And in 1937, in the midst of the Spanish Civil War, bombing of civilian targets escalated when Germany dropped fire bombs on Guernica, Spain, in a 3-hour assault that destroyed the entire town and killed approximately 1,000 civilians.

Intensity and frequency of aerial bombing increased during the Second World War, destroying cities and injuring and killing millions of people. In 1940, Germany bombed Rotterdam, killing tens of thousands of people. From September 1940 through May 1941, it carried out nighttime bombing raids on London, killing approximately 40,000 people. Subsequently, Great Britain bombed military and industrial targets in German cities; in one night in 1943, it dropped firebombs on Hamburg that created a huge firestorm, which killed 40,000 people. Germany retaliated with rocket attacks on London. Then Britain responded

From Horror to Hope. Barry S. Levy, Oxford University Press. © Oxford University Press 2022.
DOI: 10.1093/oso/9780197558645.003.0011

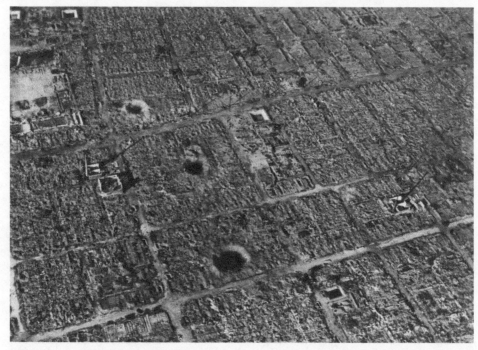

FIGURE 6-1 Damage to Osaka in 1945 as a result of a series of attacks by American B-29 bombers. Their bombloads included a high percentage of incendiaries, which destroyed the city's large wooden houses by fire. (Library of Congress, Negative LC-USZ 62-104726.)

with extensive bombing of Dresden, killing 35,000 civilians and totally destroying the city. In 1944 and 1945, U.S. bombers attacked cities in Japan, including Osaka (Figure 6-1) and Tokyo, where they created a firestorm that killed at least 80,000 people. And in August 1945, the United States dropped atomic bombs at Hiroshima and Nagasaki, killing hundreds of thousands of people.[1] (See Chapter 5.)

Since the Second World War, extensive bombing during war has continued to injure and kill millions of civilians. During the Vietnam War, the U.S. military dropped 6.2 million tons of bombs (an average of 44,000 tons a month), mainly on North Vietnam, injuring and killing many civilians (Figure 6-2). Over 37 days in the Gulf War in 1991, the United States bombed even more intensively, dropping 88,500 tons of bombs on Iraq and occupied Kuwait. Seventy percent of these bombs missed their military targets.[2]

In the first 6 years of the Syrian Civil War, the Bashar al-Assad regime dropped almost 70,000 barrel bombs on its own people in hospitals, schools, and elsewhere.[3,4] (Such government actions, which are designed to kill people "with an intentional or known reckless and depraved disregard for life," have been described as *democide*.[5]) The fight against ISIS also involved intensive bombing in Syria; during 4 months in 2013, the U.S.-led coalition dropped 10,000 bombs on Raqqa, destroying more than three-fourths of this city where 300,000 people lived.[6]

Since 2004, the United States, as part of its "war on terror," has conducted more than 14,000 aerial strikes in Afghanistan, Pakistan, Somalia, and Yemen using armed drones

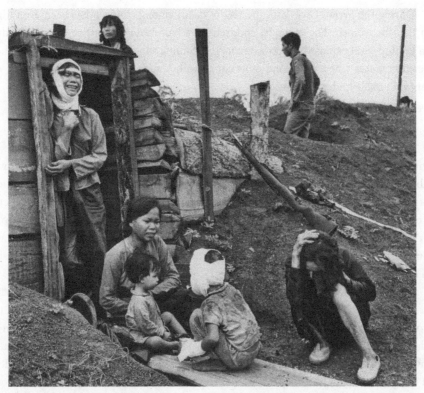

FIGURE 6-2 Wounded and shocked civilian survivors of the battle at Dong Xoai, Vietnam, in 1965, outside of the fort/bunker where they had survived the ground fighting and air bombardments of the previous 2 days. (AP Photo/Horst Faas.)

(unmanned aerial vehicles), reportedly killing more than 8,800 alleged terrorists. These attacks have also killed at least 910 civilians, including 283 children.[7,8]

Other types of weapons also indiscriminately injure and kill civilians during war, including small arms and light weapons, improvised explosive devices (IEDs), and landmines and unexploded ordnance (Chapter 4). Easy to produce and deploy, IEDs accounted for 42% of the almost 29,000 incidents of explosive violence worldwide between 2010 and 2020. These attacks killed or injured more than 136,000 civilians.[9]

Suicide bomb attacks have accounted for much injury and death in some wars. Between 2011 and 2020, there were more than 2,100 suicide attacks with explosive devices worldwide.[9] In the first 7 years of the Iraq War, from 2003 to 2010, there were 1,003 documented suicide bomb events, accounting for 26% of all injured civilians and 11% of all civilian deaths. An average of 19 civilians died in each suicide bomb attack that targeted civilians; for every person killed in a suicide bomb attack, there were, on average, 2.5 more people injured.[10]

Women and children have been at especially high risk of dying from indiscriminate explosions during war. Women and children were victims in one-fourth of suicide bomb attack deaths in Iraq between 2003 and 2010.[10] And women and children accounted for 79% of civilian deaths from mortar fire, 54% of civilian deaths from non-suicide-vehicle bomb attacks, and 69% of civilian deaths from Coalition air attacks there in the mid-2000s.[11]

During the Syrian Civil War, the risk of death among children has been even higher than that for women. For example, children have had more than twice the risk of dying from ground-level explosives than women. This finding suggested that children were being targeted in places where they were most concentrated, such as schools, and that they were highly vulnerable to these explosions.[12]

INJURIES

During war, intentional and unintentional injuries increase, leading to much death and disability. For example, a study in Baghdad during the Iraq War found that intentional injuries, which were frequently due to gunshots and explosions, killed 39% of victims and disabled 56% of them. However, *unintentional* injuries accounted for 90% of reported injuries during the war. The study found that major unintentional injuries, which were frequently due to falls and traffic-related accidents, killed 7.3% of victims and disabled 77% of them.[13,14]

For every child who dies during armed conflict, three additional children are either injured or permanently disabled. During war, children often sustain wounds from bullets, explosive weapons, and shrapnel. Adequate healthcare for injured children is often not available or accessible because of damage to hospitals, clinics, and transportation systems. Many children die from blood loss, wound infections, or other preventable causes of death. And many injured children who survive develop permanent disabilities, for which adequate healthcare is often not available.[15]

Many children are seriously injured by *explosive remnants of war*, which include antipersonnel landmines and *unexploded ordnance* (UXO)—grenades, mortar shells, bombs, and cluster munitions that have failed to detonate. Children are often injured or killed by landmines or UXO when they cultivate fields, herd animals, or search for firewood.[16] Attracted to the bright color of some landmines and UXO and not being aware of the danger, children are often tempted to touch them. Detonated landmines and UXO damage limbs and cause facial injuries, resulting in deafness, blindness, and other impairments. In Cambodia, approximately 20% of children injured by landmines and UXO died. (See Chapter 4.)

For children who survive injuries from landmines and UXO, amputation of limbs is often necessary. After surgery, victims face additional challenges. Limb prostheses may not be properly fitted and may not be replaced frequently, as is necessary for growing children. And limb prostheses may not be available at all.[16] Even when children are not injured, their families may be adversely affected by the presence of landmines and UXO in fields, making growing crops or raising animals difficult or impossible.

Displaced people are at increased risk of injuries from gunfire and explosions of bombs, IEDs, landmines, and unexploded ordnance. At especially high risk are people trapped within war zones and internally displaced persons. Among the millions of Afghan refugees in Pakistan, most war-related injuries have been caused by explosions—33% from landmines, 33% from shrapnel and other fragments, and 27% from firearms—and 1% of injured refugees have died.[17]

GENOCIDE AND MASS KILLING

Genocide and mass killing have often been associated with war. In the 20th century, genocides and mass killings included, but were not limited to, the Armenian massacre by the Ottoman Empire; the almost complete extermination of European Jews, Roma (Gypsies), gays and lesbians, and other groups by Nazi Germany during the Second World War; the mass killing of Cambodians by the Khmer Rouge in the late 1970s; and the genocide in Rwanda in 1994 (Table 6-1).[18,19] There have been many instances of mass killing. For example, Bosnian Serbs killed more than 8,300 Muslim men and boys in Srebrenica, a town in Bosnia and Herzegovina, in 1995 (Figure 6-3).

The Rohingya people of Myanmar, the vast majority of whom have been stripped of their citizenship, are stateless people. They have been attacked by Myanmar military forces, who have killed at least 25,000 of them since 2017, and the survivors have been forced to flee to other countries. They have suffered malnutrition, poor health, waterborne illness, and lack of obstetric care.[20,21]

Genocide results not only in the deaths of many individuals, but also in *social death*—the condition of people not being accepted as fully human by wider society, as if they were dead or nonexistent.[22,23] Genocide can produce long-lasting impacts on mental health among survivors and relatives of victims. Exposure to traumatic episodes during the Rwandan genocide was associated, 17 years later, with major depression and suicidality, especially in men.[24] Among mothers and children in Rwanda 25 years after the genocide, 30% had posttraumatic stress disorder (PTSD).[25]

TABLE 6-1 Some Genocides and Mass Killings in the 20th Century

Period	Description
1915–1923	1 million ethnic Armenians, Assyrians, and Greeks were killed in the Ottoman Empire.
1933–1945	6 million Jews and 5 million Slavs, Roma, people with disabilities, Jehovah's Witnesses, gays and lesbians, and political and religious dissidents were killed in the Holocaust in Europe.
1965–1966	Between 500,000 and 1 million people were killed in mass killings and civil unrest in Indonesia.
1971	Pakistani troops killed between 1 and 2 million Bengalis in what was then East Pakistan.
1972	Tutsis killed between 100,000 and 150,000 Hutus in Burundi.
1975	Indonesia invaded East Timor and killed between 100,000 and 200,000 civilians.
1975–1979	An estimated 1.5 million Cambodians died during the Khmer Rouge regime.
1981–1983	The Guatemalan military government massacred Maya civilians during counterinsurgency operations, killing at least 45,000 adults.
1987–1988	Saddam Hussein's forces killed approximately 100,000 Iraqi Kurds.
1992–1995	The army of Republika Srpska and Serb paramilitary groups killed large numbers of Bosnian Muslims and Bosnian Croats, including more than 8,300 in the Srebrenica massacre in 1995.
1994	800,000 Tutsis and moderate Hutus were killed in the Rwandan genocide.

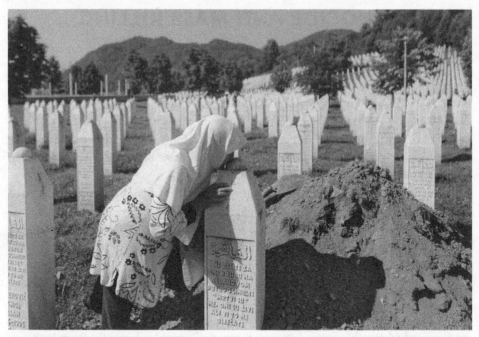

FIGURE 6-3 Over 10 days in 1995, Bosnian Serb forces attacked Srebrenica, Bosnia, and killed more than 8,300 Bosnian Muslims during the closing months of the country's civil war. It was the worst massacre in Europe since the end of the Second World War. In this photograph, a woman kisses a gravestone in Potocari, near Srebrenica, in 2020 during the 25th anniversary of the massacre. (AP Photo/Kemal Softic.)

How do societal conditions lead to genocide? There is no simple answer. But one analysis concludes that difficult life conditions can create social disorganization and activate basic human needs—security, a positive identity, and a need to connect with other people for mutual support. If societal collapse or social change makes people challenge their traditional ways of viewing the world, they may try to develop a new framework of reality and their place in it. As individuals and groups develop new ideologies, they may blame other people for their own problems and increasingly commit violence against other people.[26]

The U.S. government has generally not intervened in genocides. For example, it did little to stop the Rwandan genocide, possibly because it lacked the will to invest the military, financial, or political capital to do so. Short of direct intervention, the United States and other countries could have condemned the perpetrators, cut off external aid, and implemented other measures to stop the genocide. The lack of U.S. action to intervene in genocide is contrary to popular opinion in the United States; most Americans support U.S. participation in multilateral campaigns to stop genocide.[27]

One reason offered as to why some people have not been intensely concerned about genocide is the *collapse of compassion* (*psychophysical numbing*), which is ingrained in human cognitive and perceptual systems. When a single victim is made into a cause, people are generally compassionate and generous. But when a need is very large and victims are not identified, people are generally less interested. As Mother Teresa once observed: "If I look at the mass, I will never act. If I look at the one, I will."[28-31]

TARGETED ATTACKS ON CIVILIANS

Although attacks on civilians violate human rights and international humanitarian law, they occur frequently during war, especially intrastate armed conflict. Military forces intentionally injure and kill civilians to seek revenge, to reduce the size of the enemy population, to terrorize civilian supporters of enemy forces, or to make the enemy surrender. In some instances, they kill civilians to cover up their own illegal activities, such as stealing assets from civilians.[32,33] Often, military forces refrain from attacking civilians because they choose to comply with international humanitarian law and because they need assistance or support from other countries and international organizations.[34]

It may be difficult to distinguish civilians from combatants during war, especially intrastate war. Some civilians play economic roles that support a war (*economic ambiguity*). Some are part-time combatants (*military ambiguity*). Some assist or comfort members of the military (*social ambiguity*). And some voice political views or play political roles related to a war (*political ambiguity*).[32] However, during war, *all civilians* are protected under the Geneva Conventions, except when they are playing active combat roles.

Among the most severe forms of violence against civilians are massacres, scorched-earth policies, deliberate bombing and shelling of civilian targets, and forced expulsion. In civil wars from 1989 to 2010, 58% of rebel groups and 51% of governments committed at least one of these severe forms of violence (Table 6-2).[34]

How do governments and military forces motivate people during war to participate or collude in killing others? They do this by social conditioning, creating justifications for killing, dehumanizing the enemy, exerting coercive obedience, and mobilizing hatred from previous grievance or humiliation.[32]

Gender-Based Violence

Gender-based violence includes rape and other forms of sexual assault, intimate partner violence, early and forced marriage, forced impregnation, forced abortion, strip searches and

TABLE 6-2 Percentage of Rebel Groups and Governments That Committed the Most Severe Forms of Violence Directed Against Civilians, by Form of Violence, All Civil Wars, 1989–2010

Severe Form of Violence	Perpetrators	
	Rebel Groups	Governments
Massacres	30%	25%
Scorched-earth policies	27%	47%
Deliberate bombing or shelling of civilian targets	29%	22%
Forced expulsion	11%	14%
One or more of these four forms of violence	58%	51%
None of these four forms of violence	42%	49%

(Source: Stanton JA. Violence and Restraint in Civil War: Civilian Targeting in the Shadow of International Law. Cambridge, UK: Cambridge University Press, 2016, pp. 4–5.)

other humiliating violating acts, torture, and abduction and slavery.[35,36] Women and adolescent girls are constantly vulnerable to gender-based violence during war and its aftermath.[37-39] As a study in the Democratic Republic of the Congo (DRC) concluded: "From the victims' perspective, sexual violence is not only a part of . . . war, it *is* war."[40]

An extensive review of health outcomes of sexual violence on civilians in conflict zones found that the most common physical outcomes were pregnancy, traumatic genital injuries/tears, rectal and vaginal fistulae, sexual problems/dysfunction, and sexually transmitted infections. It also found that the most frequent mental health outcomes were PTSD, anxiety, and depression, and that the most common social outcomes were rejection by family and/or community and spousal abandonment.[41]

During war, rape has often been part of a systematic strategy to destabilize and humiliate the population and to create an atmosphere of fear and submission. Because military forces often perceive women and girls as reproducers of "the enemy," they frequently make women and girls prime targets during war.[35,42]

In 2019, the United Nations documented rape and other forms of sexual violence in 37 current conflicts—in the DRC, Myanmar, Somalia, South Sudan, Syria, and elsewhere.[43] It also estimated the occurrence of rape in earlier conflicts: at least 200,000 in the DRC since 1998, 100,000 to 250,000 in Rwanda in 1994, 60,000 in Sierra Leone between 1991 and 2002, and up to 60,000 in former Yugoslav republics between 1992 and 1995.[43,44] A survey in the DRC in 2007 found a much higher occurrence—more than 400,000 women there had been raped during the previous 12 months.[45] Reports generally underestimate the actual incidence of rape because victims are often frightened to report it.

DRC obstetrician-gynecologist Denis Mukwege, in 2009, called attention to the destructive sadistic behavior systematically perpetrated by armed groups in the Eastern DRC over the previous 10 years, which he described as "rape with extreme violence."[46] In addition to treating many victims at the Panzi Hospital in Bukavu, South Kivu, he and his colleagues performed several clinical and epidemiological studies on this sexual violence. For the 2004–2008 period, they found that 52% of perpetrators were identified as armed combatants and many of the rest were suspected as being armed combatants.[47] They also found that, over the course of this 5-year period, the number of sexual assaults allegedly perpetrated by armed combatants decreased by 77% and the number allegedly perpetrated by civilians increased 17-fold.[48] And they also found that the mean time between sexual assault and seeking care was 10.4 months; reasons included women waiting for symptoms to develop or worsen before they sought medical attention, no access to medical care, concern that family members would learn about the sexual assault, stigma related to sexual violence, and women having been abducted into sexual slavery for prolonged periods of time.[49] (See Profile 6.)

British journalist and author Christina Lamb, in her landmark book *Our Bodies Their Battlefield: What War Does to Women*, documented the experiences of rape victims during war and concluded that rape is the most neglected war crime. "It turns young girls into outcasts who wish their lives over when they are hardly begun," she observed. "It begets children who are daily reminders to their mothers of their ordeal and are often rejected by their community as 'bad blood'. And it's almost always ignored in the history books."[50]

As a woman who survived rape during the Bangladesh Liberation War in 1971 said: "We have given our most precious thing and have died inside many times but you won't find our names engraved on any monument or war memorial."[51]

Rape victims suffer physical and psychological consequences, including humiliation, shame, and anguish. Because of unwanted pregnancies, they have abortions—often unsafe abortions, with consequent health risks. They have flashbacks, ongoing fear, problems in establishing intimate relationships, and blunting of enjoyment in life. They have an increased risk of suicide. They are at increased risk of acquiring and dying from HIV/AIDS or other sexually transmitted infections. Adolescent girls are often at very high risk of being raped by soldiers because they are perceived as being physically weaker than adult women and less likely to have HIV/AIDS or other sexually transmitted infections.[52]

War adversely affects the societal structures and mechanisms that promote justice, stable governance, and policing, all of which protect young women and girls from sexual violence and coercion. War adversely affects health systems and policies that facilitate access to sexual and reproductive health services. War disrupts political processes that give women a voice in the decisions that affect their lives. And war damages the social safety net.[53]

Women and girls who have been displaced by war are at even higher risk of sexual violence—21% in one study.[51] In war zones and camps, they fear rape by militias, men who distribute aid in exchange for sex, husbands who demand that they replace dying children by producing still more children, and even neighbors and strangers.[54] And they worry that militias will abduct and enslave their children.

War disrupts agricultural livelihoods and forces young women into performing transactional sex in order to raise money to support their families—a survival strategy.[53] And war increases women's and girls' vulnerabilities to sex trafficking.[55,56]

Intimate partner violence increases during war and, often even more, in the aftermath of war.[57] Among displaced people, intimate partner violence has been a major problem, which has been largely overlooked by humanitarian aid agencies.[58,59]

Sexual Violence Against Children

During war and its aftermath, children are often sexually assaulted and abused. For example, in South Sudan, direct exposure to war increased by sevenfold adolescent girls' risk of non-partner sexual violence.[60]

A study in post-conflict northern Uganda found that most assaulted and abused children did not have caring and loving caregivers. Family breakdown and alcoholism were contributing factors. Children who yearned to be loved and cared for made them vulnerable to sexual assault. In some cases, perpetrators knew the children and pretended to be helping them, even sometimes promising to marry them; they often forced girls into sexual acts and then intimidated them to remain silent. In other cases, children became vulnerable when they walked alone to distant locations to obtain water or perform other errands.[61]

Adolescent boys are also vulnerable to sexual violence, especially during war-related displacement. Sexual violence against boys (and men) has been widespread during wars in Sudan, Liberia, the DRC, and former Yugoslavia republics.[62]

Children who have been sexually assaulted have faced stigma in their communities and many have dropped out of school as a result. Girls who have been sexually assaulted may be unable to marry or have children.[61]

Child Soldiers

Globally, there are estimated to be more than 250,000 children under age 18 who are involved in armed forces or armed groups (Figure 6-4). Over the course of decades, child soldiers have been deployed in 87 countries, with the largest number in Africa. Since 1998, there have been armed conflicts with child soldiers in at least 36 countries.

Child soldiers bear many of the physical, psychological, and social burdens of war. They have high rates of depression, anxiety, and posttraumatic stress symptoms.[63] Because children can be easily manipulated, child soldiers are frequently directed to perform crimes and atrocities—often not questioning their superiors. Child soldiers participate in combat, deploy antipersonnel landmines and other explosive weapons, scout and spy, act as couriers or guards, and perform support tasks for military forces. And they are often forced to become human shields and to perform sexual acts.

A typical child soldier is an orphaned boy between 8 and 18 years of age, bonded with a group of armed peers, who are addicted to drugs or alcohol, amoral, merciless, illiterate, and dangerous.[64] Child soldiers often come from low-income and disadvantaged families. Children are kidnapped or enticed into becoming child soldiers by propaganda, financial

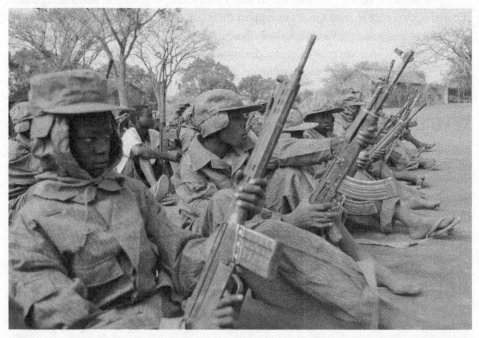

FIGURE 6-4 Child soldiers of the rebel Sudan People's Liberation Army (SPLA) wait for their commander at a demobilization ceremony at their barracks in Malou, southern Sudan, in February 2001. Under an agreement with the United Nations Children's Fund (UNICEF), the SPLA demobilized 2,500 child soldiers between 8 and 18 years of age. (AP Photo/Sayyid Azim.)

rewards, a strong personal belief in the goal of the conflict, the thrill of adventure, entrapment, and/or attraction to identify with a military group. Some children choose to become child soldiers after their parents or other relatives have been killed or after their homes or communities have been destroyed. Others have been forcibly displaced or have faced economic hardship, political oppression, or harassment.

Studies of former Ugandan and Congolese child soldiers confirmed this typical profile. On average, they had been violently recruited or abducted at about age 12, had served for about 2 to 3 years, and had been exposed to multiple potentially traumatic events, such as having witnessed shooting or having been seriously beaten. More than half of them reported killing someone, and more than one-fourth reported that they were forced to engage in sexual acts.[65,66]

A study in Sri Lanka provided a similar picture of adolescent soldiers: 32% had experienced a war-related death of a relative, 25% had witnessed violence, and 25% had their lives threatened. Many had psychosocial problems, including hostility, anxiety, and PTSD. And many had cognitive problems, including decreased concentration and memory.[67] After armed conflict ends, former child soldiers experience problems with psychosocial adjustment and social reintegration.[68,69]

TORTURE

The United Nations has defined *torture* as an act by which severe pain or physical or mental suffering is intentionally inflicted on a person to obtain information or a confession, to provide punishment for a committed or suspected act, to produce intimidation or coercion, or for any reason based on discrimination.[70] Torture takes several forms: physical torture, such as beatings and electric shocks; sexual torture, such as rape and sexual humiliation; and psychological torture, such as deprivation, prolonged solitary confinement, and ways to instill fear (Figure 6-5).

Torture is most prevalent in war-torn countries and parts of countries where human rights have been violated. In 2019, of the 22.5 million refugees uprooted by war, about one-third reported that they had been tortured.[71] Torture of detainees during war has usually been done to establish a state of terror among populations. Contrary to the UN definition, it has generally not been done to obtain information or confessions.

From 2009 to 2013, Amnesty International received reports of torture in 141 countries. High-profile cases of torture, such as the U.S. Central Intelligence Agency's secret detention program, have been justified by the false impression that torture is necessary to protect national security or to provide effective counterterrorism. People of many different types in many different situations have been tortured, including activists and protesters, petty criminals, and members of ethnic minorities. But most torture victims have been poor and marginalized people.[72]

Under President Bashar al-Assad, the Syrian government has tortured tens of thousands of detainees. Between March 2011 and February 2021, the Syria Network for Human Rights documented 14,451 deaths due to torture and 84,371 enforced disappearances of people who are presumed to be dead or still detained.[73] In 2012, Human Rights Watch

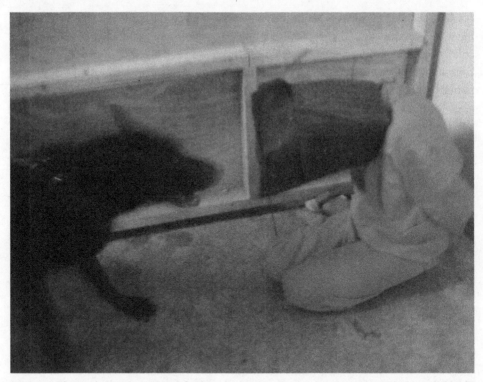

FIGURE 6·5 Dog being used to instill fear in a prisoner at the U.S.-operated Abu Ghraib prison in Iraq in 2006. (AP Photo.)

identified and mapped 27 detention centers in Syria and, in 2015, it obtained photographs of 6,786 individuals who died in custody.[74] In 2019, *New York Times* correspondent Anne Barnard wrote a detailed account of torture in Syria's secret prisons, by which President al-Assad had crushed dissent.[75]

Torture causes serious physical injuries and mental disorders that can have long-term consequences. PTSD has been documented in up to 88% of torture survivors from the Middle East, Central Africa, South Asia, and Southeast Europe; depression in up to 95% of African torture survivors; and anxiety in up to 91% of South African torture survivors. Torture severity and delay in receiving treatment are associated with a high rate of mental symptoms.[72]

Many displaced people have experienced torture or cruel and inhumane treatment and developed mental disorders as a result. In the Middle East, Central Africa, South Asia, and Southeast Europe, more than 80% of refugees who had been tortured subsequently developed PTSD, depression, anxiety, and other psychological disorders.[71]

Although 173 countries are states parties to the International Covenant on Civil and Political Rights, which prohibits torture and other forms of ill-treatment, and 171 countries are states parties to the UN Convention Against Torture, many countries have failed to criminalize torture as a specific offense in their national laws. And many countries have committed torture. (See Chapter 3.)

PROTECTING CIVILIANS AND CIVILIAN INFRASTRUCTURE

Transforming Protection of Civilians

Governments and humanitarian aid organizations can transform the way civilians are protected during war. They can rigorously prosecute targeting of civilians as a war crime. They can protect civilian infrastructure during war. They can ensure medical neutrality. They can evacuate civilians from war zones to safe areas, when necessary. They can transform the public mindset about the plight of civilians during war by enabling the public to see that civilians are not supporters or members of opposing military forces. And they can address the social and psychological forces that permit and encourage military forces to injure and kill civilians and to destroy civilian communities.[76]

Planning Military Operations to Minimize Harm

Violence against civilians can be prevented by planning military operations to minimize harm to civilians, training soldiers to distinguish between military and civilian targets, and punishing soldiers who commit violence against civilians. Deploying UN peacekeeping forces, placing human rights monitors, and delivering humanitarian aid can also protect civilians. Governments must address the widely held belief by military forces that many civilians in the country of an "enemy" are supporters or members of the enemy's military. Governments must also address the social and psychological forces that allow—and encourage—military forces to injure and kill civilians and to destroy civilian communities.[76]

Protecting Women from Rape and Other Gender-Based Violence

Some international standards have helped to prevent sexual violence against women. These standards promote reporting of gender-based violence, reduction of the social stigma against rape victims, prompt and thorough investigation of sexual violence, improved security for women, and removal of corruption and increased accountability in judicial systems. Governments and humanitarian aid organizations need to include women in the design and implementation of these measures.[77] And they need to provide greater support, assistance, and reparation to survivors of violence.[78]

In 1998, rape was officially established as a war crime in the Rome Statute, which created the International Criminal Court (ICC). In 2008, the UN Security Council adopted Resolution 1820, which stated that "Rape and other forms of sexual violence can constitute a war crime." But between 1998 and 2019, the ICC made no convictions for rape during war.[50]

Governments have an obligation, under international human rights law, to protect women and children from domestic and family violence in the aftermath of war. If a government is aware of domestic and family violence but does not take reasonable measures to ensure the safety of victims and to investigate complaints, it is failing to meet this obligation.[79]

During war, gender inequalities that are structurally present in many countries are exacerbated and progress regarding women's rights is often reversed. Empowerment of women may only be achieved by transforming the social norms that perpetuate patriarchal systems.[80]

There is a significant gap in research needed to guide programs providing protection for women and girls during war and its aftermath.[81] UN agencies, governments, and non-governmental organizations, in partnership with academic institutions, need to promote, support, and broaden this research.

Rigorously Prosecuting Those Who Target Civilians

Targeting of civilians during war needs to be rigorously prosecuted as a war crime. Impunity for perpetrators must end. The international community needs to hold parties to conflicts accountable for respecting medical neutrality during war and for protecting healthcare workers and facilities from attack.[82] And it needs to denounce and punish unlawful behavior and ensure compliance with the Geneva Conventions and other elements of international humanitarian law.[83]

Documenting and Publicizing Attacks on Civilians and Other Prohibited Activities

Governments, international organizations, and health professional organizations can document and publicize attacks on civilians and civilian infrastructure and other prohibited acts during war. The Dirty War Index is a tool that can be used to translate these prohibited acts into human rights protection, policy development, and compliance with international health law.[84]

There is a need to improve data on traumatic injuries among civilians during war in order to improve systems to respond to and prevent these injuries. A systematic review of conflict-related injuries sustained by civilians and local combatants between 2001 and 2019 found that fewer than 25% of reports on injuries in armed conflicts included measures of injury severity, resource utilization, and outcomes other than mortality. Establishment of a global humanitarian trauma registry could help improve capabilities of humanitarian aid organizations to respond better to civilian injuries during war.[85]

In 2016, the UN Security Council adopted Resolution 2286 regarding measures to prevent acts of violence, attacks, and threats against wounded and sick individuals as well as medical and humanitarian personnel.[86] As a follow-up to that resolution, the UN Secretary-General made recommendations to improve protection of these individuals under international law, including that UN member states should:

- Ratify all international treaties concerning the protection of medical care in armed conflict
- Undertake comprehensive reviews of their domestic laws and adopt necessary reforms to ensure that they fully incorporate international legal obligations regarding the protection of medical care in armed conflict
- Adopt legal and practical measures to guarantee the ability of personnel exclusively engaged in medical duties to treat patients without any distinction other than on medical grounds.[87] (See Chapter 2.)

Supporting Civilians Who Are Protecting Themselves

Civilians have learned to protect themselves against heavily armed military forces in several countries, such as Colombia, Afghanistan, and Syria. Their effectiveness has relied on social organization and cohesion, which has enabled them to avoid attacks, resolve disputes, deceive military forces, organize protests, and negotiate with armed groups.[88] UN agencies, governments of other countries, and nongovernmental organizations should support these efforts.

SUMMARY POINTS

- Civilians are frequently injured and killed during war by indiscriminate use of weapons and by targeted attacks.
- Civilian populations have often suffered from genocides and mass killings during war.
- Gender-based violence causes profound physical and psychological impacts on women.
- Torture causes physical injuries and mental disorders, often with long-term consequences.
- Protection of civilians and civilian infrastructure during war is essential.

REFERENCES

1. Constitutional Rights Foundation. Firestorms: The Bombing of Civilians in World War II. Available at: https://www.crf-usa.org/bill-of-rights-in-action/bria-15-3-a-firestorms-the-bombing-of-civilians-in-world-war-ii. Accessed on December 7, 2020.
2. Gellman B. U.S. bombs missed 70% of the time. Washington Post, March 16, 1991. Available at: https://www.washingtonpost.com/archive/politics/1991/03/16/us-bombs-missed-70-of-time/9ba41e93-dbd8-4064-be39-37ccfe8888d6/. Accessed on January 13, 2021.
3. Syrian Network for Human Rights. The Syrian regime has dropped nearly 70,000 barrel bombs on Syria: The ruthless bombing. December 25, 2017. Available at: https://reliefweb.int/sites/reliefweb.int/files/resources/The_Syrian_Regime_Has_Dropped_Nearly_70%2C000_Barrel_Bombs_en.pdf. Accessed on January 13, 2021.
4. Browne M, Triebert C, Hill E, et al. Hospitals and schools are being bombed in Syria. A U.N. inquiry is limited. We took a deeper look. New York Times, December 31, 2019. Available at:https://www.nytimes.com/interactive/2019/12/31/world/middleeast/syria-united-nations-investigation.html. Accessed on January 13, 2021.
5. Rummel RJ. Death by Government. New Brunswick, NJ: Transaction Publishers, 1994.
6. Gopal A. America's war on Syrian civilians. New Yorker, December 14, 2020. Available at: https://www.newyorker.com/magazine/2020/12/21/americas-war-on-syrian-civilians. Accessed on January 13, 2021.
7. Renic NC. Asymmetric Killing: Risk Avoidance, Just War, and the Warrior Ethos. Oxford: Oxford University Press, 2020.
8. Bureau of Investigative Journalism. Drone warfare. Available at: https://www.thebureauinvestigates.com/projects/drone-war. Accessed on January 15, 2021.
9. Overton I, Davies R, Tumchewics L. Improvised explosive devices: Past, present and future. Action on Armed Violence, October 15, 2020. Available at: https://reliefweb.int/report/world/improvised-explosive-devices-past-present-and-future. Accessed on January 30, 2021.

10. Hicks MH, Dardagan H, Bagnell PM, et al. Casualties in civilians and coalition soldiers from suicide bombings in Iraq, 2003-10: A descriptive study. Lancet 2011; 378: 906-914.

11. Hicks MHR, Dardagan H, Serdán GG, et al. Violent deaths of Iraqi civilians, 2003–2008: Analysis by perpetrator, weapon, time, and location. PLoS Medicine 2011; 8: e1000415. doi: 10.1371/journal.pmed.1000415.

12. Guha-Sapir D, Rodriguez-Llanes J, Hicks MH, et al. Civilian deaths from weapons used in the Syrian conflict. British Medical Journal 2015; 351: h4736. doi: 10.1136/bmj.h4736.

13. Lafta R, Al-Shatari S, Cherewick M, et al. Injuries, death, and disability associated with 11 years of conflict in Baghdad, Iraq: A randomized household cluster survey. PloS ONE 2015; 10: e0131834. https://journals.plos.org/plosone/article?id=10.1371/journal.pone.0131834

14. Donaldson RI, Hung YW, Shanovich P, et al. Injury burden during an insurgency: The untold trauma of infrastructure breakdown in Baghdad, Iraq. Journal of Trauma 2010; 69: 1379-1385.

15. United Nations Children's Fund. Impact of armed conflict on children: Patterns in conflict: Civilians are now the target. Available at: https://sites.unicef.org/graca/patterns.htm. Accessed on October 21, 2020.

16. Machel G. Impact of armed conflict on children. Report of the expert of the Secretary-General, Ms. Graca Machel, submitted pursuant to General Assembly resolution 48/157. New York: United Nations General Assembly, 1996. Available at: https://www.un.org/ga/search/view_doc.asp?symbol=A/51/306. Accessed on April 21, 2020.

17. Nasir K, Hyder AA, Shahbaz CM. Injuries among Afghan refugees: Review of evidence. Prehospital and Disaster Medicine 2004; 19: 169-173.

18. Blum R, Stanton GH, Sagi S, Richter ED. "Ethnic cleansing" bleaches the atrocities of genocide. European Journal of Public Health 2007; 18: 204-209.

19. Gourevitch P. We Wish to Inform You That Tomorrow We Will Be Killed With Our Families: Stories From Rwanda. New York: Picador USA, 1998.

20. Mahmood SS, Wroe E, Fuller A, Leaning J. The Rohingya people of Myanmar: Health, human rights, and identity. Lancet 2017; 389: 1841-1850.

21. Beyrer C, Kamarulzaman A. Ethnic cleansing in Myanmar: The Rohingya crisis and human rights. The Lancet 2017; 390: 1570–1573.

22. Patterson O. Slavery and Social Death: A Comparative Study, with a new Preface (2nd edition). Cambridge, MA: Harvard University Press, 2018.

23. Card C. Genocide and social death. Hypatia 2003; 18: 63-79.

24. Rugema L, Mogren I, Ntaganira J, Krantz G. Traumatic episodes and mental health effects in young men and women in Rwanda, 17 years after the genocide. BMJ Open 2015; 5: e006778. doi: 10.1136/bmjopen-2014-00678.

25. Mutuyimana C, Sezibera V, Nsabimana E, et al. PTSD prevalence among resident mothers and their offspring in Rwanda 25 years after the 1994 genocide against the Tutsi. BMC Psychology 2019; 7: 84. doi: https://doi.org/10.1186/s40359-019-0362-4.

26. Staub E. Cultural-societal roots of violence: The examples of genocidal violence and of contemporary youth violence in the United States. American Psychologist 1996; 51: 117-132.

27. Power S. "A Problem from Hell": America in the Age of Genocide. New York: Basic Books, 2002.

28. Leidner B. America and the age of genocide: Labeling a third-party conflict "genocide" decreases support for intervention among ingroup-glorifying Americans because they down-regulate guilt and perceived responsibility to intervene. Personality and Social Psychology Bulletin 2015; 41: 1623-1645.

29. Small DA, Loewenstein G, Slovic P. Sympathy and callousness: The impact of deliberative thought on donations to identifiable and statistical victims. Organizational Behavior and Human Decision Processes 2007; 102: 143-153.

30. Cameron CD, Payne BK. Escaping affect: How motivated emotion regulation creates insensitivity to mass suffering. Journal of Personality and Social Psychology 2011; 100: 1-15.

31. Fetherstonhaugh D, Slovic P, Johnson SM, Friedrich J. Insensitivity to the value of human life: A study of psychophysical numbing. Journal of Risk and Uncertainty 1997; 14: 283-300.

32. Slim H. Killing Civilians: Method, Madness, and Morality of War. New York: Columbia University Press, 2008.

33. Hedges C, Al-Arain L. Collateral Damage: America's War Against Iraqi Civilians. New York: Nation Books, 2008.
34. Stanton JA. Violence and Restraint in Civil War: Civilian Targeting in the Shadow of International Law. Cambridge, UK: Cambridge University Press, 2016.
35. Mazurana D. "Women, girls and armed conflict" in U.S. Department of State, Bureau of International Information Programs. Global Women's Issues: Women in the World Today, Extended Version, 2012, pp. 68-69. Available at: https://static.america.gov/uploads/sites/8/2016/05/Global-Womens-Issues_Women-in-the-World-Today_English_508.pdf. Accessed on October 21, 2020.
36. Kozina S, Vlastelica M, Borovac JA, et al. Violence without a face: The analysis of testimonies of women who were sexually assaulted during the war in Croatia and Bosnia and Herzegovina. Psychiatria Danubina 2019; 31: 440-447.
37. Amnesty International. Casualties of War: Women's Bodies, Women's Lives: Stop Crimes Against Women in Armed Conflict. 2004. Available at: https://www.amnesty.org/en/documents/act77/072/2004/en/. Accessed on September 16, 2021.
38. The erosion of women's sexual and reproductive rights (Editorial). Lancet 2019; 393: 1773.
39. Petchesky RP. Conflict and crisis settings: Promoting sexual and reproductive rights. Reproductive Health Matters 2008; 16: 4-9.
40. Maedl A. Rape as a weapon of war in the Eastern DRC?: The victims' perspective. Human Rights Quarterly 2011; 33: 128-147.
41. Ba I, Bhopal RS. Physical, mental and social consequences in civilians who have experienced war-related sexual violence: A systematic review (1981–2014). Public Health 2017; 142: 121-135.
42. Seifert R. "Rape: The Female Body as a Symbol and a Sign: Gender-Specific Violence and the Cultural Construction of War" in I Taipale, PH Mäkelä, K Juva, et al. (Eds.). War or Health?: A Reader. Dhaka, Bangladesh: University Press, Bangkok, Thailand: White Lotus, Cape Town, South Africa: NAE, London and New York: Zed Books in association with Physicians for Social Responsibility (Finland) and the International Physicians for the Prevention of Nuclear War, 2002, pp. 280-294.
43. United Nations. Conflict-related sexual violence: Report of the United Nations Secretary-General. March 29, 2019. Available at: https://www.un.org/sexualviolenceinconflict/wp-content/uploads/2019/04/report/s-2019-280/Annual-report-2018.pdf. Accessed on April 23, 2020.
44. Kabengele Mpinga E, Koya M, Hasselgard-Rode J, et al. Rape and armed conflicts in the Democratic Republic of Congo: A systematic review of the scientific literature. Trauma, Violence & Abuse 2017; 18: 581-592.
45. Peterman A, Palermo T, Bredenkamp C. Estimates and determinants of sexual violence against women in the Democratic Republic of Congo. American Journal of Public Health 2011; 101: 1060-1067.
46. Mukwege DM, Nangini C. Rape with extreme violence: The new pathology in South Kivu, Democratic Republic of Congo. PLoS Medicine 2009; 6: e1000204.
47. Bartels S, Kelly J, Scott J, et al. Militarized sexual violence in South Kivu, Democratic Republic of Congo. Journal of Interpersonal Violence 2013; 28: 340-358.
48. Bartels S, Scott J, Leaning J, et al. Sexual violence trends between 2004 and 2008 in South Kivu, Democratic Republic of Congo. Prehospital Disaster Medicine 2011; 26: 408-413.
49. Bartels S, Scott J, Leaning J, et al. Demographics and care-seeking behaviors of sexual violence survivors in South Kivu, Democratic Republic of Congo. Disaster Medicine and Public Health Preparedness 2012; 6: 393-401.
50. Lamb C. Our Bodies Their Battlefield: What War Does to Women. London: William Collins, An Imprint of HarperCollins Publishers, 2020.
51. Clark H. A commitment to support the world's most vulnerable women, children, and adolescents (Comment). Lancet 2021; 397: P450-P452. doi: 10.1016/S0140-6736(21)00137-9.
52. McKay S. The effects of armed conflict on girls and women. Peace and Conflict: Journal of Peace Psychology 1998; 4: 381-392.
53. Hutchinson A, Waterhouse P, March-McDonald J, et al. Understanding early marriage and transactional sex in the context of armed conflict: Protection at a price. International Perspectives on Sexual and Reproductive Health 2016; 42: 45-49.
54. Macklin A. "Like Oil and Water, with a Match: Militarized Commerce, Armed Conflict, and Human Security in Sudan" in W Giles, J Hyndman (eds.). Sites of Violence: Gender and Conflict Zones. Oakland: University of California Press, 2004, pp. 75–107.

55. United Nations Office on Crime and Drugs. Human trafficking. Available at: https://www.unodc.org/unodc/en/human-trafficking/what-is-human-trafficking.html. Accessed on September 9, 2020.

56. McAlpine A, Hossain M, Zimmerman C. Sex trafficking and sexual exploitation in settings affected by armed conflicts in Africa, Asia and the Middle East: Systematic review. BMC International Health and Human Rights 2016; 16: 34. doi: 10.1186/s12914- 016-0107-x.

57. Kinyanda E, Weiss HA, Mungharera M, et al. Intimate partner violence as seen in post-conflict eastern Uganda: Prevalence, risk factors and mental health consequences. BMC International Health and Human Rights 2016; 16: 5. doi 10.1186/s12914-016-0079-x.

58. Goessmann K, Ibrahim H, Saupe LB, et al. The contribution of mental health and gender attitudes to intimate partner violence in the context of war and displacement: Evidence from a multi-informant couple survey in Iraq. Social Science & Medicine 2019; 237: 112457.

59. Al-Natour A, Al-Ostaz SM, Morris EJ. Marital violence during war conflict: The lived experience of Syrian refugee women. Journal of Transcultural Nursing 2019; 30: 32-38.

60. Murphy M, Bingenheimer JB, Ovince J, et al. The effects of conflict and displacement on violence against adolescent girls in South Sudan: The case of adolescent girls in the Protection of Civilian sites in Juba. Sexual and Reproductive Health Matters 2019; 27: 181-191.

61. Nyangoma A, Ebila F, Omona J. Child sexual abuse and situational context: Children's experiences in post-conflict northern Uganda. Journal of Child Sexual Abuse 2019; 28: 907-926.

62. Chynoweth S, Freccero J, Touquet H. Sexual violence against men and boys in conflict and forced displacement: Implications for the health sector. Reproductive Health Matters 2017; 25: 90-94.

63. Song SJ, de Jong J. Child soldiers: Children associated with fighting forces. Child and Adolescent Psychiatric Clinics of North America 2015; 24: 765-775.

64. Pearn J. Children and war. Journal of Pediatrics and Child Health 2003; 39: 166-172.

65. Bayer CP, Klasen F, Adam H. Association of trauma and PTSD symptoms with openness to reconciliation and feelings of revenge among former Ugandan and Congolese child soldiers. Journal of the American Medical Association 2007; 298: 555-559.

66. Derluyn I, Broekaert E, Schuyten G, De Temmerman E. Post-traumatic stress in former Ugandan child soldiers. Lancet 2004; 363: 861-863.

67. Somasundaram D. Child soldiers: Understanding the context. British Medical Journal 2002; 324: 1268-1271.

68. Betancourt TS, Khan KT. The mental health of children affected by armed conflict: Protective processes and pathways to resilience. International Review of Psychiatry 2008; 20: 317-328.

69. Betancourt TS, Borisova I, Williams TP, et al. Research review: Psychosocial adjustment and mental health in former child soldiers: A systematic review of the literature and recommendations for future research. Journal of Child Psychology and Psychiatry 2013; 54: 17-36.

70. United Nations Human Rights, Office of the High Commissioner. Convention against Torture and Other Cruel, Inhuman or Degrading Treatment or Punishment, June 26, 1987. Available at: https://www.ohchr.org/en/professionalinterest/pages/cat.aspx. Accessed on December 18, 2020.

71. Suhaiban HA, Grasser LR, Javanbakht A. Mental health of refugees and torture survivors: A critical review of prevalence, predictors, and integrated care. International Journal of Environmental Research and Public Health 2019; 16: 2309. doi: 10.3390/ijerph16132309.

72. Amnesty International. Torture. Available at: amnesty.org/en/what-we-do/torture/. Accessed on July 14, 2020.

73. Syria Network for Human Rights. Available at: https://sn4hr.org/. Accessed on February 6, 2021.

74. Human Rights Watch. If the Dead Could Speak: Mass Deaths and Torture in Syria's Detention Facilities, December 16, 2015. Available at: https://www.hrw.org/report/2015/12/16/if-dead-could-speak/mass-deaths-and-torture-syrias-detention-facilities. Accessed on February 6, 2021.

75. Barnard A. Inside Syria's secret torture prisons: How Bashar al-Assad crushed dissent. New York Times, May 11, 2019. Available at: https://www.nytimes.com/2019/05/11/world/middleeast/syria-torture-prisons.html. Accessed on February 6, 2021.

76. Levy BS, Sidel VW. Protecting non-combatant civilians during war (Commentary). Medicine, Conflict and Survival 2015; 31: 88-91.

77. Manjoo R, McRaith C. Gender-based violence in justice and post-conflict areas. Cornell International Law Journal 2011; 44: 11-31.

78. Amnesty International. Combating sexual violence in conflict: Recommendations to states at the Global Summit to End Sexual Violence in Conflict (10–13 June 2014). London: Amnesty International Publications, 2014. Available at: https://www.amnesty.org/en/documents/ior53/006/2014/en/. Accessed on September 16, 2021.

79. Bradley S. Domestic and family violence in post-conflict communities: International human rights law and the state's obligation to protect women and children. Health and Human Rights 2018; 20: 123-136.

80. San Pedro P. Women in conflict zones. Oxfam International, April 3, 2019. Available at: https://www.oxfam.org/en/research/women-conflict-zones. Accessed on May 18, 2021.

81. Noble E, Ward L, French S, Falb K. State of the evidence: A systematic review of approaches to reduce gender-based violence and support the empowerment of adolescent girls in humanitarian settings. Trauma, Violence & Abuse 2019; 20: 428-434.

82. Rubenstein LS, Bittle MD. Responsibility for protection of medical workers and facilities in armed conflict. Lancet 2010; 375: 329-340.

83. Trelles M, Stewart BT, Kushner AL. Attacks on civilians and hospitals must stop (Correspondence). Lancet 2016; 4: e298-e299.

84. Hicks MH-R, Spagat M. The Dirty War Index: A public health and human rights tool for examining and monitoring armed conflict outcomes. PLoS Medicine 2008; 5: 1658-1664.

85. Wild H, Stewart BT, LeBoa C, et al. Epidemiology of injuries sustained by civilians and local combatants in contemporary armed conflict: An appeal for a shared trauma registry among humanitarian actors. World Journal of Surgery 2020; 44: 1863-1873.

86. United Nations Security Council. Resolution 2286 (2016). Available at: https://digitallibrary.un.org/record/827916?ln=en. Accessed on March 5, 2021.

87. United Nations Security Council Letter dated 18 August 2016 from the Secretary-General addressed to the President of the Security Council. Available at: https://reliefweb.int/sites/reliefweb.int/files/resources/N1626255.pdf. Accessed on March 5, 2021.

88. Kaplan O. Resisting War: How Communities Protect Themselves. Cambridge, UK: Cambridge University Press, 2017.

Profile 6:
Denis Mukwege, M.D., Ph.D.
Preventing Sexual Violence

Denis Mukwege, an obstetrician-gynecologist in the Democratic Republic of the Congo (DRC), has made extraordinary contributions to diagnosing, treating, and preventing sexual violence, both locally and throughout the world.

After completing his residency training in obstetrics and gynecology, he focused much of his work on reducing extremely high maternal mortality in the DRC. In 1996, at the beginning of the First Congo War, the hospital where he was working was attacked. He fled to Bukavu, where 3 years later he established the Panzi Hospital.

There, Dr. Mukwege and his colleagues began treating many women who were victims of sexual violence during war. Between 1999 and 2021, they treated more than 69,000 women and girls with complex gynecological injuries, about 60% of whom were survivors of sexual violence—most of them from zones of armed conflict. He performed reconstructive surgery on them, and he established a holistic healing process in which they also received psychological counseling, assistance and support with socioeconomic reintegration into their communities, and access to legal services. He co-founded the Panzi Foundation to support this program.

Dr. Mukwege observes: "When rape is used as a weapon of war, it is intended to destroy entire families and communities. Survivors often face not only physical trauma, but also stigmatization and isolation that causes severe psychological pain. They are often abandoned by their families and have no means to support themselves. Moreover, in the DRC, seeking justice is often difficult due to rampant impunity."

Dr. Mukwege and his colleagues have also trained many others in their holistic healing process for victims of sexual violence. And they have performed clinical and epidemiological research to study and document sexual violence and have established the International Mukwege Chair at the University of Liège in Belgium and at the Evangelical University of Africa in Bukavu.

From Horror to Hope. Barry S. Levy, Oxford University Press. © Oxford University Press 2022.
DOI: 10.1093/oso/9780197558645.003.0012

Dr. Mukwege recognized that treating his patients one at a time would not prevent sexual violence. And so he has raised awareness within the DRC and globally about sexual violence and he has been an effective advocate for measures to prevent sexual violence.

The United Nations reported on 617 serious human rights violations in the DRC between 1993 and 2003, which could be determined to be war crimes, crimes against humanity, or possibly crimes of genocide. The perpetrators have not been punished. Dr. Mukwege and his colleagues have advocated for the creation of an international criminal tribunal for the DRC; they believe that violence will continue to occur until the perpetrators are held accountable for their crimes.

The Panzi Hospital is still treating 120 to 150 new victims of sexual violence monthly. Its staff includes 52 physicians, 103 nurses, and 238 other workers. Its programs now extend to other countries, including the Central African Republic, Guinea, Burkina Faso, and Iraq, through the support of its sister organization, the Dr. Denis Mukwege Foundation. Dr. Mukwege's work has awakened the global community to sexual violence as a weapon of war. He is gratified to see sexual violence receiving greater attention and being more effectively addressed in the DRC and throughout the world.

In 2018, Dr. Mukwege and Nadia Murad, an Iraqi Yazidi human rights activist, were jointly awarded the Nobel Peace Prize. In his Nobel Lecture, the text of which is available on the Internet, Dr. Mukwege said: "The Nobel Peace Prize . . . will be of value only if it leads to concrete change in the lives of victims of sexual violence all over the world and the restoration of peace in our countries. . . . If there is a war to be waged, it is the war against the indifference which is eating away at our societies."

Dr. Mukwege is Medical Director and Founder of the Panzi Hospital and Co-Founder of the Panzi Foundation in Bukavu, Democratic Republic of the Congo.

7

Malnutrition and Communicable Diseases

Peace we want because there is another war to fight—against poverty, disease, and ignorance.

INDIRA GANDHI

INTRODUCTION

Two of the major health impacts of war are malnutrition and communicable diseases, which often occur in the same populations. Because malnutrition predisposes people to acquiring communicable diseases and because some communicable diseases predispose people to malnutrition, these two health impacts are addressed together in this chapter.

MALNUTRITION

Malnutrition can affect people of all ages, but children under 5 years of age are most vulnerable. Other populations vulnerable to malnutrition during war and its aftermath include women, displaced people, older people, and people with disabilities.

Definitions

Classification of malnutrition in children between 6 and 59 months of age is based on body size and the presence of diffuse peripheral edema. The main categories are *stunting* (reduced linear growth), *wasting* (low body tissue mass), and *kwashiorkor* (diffuse peripheral edema). In addition, children (and adults) can develop deficiencies of iron; vitamins A, C, and D; and other micronutrients.

Criteria that define the main categories of childhood malnutrition are based on middle-upper arm circumference (MUAC) and weight-for-height *Z-score* (based on the number of standard deviations away from the median of a reference population). *Severe wasting* is defined as either a weight-for-height Z-score less than −3 (three standard deviations below the median), or an MUAC less than 115 mm in the absence of nutritional edema. *Severe acute*

From Horror to Hope. Barry S. Levy, Oxford University Press. © Oxford University Press 2022.
DOI: 10.1093/oso/9780197558645.003.0013

malnutrition is defined as severe wasting and/or kwashiorkor. *Moderate acute malnutrition* is defined as a weight-for-height Z-score between −3 and less than −2, or an MUAC between 115 mm and less than 125 mm in the absence of nutritional edema. *Global acute malnutrition* is defined as the sum of severe and moderate acute malnutrition.[1]

Acute food insecurity is defined as "any manifestation of food insecurity at a specific point in time of a severity that threatens lives, livelihoods or both, regardless of the causes, context or duration."[2] *Chronic food insecurity* is defined as "the long-term or persistent inability to meet dietary energy requirements (lasting for a significant period of time during the year)."[2] The Food and Agriculture Organization defines chronic food insecurity as "undernourishment."

Causes

Multiple factors generally cause or contribute to the development and persistence of malnutrition. Forced displacement is a major cause of malnutrition, especially among internally displaced persons. Concomitant diseases often cause or contribute to malnutrition, especially among infants and young children. For example, diarrheal diseases and infestations with intestinal parasites may impede absorption of essential nutrients. Diarrheal diseases often cause dehydration, which further weakens individuals. Individuals affected by communicable diseases may lose their appetite or be too weak to eat adequate amounts of food.

During war and its aftermath, malnutrition often occurs because of breakdowns in the food supply, healthcare, and other parts of civilian infrastructure:

- Reduced food production: Warfare damages farmland, farm equipment, and farm animals. Ongoing local warfare or the presence of antipersonnel landmines and unexploded ordnance make farmland unusable. War reduces availability of seeds, fertilizers, and pesticides—and water. And war disables or kills farmworkers or forcibly displaces them.
- Damaged storage and transport infrastructure: War damages silos and other food storage facilities. It destroys transport vehicles as well as roads and railroads. It reduces availability of fuel for transport. And it impedes transport of food.
- Damaged markets: War damages the physical structures of markets and the economic systems that enable them to operate. In addition, because of food shortages, prices rise, making food unaffordable for many people.
- Diversion or delay in food supply: Military forces and corrupt government officials may divert food. Bandits may steal food. Underfunded and understaffed government agencies may be unable to provide food assistance. And military forces may use food as a weapon, consciously reducing food access for the civilian population of the adversary party (see next page).
- Restricted import of food: Food embargoes or economic sanctions, imposed by the United Nations or groups of countries, restrict or prevent import of food, typically causing their most detrimental effects on vulnerable or disadvantaged people.
- Inadequate humanitarian food aid: An insufficient amount of food may have been provided. This shortfall may arise from inadequate needs assessment, delays at international

borders or points of entry, and, as already described, diversion and inadequate storage or transport.

- Failure to utilize available food: Because of poverty, lack of information, or other factors, caregivers of children may not be able to provide them with an adequate amount of essential nutrients. Infants and very young children may not be able to breastfeed because their mothers are malnourished or their mothers are not aware of the benefits of breastfeeding. Infant formula may have been made with contaminated water, causing diarrheal disease and subsequent malnutrition. Mothers may have been injured, made ill, or killed. And children may have been separated from their parents and other caregivers.

- Unavailable or inaccessible health services: Malnutrition and communicable diseases that contribute to malnutrition are not diagnosed, treated, or prevented because healthcare facilities have been damaged and healthcare providers and public health workers have been injured, made ill, killed, or forced to flee.

- Other causative and contributing factors: These factors may include racism and other forms of discrimination, inequities and poverty, occurrence of endemic or epidemic disease, and damage to systems for water treatment and supply. In addition, marginalization of affected populations, including their limited political power, is often a contributing factor.[3]

Use of Food as a Weapon

Food has been used a weapon of war, causing famine and mass starvation. Withholding of food, which most severely affects those who are young, old, sick, or poor, is a crime against humanity. Using food as a weapon violates principles of international humanitarian law: the principles of *distinction* (or *discrimination*, between civilians and combatants) and *proportionality* (the requirement of a reasonable relationship between unplanned damage to civilians and military advantage gained by using a method of warfare) (Chapter 3).[4]

Famine has been defined as "a food crisis that causes increased mortality for a specific period of time."[5] *Great famines* are associated with 100,000 or more excess deaths. Between 1870 and 2010, about 34% of the 104,000 deaths that occurred during great famines took place during wartime and another 2% in countries emerging from armed conflict. The most recent war-related great famines have occurred in the Democratic Republic of the Congo (DRC), Sudan (Darfur), South Sudan, Uganda, and Somalia.[5]

Famines are generally perpetrated in pursuit of genocide, imperial conquests, counterinsurgency, or totalitarian social transformation. They are considered to be a "form of political crime [that is] committed by governments and other political authorities that regard human lives as without value, or to be subordinated to other ends."[6] Many famine-related deaths have occurred when "governments or other authorities deliberately use famine as a tool of extermination or as a means of forcing a population to submit to their control."[5,7] But 61% of deaths in great famines have been those in which "public authorities pursue policies that are the principal cause of famine and continue to do so even after becoming aware that they result in famine."[5,7]

Since 1990, there have been eight famines with 50,000 or more deaths, seven of which have been associated with armed conflict. In early 2019, there were four countries with emergency situations associated with acute food insecurity (Afghanistan, Nigeria, South Sudan, and Yemen), all of which were experiencing or had experienced recent armed conflicts.[8]

In the Yemeni Civil War, food has been the primary weapon, accounting for more deaths than any other cause. Between March 2015 and March 2018, there were more than 16,700 air attacks by a coalition of countries led by Saudi Arabia and the United Arab Emirates that targeted farms, port facilities, and other infrastructure that was essential for food production and transport. The air attacks destroyed and diverted food aid. Air and naval blockades severely restricted the import of food. There was more than a doubling of severe acute malnutrition, affecting more than 400,000 children.[9] By December 2020, there were 131,000 war-related deaths from indirect causes, including lack of food, health services, and damage to infrastructure.[10] In February 2021, four UN agencies projected that there would be more than 2.25 million cases of acute malnutrition in children under age 5 during 2021.[11] Major contributing factors for acute malnutrition in Yemen were high prevalence of diarrhea and "malaria/fever"; elevated levels of acute food insecurity; poor infant and young child feeding practices; poor access to nutrition and health services; and poor water, sanitation, and hygiene services.[11] Disease and famine have been used as weapons of war in the Yemeni Civil War, a humanitarian disaster that has been woefully underreported.[12]

Food has also been used as a weapon in the Syrian Civil War. All sides in the war have regularly used violence to capture agriculture in order to control cropland and harvests. In addition, combatants have attempted to deny opposing forces access to cropland and harvests by using violence to destroy agriculture.[13]

Health Consequences of Malnutrition in High-Risk Populations

This section focuses on three populations at increased risk of malnutrition and its consequences during war and its aftermath: women, children, and displaced people (most of whom are women and children).

Women

Maternal malnutrition is related not only to the amount and quality of food ingested, but also to the amount of energy that mothers need to carry out their many responsibilities. These responsibilities include caring for their children, cooking meals, washing clothes, cleaning their homes, gathering firewood, and performing other activities.

Micronutrient deficiencies sometimes occur in pregnant women during war and its aftermath. These deficiencies are associated with adverse outcomes for both pregnant women and their offspring, including maternal anemia, maternal and perinatal mortality, low birthweight, preterm birth, intrauterine growth restriction, and altered immune response and cognitive deficits in their infants.[14] Consequences of maternal undernutrition are summarized in Table 7-1. Iron-deficiency anemia, which may be caused by low consumption or

TABLE 7-1 Some Consequences of Maternal Undernutrition

Deficiency	Consequence
Iron	Anemia Increased risk of maternal death Low-birthweight infants
Calcium	Increased risk of maternal death Gestational hypertensive disorders Preterm birth and fetal growth restriction
Iodine	Adverse effects on fetal development Intelligence (IQ) deficits in children
Folate	Increased risk of neural tube defects (congenital malformations of the spinal cord and brain)
Vitamin D	Severe preeclampsia, leading to increased risk of perinatal morbidity and mortality

(Source: Black RE, Victora CG, Walker SP, et al. Maternal and child undernutrition and overweight in low-income and middle-income countries. Lancet 2013; 382: 427–451.)

absorption of iron or by blood loss, such as from intestinal worms, increases the risk of maternal mortality.[15]

Malnourished pregnant women are at increased risk of dying during childbirth as well as having a miscarriage and giving birth to premature or low-birthweight infants. Their infants are at increased risk of stunted growth and communicable diseases.[16]

In Yemen, immediately before and during the civil war, many women suffered from malnutrition and its consequences. From 2013 to 2016, approximately 25% of women of reproductive age were underweight.[17] The number of pregnant and breastfeeding women treated for acute malnutrition increased from almost 220,000 in 2016 to almost 410,000 in 2018. In addition, an estimated 150,000 pregnant and breastfeeding women with acute malnutrition in 2018 were not treated because of brutal fighting, lack of access to care, and underfunding of health and nutrition services.[18] (See Chapter 9.)

Children

During war and its aftermath, children are at greatly increased risk of malnutrition and its adverse consequences (Figure 7-1). In low-income countries, where most wars occur, young children are twice as likely to die if they are mildly malnourished, more than four times more likely to die if they are moderately malnourished, and more than eight times more likely to die if they are severely malnourished.[19]

Stunting is associated with abnormal child development. Stunted children exhibit behavioral abnormalities in early childhood, including apathy; more negative affect; and reduced activity, play, and exploration.[15] Children who are breastfeeding are at increased risk of becoming malnourished if their mothers are malnourished. Childhood malnutrition reduces cognitive function in both the short and long term.[20,21] Malnourished children are at increased risk during adulthood of developing type 2 diabetes mellitus[22] and metabolic syndrome,[23] smoking cigarettes, and becoming physically inactive (Chapter 10).[24] Malnutrition

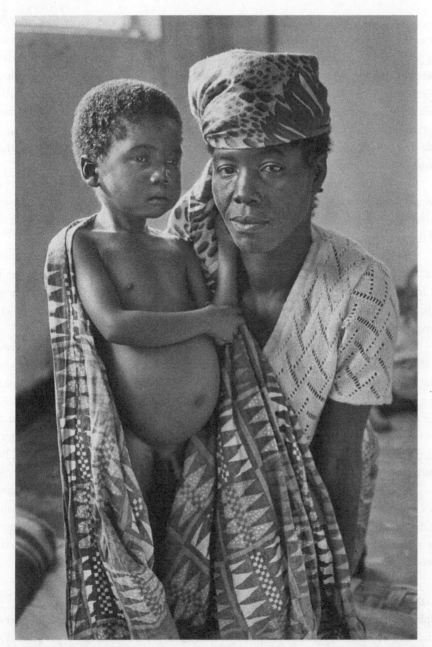

FIGURE 7-1 Malnourished child and mother in Kuito, Angola, in 1997, in the midst of the Angolan Civil War, which began in 1975. (Photograph by Sebastião Salgado.)

in early childhood may be associated with worse economic status in adulthood.[25] And malnutrition induced by war shortens life expectancy.[26]

Deficiencies of micronutrients adversely affect children. Deficiencies of vitamin A and zinc increase the risk of death in children. Deficiencies of iodine and iron can contribute to children not reaching their full development potential.[15]

Malnourished children are at increased risk of acquiring and dying from diarrheal diseases, acute respiratory infections, measles, and possibly malaria.[27] Reduced immunity and poor sanitation and consumption of water contaminated with microorganisms increase children's risk for cholera, bacillary dysentery (shigellosis), and gastroenteritis due to *Escherichia coli*, salmonella, rotavirus, and other pathogens. Crowded living conditions facilitate the spread of gastrointestinal and respiratory pathogens. Because war damages healthcare facilities and adversely affects public health services, many cases of communicable diseases are not diagnosed or treated and measures are not taken to prevent transmission of disease agents.

Diarrhea in children predisposes to malnutrition. For example, nutrition surveys in Ethiopia found that diarrhea during the previous 2 weeks was associated with higher levels of wasting. Diarrhea can cause malnutrition from a loss of nutrient intake, malabsorption, and the effect of inflammation in the gastrointestinal tract.[28]

Childhood malnutrition during war and its aftermath has been documented for decades. During the First World War, long-term food shortages seriously affected growth of children and adolescents in Germany. Shortly after the war ended, 89% of children were underweight and about 50% were below their expected height. The average weight deficit of younger children was 20% and that of older children was 33%.[29]

In recent years, malnutrition has continued to be prevalent in war-torn countries. In Mozambique and Ethiopia, up to 53% of young children had stunted growth due to chronic or long-term undernutrition and up to 7% had severe wasting due to acute nutritional deficiency.[30,31] In Sudan in 2014, young children affected by armed conflict were at substantially increased risk of being moderately or severely underweight.[32] In 2018, UNICEF and its partners treated more than 3.4 million children with severe malnutrition in humanitarian settings, including Afghanistan, Yemen, Nigeria, and South Sudan—all of which had been affected by recent armed conflict.[33]

Prevalence of acute malnutrition can increase very sharply during the first weeks of a crisis. For example, Kurdish refugee children along the Turkey–Iraq border in 1991 sustained significant weight loss and developed a threefold increase in acute malnutrition during the first month of the crisis. Half of the children had diarrheal disease, which contributed to their risk of malnutrition and death.[34]

Displaced People

Displaced people, especially internally displaced persons, are often malnourished. Physical, social, and economic barriers may make it difficult to access culturally appropriate food. Food preservation and preparation may be constrained. And armed conflict interrupts access to food.[35]

Internally displaced children are especially vulnerable to malnutrition and related disorders. So are refugee children living in camps or informal tented settlements.[36] Some studies of malnutrition in displaced children are summarized in Table 7-2.

TABLE 7-2 Selected Studies Documenting Malnutrition in Displaced Children

Location (Year)	Main Findings
Horn of Africa (1997–2009)[a]	9.2% of displaced young children from agriculturist families and 19.1% from pastoralist families had acute malnutrition.
Eritrea (1998–2000)[b]	War-exposed children had lower height-for-age Z-scores, with similar effects for children born before or during the war.
Chad (2007)[c]	Prevalence of acute malnutrition in young children was 21% in camps for internally displaced persons, compared with 16% in nearby villages and 10% in a nearby town.
Uganda (2008)[d]	Prevalence of global stunting was 52%, with male children at increased risk. Prevalence of global acute malnutrition was 6%, with children 3 to 24 months of age at increased risk.

[a] Mason JB, White JM, Herron L, et al. Child acute malnutrition and mortality in populations affected by displacement in the Horn of Africa, 1997-2009. International Journal of Environmental Research and Public Health 2012; 9: 791-806.
[b] Akresh R, Lucchetti L, Thirumurthy H. Wars and child health: Evidence from the Eritrean-Ethiopian conflict. Journal of Development Economics 2012; 99: 330-340.
[c] Guerrier G, Zounoun M, Delarosa O, et al. Malnutrition and mortality patterns among internally displaced and non-displaced population living in a camp, a village or a town in Eastern Chad. PLoS ONE 2009; 4: e8077. doi: 10.1371/journal.pone.0008077.
[d] Olwedo MA, Mworozi E, Bachou H, Orach CG. Factors associated with malnutrition among children in internally displaced person's camps, northern Uganda. African Health Sciences 2008; 8: 244-252.

COMMUNICABLE DISEASES

Categories

Major categories of communicable diseases during war and its aftermath are:

- Diseases related to contaminated water and to poor sanitation and hygiene: Diarrheal diseases (cholera, bacillary dysentery [shigellosis], and gastroenteritis caused by salmonella and toxigenic *E. coli*), which occur mainly due to contaminated water, substandard sanitation, and poor hygiene
- Respiratory diseases associated with overcrowding: Measles, tuberculosis (TB), meningococcal meningitis, and acute respiratory infections (for which indoor exposure to smoke from cookstoves can be a contributing factor)
- Vector-borne diseases: Malaria, dengue, and other diseases spread by mosquitoes and other vectors (which are endemic in specific regions)
- Other diseases: Including hepatitis A, hepatitis E, leptospirosis, tetanus, and leishmaniasis.[37]

Additional contributing factors to the occurrence of communicable diseases include poverty; damage to healthcare facilities, water treatment plants, and electrical grids; reduced numbers of healthcare and public health workers and financial resources; and import restrictions and embargoes that prevent adequate repair to infrastructure damage. War hampers humanitarian aid organizations from delivering equipment and supplies and from providing technical assistance to control disease outbreaks. War facilitates antimicrobial resistance because of misdiagnoses, inappropriate drug treatment, unregulated pharmacies, use of outdated drugs, and patients' noncompliance with prescribed treatment—and weakened capacity of public health agencies.

Some Examples of War-Related Communicable Diseases

Tuberculosis

Disruption of living conditions by war often creates ideal environments for the development of TB. Displaced people from conflict-affected areas are at high risk of acquiring and transmitting TB. During the First World War, there was a marked increase in TB mortality rates in countries engaged in the war, primarily by conversion of latent tubercle bacillus infection to active TB. In more recent wars in Bosnia and Herzegovina, Guinea Bissau, the DRC, Afghanistan, and Somalia, there have been substantial increases in TB incidence and mortality.[38] TB incidence or prevalence is frequently increased twofold or more in crisis-affected populations.[39]

Multidrug-resistant tuberculosis (MDR-TB) is a challenging problem in Africa and the Middle East, accounting for 5.2% of newly diagnosed cases and 41% of previously treated cases. War-torn Somalia has experienced the highest rates.[40]

Since the start of the Syrian Civil War in 2011, overcrowding of displaced persons and destruction of civilian infrastructure has adversely affected diagnosis, contact tracing, directly observed therapy, and follow-up of TB patients.[41] These factors have led to a substantial increase in reported TB cases in countries bordering Syria, including Turkey, Jordan, Lebanon, and Iraq, which has been attributed to the massive displacement of the Syrian population.[39,40,42]

Cholera and Bacillary Dysentery

These diseases have occurred frequently among displaced populations, such as in the following three situations:

- In 1990, an epidemic of cholera occurred among Mozambican refugees in Malawi, with almost 2,000 cases and 68 deaths; 63% of the deaths occurred within 24 hours of hospital admission, indicating delays in seeking healthcare and inadequate rehydration. The mortality rate was highest in children under age 4. A significant risk factor was drinking river water.[43]
- In 1994 in the former Zaire (now the DRC), an outbreak of cholera and dysentery killed more than 12,000 refugees who had fled the genocide in Rwanda.[44]
- During the Yemeni Civil War, a large outbreak of cholera occurred, with more than 1.2 million cases (58% in children) and more than 3,000 deaths in the first 6 months. A contributing factor was extensive bombing of water, sanitation, and hygiene facilities; hospitals and other healthcare facilities; the country's main seaport; and a bridge on the main supply route to the capital. The outbreak was worsened by chronic malnutrition and lack of basic supplies. The initial response by major humanitarian aid organizations did not focus sufficiently on preventive measures, such as establishing community isolation facilities with proper sanitation, reliable sewage disposal systems, and clean water supplies.[45,46]

Measles

The measles virus is among the most contagious viruses. It is transmitted by respiratory droplets that can remain in the air for hours. The case-fatality rate in low-income countries generally ranges between 3% and 6%, but it can increase to as high as 30% in some out-breaks. Those who survive can be left with permanent blindness, hearing impairment, or brain damage. Increased incidence and mortality rates due to measles among unimmunized children in war-torn countries have occurred for many years.

In the past few years, there has been a marked increase in measles cases. In 2018, measles cases increased to an estimated 10 million cases worldwide, 140,000 of which were fatal—a 58% increase since 2016. In low-income countries, underfunding of public health systems has made it difficult to deliver measles vaccine to unimmunized children. Armed conflict adds to this challenge. The COVID-19 pandemic further worsened the situation, with many countries suspending measles vaccination campaigns as health workers responded to the pandemic.[47]

Frequently, outbreaks of measles are the first to occur among children during intrastate conflicts. Measles outbreaks in Syria and surrounding countries have increased due to the Syrian Civil War and mass displacement of Syrians within Syria and neighboring countries.[42]

Because of the serious challenges of containing measles in war-affected settings, there is a pressing need to develop, test, and implement innovative approaches to immunize un-vaccinated children in these settings. To do so will require (a) developing strong partnerships between parties at war and local communities, and (b) integrating measles immunization into primary healthcare services.[48]

Malaria

Malaria has been endemic in many tropical countries prior to armed conflict. In some of these countries, malaria had been well controlled, with bednets, measures to prevent mosquitoes from breeding, treatment of patients, and use of prophylactic medications. For example, in Afghanistan, malaria, which had been well controlled before armed conflict began in 1979, surged soon after war began. Reasons for this surge included decreased access to healthcare, which limited use of medications for prophylaxis and treatment, and reduced public health measures to control malaria.

Leishmaniasis

The incidence of both cutaneous leishmaniasis (CL) and visceral leishmaniasis (VL) has in-creased during war in countries where this disease is endemic. In countries experiencing intense armed conflict, with population displacement and deterioration of public health services, CL incidence has doubled and VL incidence has increased sixfold.[49] Large CL outbreaks have occurred in Afghanistan, Syria, Sudan, and other war-torn countries.[50,51]

Populations at High Risk for Communicable Disease

Children

During war and its aftermath, children are at increased risk of acquiring or dying from communicable diseases, especially diarrheal diseases, acute respiratory infections, and, where it is endemic, malaria. Outbreaks of meningitis, cholera, bacillary dysentery, and measles often occur.[52] Bottle-fed infants and young children are at increased risk of diarrheal disease when formula has been prepared with water that has been contaminated by microorganisms.

War adversely affects immunization rates, making children susceptible to measles and other preventable diseases. Among Syrian refugee children under age 5 at two camps in Berlin, Germany, only 28% were fully immunized; at one of these camps, 5% of children had no immunizations at all.[53] After the Angolan Civil War, children with the lowest immunization rates were those who were born and/or had grown up during the war and were living in parts of the country where fighting had been especially ferocious and devastation was most profound.[54]

Displaced People

Refugees acquire communicable diseases in their home countries, during migration, and, less frequently, in their host countries. Many cases of communicable disease among refugees are not diagnosed or treated in their countries of origin or during migration because of inadequate healthcare or language and cultural barriers.

Diarrheal diseases are often exacerbated by reduced access to safe potable water; acute respiratory infections are often exacerbated by crowding, poor ventilation, and inadequate shelter. Displaced people acquire malaria when they move from areas of low malaria prevalence through or to areas of high malaria prevalence. Displaced children who have not been vaccinated against measles are at high risk of acquiring the disease. Other frequently occurring communicable diseases in displaced people are viral hepatitis, TB, HIV/AIDS and other sexually transmitted infections, and sometimes meningococcal meningitis.[55] Outbreaks of dengue, a viral disease transmitted by *Aedes* mosquitoes, have occurred among populations displaced by war in Somalia and Yemen.[56]

A study among internally displaced persons in Africa between 2000 and 2016 found that the most frequently occurring communicable diseases were "fever/malaria" (prevalent in 85% of children and 48% of adults), diarrhea (in 62% of children and 22% of adults), and acute respiratory infections (in 45% of the population).[57]

Communicable diseases have often emerged or reemerged in countries hosting displaced populations. For example, in Jordan, which has hosted many people displaced from the war in Syria, outbreaks of CL and gastroenteritis due to *E. coli* and rotavirus have occurred frequently. These outbreaks have created additional problems for the healthcare systems in host countries. For example, healthcare officials in Jordan, who have been challenged by the substantial increase in the number of displaced people, have had to restrict immunization programs, leaving many children and adults susceptible to communicable diseases.[58]

Refugees often have lower immunization rates than residents of their host countries because of low vaccination coverage in their home countries, the challenge of administering multiple-dose vaccines, and the need to keep some vaccines refrigerated during storage and transport. In addition, refugees often do not seek healthcare in their host countries because they fear that healthcare workers will share their personal information with immigration officials.[59,60]

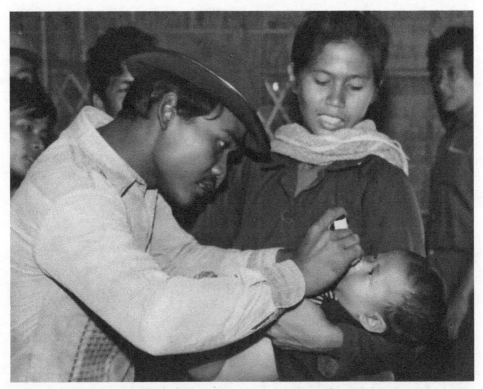

FIGURE 7-2 Public health worker administers oral polio vaccine to a child in Khao-I-Dang camp in Thailand in 1980 to control an outbreak of nine cases of polio. (Photograph by Barry S. Levy.)

For more than 60 years, there has been effective oral immunization against polio (Figure 7-2). The incidence of polio has decreased by more than 99.9% since 1988. The only two countries in which polio is endemic—that is, without interruption of transmission of indigenous wild poliovirus type 1—are war-torn Afghanistan and neighboring Pakistan, which hosts more than 2.5 million people displaced from Afghanistan.[61,62] During the Syrian Civil War, a major polio outbreak, which began in 2013, paralyzed at least 37 children.[63] By the time the outbreak was controlled with an 18-month intensive vaccination campaign, 74 cases had been reported.[64]

The COVID-19 pandemic has brought new risks for refugees and internally displaced persons. In unsanitary and overcrowded shelters and in multigenerational inner-city housing, where refugees typically live, they cannot socially distance. They are less likely to have access to masks. If one of them develops symptoms, other family members may already be infected. And they typically have poor access to healthcare because of limited services, lack of health insurance, and fear of identification by law enforcement officials.[65]

Refugees often have a high prevalence of some chronic communicable diseases, such as TB, HIV/AIDS, hepatitis B, and hepatitis C, reflecting the prevalence of these diseases in their countries of origin and in refugee camps. As a result, host countries generally screen for some chronic communicable diseases before permitting refugees to legally enter. And refugees sometimes travel back to their countries of origin without seeking advice on immunizations or other preventive measures, thereby exposing themselves to communicable diseases.[66]

ADDRESSING MALNUTRITION AND COMMUNICABLE DISEASES

Addressing malnutrition and communicable diseases during war requires an integrated approach at the local, regional, and national level. Governments, humanitarian aid organizations, and UN agencies ideally coordinate their work in providing food, water, sanitation, shelter, healthcare, and public health measures, including disease surveillance, immunizations, and health education. They need to implement interventions more systematically, with better coordination. After war ends, they need to transition from providing emergency humanitarian aid to supporting the development of locally operated sustainable programs to monitor and address malnutrition and communicable diseaes.[67]

Malnutrition

Efforts to address malnutrition during war and its aftermath need to focus on children and other vulnerable populations, including women, older people, and people with disabilities. Measures need to be tailored to the setting and the specific population. For example, programs to achieve optimal infant and child nutrition include the following components:

- Growth monitoring of infants and children to detect malnutrition
- Ensuring food security, including availability of and accessibility to food
- Ensuring feeding and caregiving resources at the maternal, household, and community levels
- Promoting breastfeeding and the use of nutrient-rich foods for infants and young children
- Ensuring access to and promoting the use of health and nutrition services
- Ensuring access to a safe water supply and a safe and hygienic environment
- Preventing communicable diseases (see page 137).[15]

Addressing childhood malnutrition and related disorders includes adequately assessing the nutritional status of and providing food for malnourished children. It also includes providing supplemental feeding and medical care for severely malnourished children, addressing the effects of malnutrition on child growth and development, and assisting households in being socially and economically sustainable.

Feeding programs operated by UN agencies, bilateral aid agencies, and nongovernmental organizations are most effective when they are an integral part of a comprehensive relief or rehabilitation program that addresses a wide range of children's needs. Progress can be impeded by political and military factors; damage to roads and other logistical problems; destruction of food storage facilities and food supply systems; and droughts, floods, and other extreme weather-related events.

Addressing malnutrition among children and other vulnerable populations usually requires a long-term commitment by international aid organizations and national and local stakeholders. It also requires establishing sustainable programs based on locally available resources.

Programs to identify malnourished children and respond to their needs have often been successful. For example, a 2004 study of young Iraqi children found that 23% suffered from chronic malnutrition and 8% from acute malnutrition.[68] Over the next few years, programs addressing this problem made substantial progress. Between 2005 and 2007, the number of people in Iraq with food insecurity decreased from 4 million to 933,000, and the percentage of people dependent on a monthly food ration decreased from 32% to 9.4%.[69]

Growth monitoring can be performed in healthcare facilities or, often more efficiently, by community health workers. Training and deploying community volunteers to perform growth monitoring of preschool children can be a practical alternative during war and its aftermath. A program in the DRC selected and trained community volunteers to monitor children's growth in their villages. Over a 2-year period, they monitored more than 5,000 children under age 5, weighing them every month and plotting their weight on weight-for-age curves. A high percentage of children participated. Over the course of the program, the median percentage of children between 12 and 59 months of age per village ranked as highly susceptible to malnutrition decreased from 4.2% to 2.8%.[70]

When the food supply is disrupted during war, civilians sometimes develop effective coping strategies. For example, during the occupation of Kuwait by Iraqi troops in 1990, access to food became difficult. As a result, an underground food network that used food recovered from local food cooperatives was established. So was a black market that used food that was imported through Iraq or locally stolen in Kuwait. In addition, 23% of people grew vegetables and 39% raised animals to supplement their nutritional needs. Nevertheless, many people had inadequate nutrition and lost weight.[71]

Communicable Diseases

Basic elements of a program to address communicable diseases include the following:

- Preparedness measures, including identifying and analyzing risks, vulnerabilities, and likely consequences; engaging in multisectoral planning for prevention, detection, and control of priority communicable diseases; and implementing relevant measures, such as immunization, heightened vector control, stockpiling of medications and other materials, and staff training
- Rapid risk assessment, including determining the capacity of international and local health entities, establishing coordination mechanisms, obtaining relevant baseline health data, identifying primary disease threats, and determining priority interventions
- Maintaining a healthy physical environment, including planning shelter to minimize overcrowding and maximize ventilation, ensuring an adequate supply of safe water, adequate sanitation and hygiene facilities and waste management, and availability of food and cooking facilities; providing essential clinical services; controlling insect vectors and

infection reservoirs; implementing mass immunization campaigns and other interventions; and providing community education on hygiene and other preventive measures

- Controlling communicable diseases in patients and contacts, with use of standard diagnostic algorithms and treatment protocols in healthcare facilities and use of simplified drug regimens, as well as ensuring a regular supply of medicines and rapid diagnostic tests
- Establishing surveillance and early warning systems, including identifying target diseases for surveillance based on risk assessment; developing case definitions for reporting; ensuring adequate laboratory confirmation services; and reporting information to participating facilities, government agencies, and humanitarian aid organizations
- Implementing epidemic measures to ensure that outbreaks are rapidly controlled, including training epidemic response teams, ensuring adequate supplies of vaccines and drugs, and ensuring appropriate risk communication.[37]

Specific communicable diseases require specific preventive measures. Measles immunization rates are often low among children in war-torn countries. Because measles has a high case-fatality rate in these populations, measles immunization often needs to be a high priority.

Preventive measures for TB include improvement of living, sanitary, and health conditions of displaced people; provision of BCG vaccine; and monitoring to determine the prevalence of latent tubercle bacillus infection to evaluate and ultimately, when possible, treat it. Curative actions need to identify potential TB patients, accurately and rapidly perform diagnostic tests, and provide treatment in order to limit disease progression and further spread of infection. Health systems need to provide reliable diagnostic tests and cover the costs of anti-TB medications. Efficient follow-up systems need to be established for TB patients who have been treated. Given the regional and global dimensions of these challenges, engagement of countries, bilateral aid organizations, and UN agencies is essential to control TB. It is also important to rehabilitate preexisting national TB control programs and to disseminate guidelines and standards in order to integrate TB treatment and control into existing healthcare programs.[39]

Prevention of cholera depends on interrupting fecal-oral transmission by ensuring access to safe, potable drinking water; appropriate sanitation and waste disposal; and proper hygiene, including handwashing. Epidemic measures include educating the population at risk regarding the need to seek immediate treatment for dehydration; providing effective treatment facilities; adopting emergency measures to ensure a safe water supply; chlorinating public water supplies or boiling water used for drinking, cooking, and washing dishes and food containers; ensuring careful preparation and supervision of food and beverages; initiating an investigation to find the main vehicles of infection and planning appropriate control measures; and providing appropriate safe facilities for sewage disposal. Oral cholera vaccines may be used but should not replace other recommended control measures.[72] Currently, there are three oral cholera vaccines that have been prequalified by the World Health Organization, each of which requires two doses for full protection.[73]

SUMMARY POINTS

- Malnutrition predisposes children to acquiring and dying from communicable diseases.
- Diarrheal diseases, which predispose children to malnutrition, frequently occur during war and its aftermath.
- Measles virus, which is highly contagious and has a high case-fatality rate, represents a grave threat to unvaccinated children in war settings.
- Control of tuberculosis, which is often weakened during war and displacement, needs to be prioritized.
- Major contributing factors to malnutrition and communicable diseases include displacement, crowding, disruption of the food supply, damage to water treatment facilities, and reduced access to healthcare and public health services.

REFERENCES

1. Bhutta ZA, Berkley JA, Bandsma RHJ, et al. Severe childhood malnutrition. Nature Reviews Disease Primers 2017; 21:3: 17067. doi: 10.1038/nrdp.2017.67.
2. Global Network Against Food Crises. 2020 Global Report on Food Crises: Joint Analysis for Better Decisions. Available at: https://www.fsinplatform.org/sites/default/files/resources/files/GRFC_2020_ONLINE_200420.pdf. Accessed on April 5, 2021.
3. Young H, Marshak A. Persistent global acute malnutrition. Boston: Feinstein International Center, Tufts University, 2017. Available at: https://fic.tufts.edu/assets/FIC-Publication-Persistent-Global-Acute-Malnutrition_web_2.26s.pdf. Accessed on March 22, 2021.
4. Provost R. Starvation as a weapon: Legal implications of the United Nations food blockade against Iraq and Kuwait. Columbia Journal of Transnational Law 1992; 30: 577-639.
5. World Peace Foundation and the Fletcher School. Famine trends dataset, tables and graphs. Available at: https://sites.tufts.edu/wpf/famine/. Accessed on March 11, 2021.
6. de Waal A. The end of famine? Prospects for the elimination of mass starvation by political action. Political Geography 2018; 62: 184-195.
7. Marcus D. Famine crimes in international law. American Journal of International Law 2003; 97: 245-281.
8. Bendavid E, Boerma T, Akseer N, et al. The effects of armed conflict on the health of women and children. Lancet 2021; 397: 522-532.
9. Runge CF, Graham L. Viewpoint: Hunger as a weapon of war: Hitler's hunger plan, Native American resettlement and starvation in Yemen. Food Policy 2020; 92: 101835.
10. UN humanitarian office puts Yemen war dead at 233,000, mostly from "indirect causes." UN News, December 1, 2020. Available at: https://news.un.org/en/story/2020/12/1078972. Accessed on March 11, 2021.
11. Food and Agriculture Organization of the United Nations, UNICEF, the World Food Programme, and the World Health Organization. Yemen: Acute malnutrition hits record levels in Yemen with a devastating toll on children under five. Issued February 2021. Available: http://www.ipcinfo.org/filead min/user_upload/ipcinfo/docs/IPC_Yemen_Acute_Malnutrition_2020Jan2021Mar.pdf. Accessed on March 22, 2021.
12. Mohareb AM, Ivers LC. Disease and famine as weapons of war in Yemen. New England Journal of Medicine 2019; 380: 109-111.
13. Linke AM, Ruether B. Weather, wheat, and war: Security implications of climate variability for conflict in Syria. Journal of Peace Research 2021; 58: 114-131.
14. Wessells KR, Ouédraogo CT, Young RR, et al. Micronutrient status among pregnant women in Zinder, Niger and risk factors associated with deficiency. Nutrients 2017; 9: 430. doi: 10.3390/nu9050430.
15. Black RE, Victora CG, Walker SP, et al. Maternal and child undernutrition and overweight in low-income and middle-income countries. Lancet 2013; 382: 427-451.

16. de Rooij SR, Wouters H, Yonker JE, et al. Prenatal undernutrition and cognitive function in late adulthood. Proceedings of the National Academy of Sciences USA 2010; 107: 16881-16886.

17. El Bcheraoui C, Jumaan AO, Collison ML, et al. Health in Yemen: Losing ground in war time. Globalization and Health 2018; 14: 42. doi: 10.1186/s12992-018- 0354-9.

18. Save the Children. Conflict in Yemen: Devastating toll on pregnant women and new mums becomes clear as malnutrition admissions soar (News and Press Release), May 3, 2019. Available at: https://relief web.int/report/yemen/conflict-yemen-devastating-toll-pregnant-women-and-new-mums-becomes-clear-malnutrition. Accessed on September 8, 2020.

19. Caulfield LE, de Onis M, Blossner M, Black RE. Undernutrition as an underlying cause of child deaths associated with diarrhea, pneumonia, malaria, and measles. American Journal of Clinical Nutrition 2004; 80: 193-198.

20. Bahwere P. Severe acute malnutrition during emergencies: Burden, management, and gaps. Food and Nutrition Bulletin 2014; 35: 547-551.

21. de Rooij SR, Caan MWA, Swaab DF, et al. Prenatal famine exposure has sex-specific effects on brain size. Brain 2016; 139: 2136-2142.

22. van Abeelen AFM, Elias SG, Bossuyt PMM, et al. Famine exposure in the young and the risk of type 2 diabetes in adulthood. Diabetes 2012; 61: 2255-2260.

23. Han C, Hong Y-C. Fetal and childhood malnutrition during the Korean War and metabolic syndrome in adulthood. Nutrition 2019; 62: 186-193.

24. Fransen HP, Peeters PHM, Beulens JWJ, et al. Exposure to famine at a young age and unhealthy lifestyle behavior later in life. PLoS ONE 2016; 11: e0156609. doi: 10.1371/journal.pone.0156609.

25. Akresh R, Lucchetti L, Thirumurthy H. Wars and child health: Evidence from the Eritrean-Ethiopian conflict. Journal of Development Economics 2012; 99: 330-340.

26. Uchendu FN. Hunger influenced life expectancy in war-torn sub-Saharan African countries. Journal of Health, Population and Nutrition 2018; 37: 11. doi: org/10.1186/s41043-018-0143-3.

27. Rice AL, Sacco L, Hyder A, Black RE. Malnutrition as an underlying cause of childhood deaths associated with infectious diseases in developing countries. Bulletin of the World Health Organization 2000; 78: 1207-1221.

28. Altare C, Delbiso TD, Guha-Sapir D. Child wasting in emergency pockets: A meta-analysis of small-scale surveys from Ethiopia. International Journal of Environmental Research and Public Health 2016; 13: 178. doi: 10.3390/ijerph13020178.

29. Hermanussen M, Bilogub M, Lindl AC, et al. Weight and height growth of malnourished school-age children during re-feeding. Three historic studies published shortly after World War I. European Journal of Clinical Nutrition 2018; 72: 1603-1619.

30. Cliff J, Noormahomed AR. The impact of war on children's health in Mozambique. Social Science and Medicine 1993; 36: 843-848.

31. Green EC, Honwa A. Indigenous healing of war affected children in Africa. Available at: http://docume nts.worldbank.org/curated/en/612131468767662523/pdf/23422-Replacement-file-IKNT10.pdf. Accessed on April 21, 2020.

32. Dahab R, Bécares L, Brown M. Armed conflict as a determinant of children malnourishment: A cross-sectional study in The Sudan. BMC Public Health 2020; 20:532. https://doi.org/10.1186/s12889-020-08665-x.

33. UNICEF. The State of the World's Children 2019: Children, Food and Nutrition: Growing Well in a Changing World. Available at: https://www.unicef.org/media/63016/file/SOWC-2019.pdf. Accessed on October 22, 2020.

34. Yip R, Sharp TW. Acute malnutrition and high childhood mortality related to diarrhea: Lessons from the 1991 Kurdish refugee crisis. Journal of the American Medical Association 1993; 270: 587-590.

35. Guerra JVV, Alves VH, Rachedi L, et al. Forced international migration for refugee food: A scoping review. Ciência & Saúde Coletiva 2019; 24: 4499-4508. doi: 10.1590/1413-812320182412.23382019.

36. Habib RR, Ziadee M, Younes EA, et al. The association between living conditions and health among Syrian refugee children in informal tented settlements in Lebanon. Journal of Public Health 2019; 42: e323-e333.

37. Gayer M. "Communicable Disease Control in Humanitarian Emergencies" in DL Heymann (ed.). Control of Communicable Diseases Manual (20th edition). Washington, DC: American Public Health Association, 2015, pp. A45-A55.

38. Ismail MB, Rafei R, Dabboussi F, Hamze M. Tuberculosis war and refugees: Spotlight on the Syrian humanitarian crisis. PLoS Pathogens 2018; 14: e1007014.

39. Kimbrough W, Saliba V, Dahab M, et al. The burden of tuberculosis in crisis-affected populations: A systematic review. Lancet Infectious Diseases 2012; 12: 950-965.

40. Sindani I, Fitzpatrick C, Falzon D, et al. Multidrug-resistant tuberculosis, Somalia, 2010–2011. Emerging Infectious Diseases 2013; 19: 478-480.

41. Abbara A, Almalla M, AlMasri I, et al. The challenges of tuberculosis control in protracted conflict: The case of Syria. International Journal of Infectious Diseases 2020; 90: 53-59.

42. Ozaras R, Leblebicioglu H, Sunbul M, et al. The Syrian conflict and infectious diseases. Expert Review of Anti-Infective Therapy 2016; 14: 547-555.

43. Swerdlow DL, Malenga G, Begkoyian G, et al. Epidemic cholera among refugees in Malawi, Africa: Treatment and transmission. Epidemiology and Infection 1997; 118: 207-214.

44. Connolly MA, Heymann DL. Deadly comrades: War and infectious diseases. Lancet Supplement 2002; 360: S23-S24.

45. Ng QX, De Deyn MLZQ, Loke W, Yeo WS. Yemen's cholera epidemic is a One Health issue. Journal of Preventive Medicine & Public Health 2020; 53: 289-292.

46. Federspiel F, Ali M. The cholera outbreak in Yemen: Lessons learned and way forward. BMC Public Health 2018; 18: 1338.

47. Roberts L. Measles is on the rise—and COVID-19 could make it worse. Nature 2020; 580: 447-448.

48. Guha-Sapir D, Moitinho de Almeida M, Scales SE, et al. Containing measles in conflict-driven humanitarian settings. BMJ Global Health 2020; 5: e003515. doi: 10.1136/bmjgh-2020-003515.

49. Berry I, Berrang-Ford L. Leishmaniasis, conflict, and political terror: A spatio-temporal analysis. Social Science & Medicine 2016; 167: 140-149.

50. Fawcett JM, Hay RJ. Cutaneous leishmaniasis and human conflict. Acta Dermato- Venereologica 2015; 95: 3-4.

51. Muhjazi G, Gabrielli AF, Ruiz-Postigo JA, et al. Cutaneous leishmaniasis in Syria: A review of available data during the war years: 2011–2018. PLoS Neglected Tropical Diseases 2019; 13: e007827.

52. Pearn J. War zone paediatrics in Rwanda. Journal of Paediatrics and Child Health 1996; 32: 290-295.

53. Fozouni L, Weber C, Lindner AK, et al. Immunization coverage among refugee children in Berlin. Journal of Global Health 2019; 9: 010432. doi: 10.7189/jogh.010432.

54. Agadjanian V, Prata N. Civil war and child health: Regional and ethnic dimensions of child immunization and malnutrition in Angola. Social Science and Medicine 2003; 56: 2515-2527.

55. United Nations Children's Fund. Lost at Home: The Risks and Challenges for Internally Displaced Children and the Urgent Actions Needed to Protect Them. New York: UNICEF, 2020. Available at: https://www.unicef.org/media/70131/file/Lost-at-home-risks-and-challenges-for-IDP-children-2020.pdf. Accessed on August 26, 2020.

56. Abdul-Ghani R, Mahdy MAK, Al-Eryani SMA, et al. Impact of population displacement and forced movements on the transmission and outbreaks of Aedes-borne viral diseases: Dengue as a model. Acta Tropica 2019; 197: 105066. doi: 10.1016/actatropica.2019.105066.

57. Owoaje ET, Uchendu OC, Ajayi TO, Cadmus EO. A review of the health problems of the internally displaced persons in Africa. Nigerian Postgraduate Medical Journal 2016; 23: 161-171.

58. Nimer NA. A review on emerging and reemerging of infectious diseases in Jordan: The aftermath of the Syrian crises. Canadian Journal of Infectious Diseases and Medical Microbiology 2018; Article ID 8679174. https://doi.org/10.1155/2018/8679174.

59. Mipatrini D, Stefanelli P, Severoni S, Rezza G. Vaccinations in migrants and refugees: A challenge for European health systems. A systematic review of current scientific evidence. Pathogens and Global Health 2017; 111: 59-68. doi: 10.1080/20477724.2017.1281374

60. Mishori R, Aleinikoff S, Davis D. Primary care for refugees: Challenges and opportunities. American Family Physician 2017; 96: 112-120.

61. Centers for Disease Control and Prevention. Our Progress Against Polio. Available at: https://www.cdc.gov/polio/progress/index.htm. Accessed on March 22, 2021.

62. Amnesty International. Afghanistan's refugees: Forty years of dispossession. June 20, 2019. Available at: https://www.amnesty.org/en/latest/news/2019/06/afghanistan-refugees-forty-years/#:~:text=Pakistan%20currently%20hosts%20more%20than,million%20Afghan%20refugees%20in%20Pakistan. Accessed on September 1, 2020.

63. Roberts L. A war within a war. Science 2014; 343: 1302-1305.

64. Polio Global Eradication Initiative. Syria polio outbreak stopped. Available at: https://polioeradication.org/news-post/syria-polio-outbreak-stopped/. Accessed on May 3, 2021.

65. Brito MO. COVID-19 in the Americas: Who's looking after refugees and migrants? Annals of Global Health 2020; 86: 69. doi: 10.5334/aogh.2915.

66. Castelli F, Sulis G. Migration and infectious diseases. Clinical Microbiology and Infection 2017; 23: 283-289.

67. Levy BS, Sidel VW. Protecting non-combatant civilians during war (Commentary). Medicine, Conflict and Survival 2015; 31: 88-91.

68. Iraq Ministry of Planning and Development Cooperation and United Nations Development Programme. Iraq Living Conditions Survey 2004, Volume II, Analytical Report. Baghdad: Ministry of Planning and Development Cooperation, 2005, p. 57.

69. UN World Food Program. Comprehensive food security and vulnerability analysis in Iraq. Rome: World Food Program, 2008, pp. 1-2. Available at: https://documents.wfp.org/stellent/groups/public/documents/ena/wfp192521.pdf. Accessed on November 9, 2020.

70. Bisimwa G, Mambo T, Mitangala P, et al. Nutritional monitoring of preschool-age children by community volunteers during armed conflict in the Democratic Republic of the Congo. Food and Nutrition Bulletin 2009; 30: 120-127.

71. Alajmi F, Somerset SM. Food system sustainability and vulnerability: Food acquisition during military occupation of Kuwait. Public Health Nutrition 2015; 18: 3060-3066.

72. Brunkard JM, Mahon B, Routh J, Mintz E. "Cholera and Other Vibrioses" in DL Heymann (ed.). Control of Communicable Diseases Manual (20th edition). Washington, DC: American Public Health Association, 2015, pp. 102-114.

73. World Health Organization. Immunization, vaccines and biologicals: Cholera. Available at: https://www.who.int/immunization/diseases/cholera/en/. Accessed on April 5, 2021.

Profile 7:
Debby Guha-Sapir, Ph.D.
Translating Epidemiology
into Social Change

Be open to possibility. Take opportunities. Learn from experience. And translate science into policy and action. These maxims have guided Dr. Debby Guha-Sapir, who over the past three decades has been—and continues to be—a leader in developing the discipline of conflict and disaster epidemiology.

After receiving her Ph.D. in epidemiology from the University of Louvain in Belgium, Dr. Guha-Sapir was employed there as a junior researcher. The professor she was assisting offered her a choice between stable, well-paid work inputting research data and exploring opportunities to apply her epidemiology skills in the wake of disasters in other countries. When she learned that Médecins Sans Frontières was seeking an epidemiologist to investigate the impact of famine in Chad, she took that opportunity.

In studying the famine, she discovered new risk factors for malnutrition. She found that, while aid groups were focusing their attention on children under age 5, malnourished children between 5 and 9 years of age were scavenging for food. She observed that families who derived their income from occupations in which clients could delay their patronage—like cutting hair, making mats, and repairing pots and pans—were at increased risk of malnutrition. Her findings helped frontline teams to identify high-risk families early.

Soon afterward, when Dr. Guha-Sapir was asked to write a book chapter about Somalia, she took the opportunity to go there. Over the next 2 months, she investigated the causes of morbidity and mortality and learned much about Somalia. Next, she worked in Darfur, Sudan, which taught her how to walk a tightrope when negotiating with local armed forces for research access. Her experiences in these settings opened her eyes to the nexus between humanitarian assistance and military intervention.

From Horror to Hope. Barry S. Levy, Oxford University Press. © Oxford University Press 2022.
DOI: 10.1093/oso/9780197558645.003.0014

By the early 1990s, she received an academic appointment at the University of Louvain, which gave her more opportunities for epidemiological research in fragile settings. In Ethiopia, she developed indicators of famine and observed how large-scale development of coffee farms interrupted the equilibrium of nomads with their environment. In Mozambique, which had almost no functioning health data systems, she set up sentinel surveillance to identify disease trends and outbreaks. And, back in Belgium, she taught medical students about health and development, enthusiastically sharing her experiences in fragile settings.

As she continued to perform -- and supervise others in performing -- many epidemiological studies about armed conflicts, natural disasters, and other humanitarian emergencies, she saw the potential benefits and opportunities to aggregate findings from epidemiological studies on these subjects worldwide. So she established two global databases, one on natural disasters (EMDAT) and one on conflict and other complex humanitarian emergencies (CEDAT), each based on strong epidemiological principles. The databases have since provided opportunities to pool data from multiple sources, to share findings widely, and to improve research methods used in disaster and conflict settings.

Dr. Guha-Sapir has recognized that it is essential to translate scientific findings into policy and action—and ultimately social change. Therefore, an important part of her work has been communicating her research findings in journal articles and the mainstream media. And she continues to do field work to stay in contact with developments at the grassroots level.

When asked why an epidemiologist should choose this type of work in unstable settings, with uncertain funding, and the potential to disrupt one's family life and the trajectory of one's career, she responds: "It is exhilarating to see how one's scientific research and resultant interventions can improve nutrition and prevent communicable disease in mothers and children."

Dr. Guha-Sapir is a Professor at the Centre for Research on Epidemiology of Disasters at the Université Catholique in Brussels, Belgium.

8

Mental Disorders

War may sometimes be a necessary evil. But no matter how necessary, it is always an evil, never a good. We will not learn how to live together in peace by killing each other's children.

JIMMY CARTER

INTRODUCTION

War-related mental disorders in civilians have generally been neglected by researchers, government agencies, and humanitarian aid organizations. There has been much less documentation and research on mental disorders in civilians than in military personnel and veterans, as described in Chapter 12. A recent PubMed search found four times more journal articles on mental health among military personnel than among civilians.

Mental disorders occur frequently during war and its aftermath. In conflict settings during the 2000–2017 period, the estimated point prevalence of mental disorders in conflict-affected populations was 22%, adjusted for comorbidity and standardized for age—13% for *mild* forms of depression, anxiety, and posttraumatic stress disorder (PTSD); 4% for *moderate* forms of these disorders; and 5% for *severe* forms of these disorders in addition to schizophrenia and bipolar disorder.[1]

War-related mental disorders among civilians are especially prevalent during intrastate wars. For example, during the Syrian Civil War, many civilians have experienced exacerbations of preexisting mental disorders, onset of new mental disorders due to violence and displacement, and psychosocial problems related to adapting to life in countries of refuge.[2]

A study in postwar communities in Algeria, Cambodia, Ethiopia, and Palestine found that the prevalence of PTSD ranged from 16% to 37% and the prevalence of anxiety disorder from 10% to 40%. Among people exposed to violence, PTSD was the most frequent disorder.[3]

Causative and contributing factors for mental disorders include physical, sexual, and psychological trauma as well as family separation, deaths of relatives and friends, damage to homes and communities, forced displacement, and witnessing torture or execution. Mental disorders are exacerbated by reduced access to mental health services because of damage to

From Horror to Hope. Barry S. Levy, Oxford University Press. © Oxford University Press 2022.
DOI: 10.1093/oso/9780197558645.003.0015

clinics, displacement or death of mental health professionals, language barriers, and stigma associated with mental illness.[4]

TYPES OF MENTAL DISORDERS

PTSD and depression occur frequently among civilians in war zones. One study found that, among adult civilian survivors who remained in war-afflicted regions, about one-fourth suffered from PTSD and one-fourth from depression.[4]

PTSD symptoms include distressing memories or recurrent dreams about a traumatic event, persistent blaming of oneself or others, estrangement from other people, sleep disturbances, hypervigilance, and aggressive, reckless, or self-destructive behavior.[5] PTSD results from a situation in which a person directly experiences or witnesses a traumatic event, learns that it affected a close family member or friend, or experiences firsthand extreme or repeated exposure to details of a traumatic event. PTSD causes substantial distress or impairment in affected individuals' social interactions and their ability to work and to perform in other areas of life.

Depression can affect anyone during war or its aftermath. Those at greatest risk have included women, older people, those with little formal education, unemployed people, impoverished people, and people who have been abused.[6]

Substance use disorders, including misuse of alcohol, opiates, or tranquilizers, are exacerbated by interruptions in healthcare and public health services during war and its aftermath. In war-affected populations, substance use disorders may increase the likelihood of communicable diseases, other behavioral and mental disorders, and gender-based violence.[7,8]

CIVILIAN POPULATIONS AT RISK
Displaced People

Displaced people are at especially high risk of developing mental disorders, including PTSD, depression, anxiety, borderline personality disorder, and dissociative disorders (conditions with disruption of identity, awareness, perception, or memory).[9-11] Alcohol abuse frequently occurs among displaced people—especially (up to 80%) in displaced men.[12] Even many years after resettlement, displaced people continue to suffer from these disorders due to both premigration trauma and post-migration stress.[13] Table 8-1 summarizes the findings of several studies of mental disorders in populations displaced by war.

Many refugees on arrival in host countries suffer from depression, anxiety, and substance use disorders. Language barriers, cultural and religious issues, racism, and unemployment often aggravate these problems. Their risk factors for mental disorders include older age, female gender, low socioeconomic status, and inadequate social support. Often refugees also find it difficult to access healthcare in host countries, including family planning services, because of legal, communication, cultural, and bureaucratic barriers.[14]

Refugees and asylum-seekers often fear that they will be forcibly repatriated—in violation of international agreements—to their countries of origin, where they would likely face

TABLE 8-1 Summary of Some Studies of Mental Disorders Among Populations Displaced by War

Group Studied	Findings
Vietnamese boat refugees in Norway[a]	62% experienced bombing, fires, and/or shooting; 48% witnessed war injuries or deaths; and 36% were wounded in war or were in life-endangering situations. War trauma was associated with decreased mental health 7 years after Vietnam War.
Displaced Bosnians who remained in their home region[b]	45% of those with PTSD, depression, or both continued to have these disorders 3 years after initial assessment.
Adult refugees from Kosovo[c]	50% had PTSD and 16% had a major depressive episode.
Internally displaced persons in Darfur region of Sudan[d]	31% had major depression. Women's mental health needs were largely unmet and their rights regarding marriage, movement, and access to healthcare were restricted.
Unaccompanied refugee minors from Sudan, about 1 year after resettlement in the United States[e]	20% had PTSD, which was associated with social isolation and history of personal injury.
Refugee children from the Middle East, most of whom had been exposed to wartime violence[f]	67% had anxiety and 30% had sleep disturbance.
Older adults in Germany who had been displaced during the Second World War[g]	Higher prevalence of PTSD, depressive, and somatoform symptoms, and lower levels of health-related quality of life
Afghan refugees (systematic review of 17 studies)[h]	Moderate to high prevalence of depressive and posttraumatic symptoms
Internally displaced persons in South Darfur[i]	62% had psychiatric disorders; 15% had PTSD, 14% had depression, and 8% had both.
Resettled Iraqi refugees[j]	Prevalence of PTSD was 8%–37% in 6 studies and prevalence of depression was 28%–75% in 7 studies.

[a] Hauff E, Vaglum P. Vietnamese boat refugees: The influence of war and flight traumatization on mental health on arrival in the country of resettlement: A community cohort study of Vietnamese refugees in Norway. Acta Psychiatrica Scandinavica 1993; 88: 162-168.
[b] Mollica RF, Sarajilic N, Chernoff M, et al. Longitudinal study of psychiatric symptoms, disability, mortality, and emigration among Bosnian refugees. Journal of the American Medical Association 2001; 286: 546-554.
[c] Turner SW, Bowie C, Dunn G, et al. Mental health of Kosovan Albanian refugees in the UK. British Journal of Psychiatry 2003; 182: 444-448.
[d] Kim G, Torbay R, Lawry L. Basic health, women's health, and mental health among internally displaced persons in Nyala Province, South Darfur, Sudan. American Journal of Public Health 2007; 97: 353-361.
[e] Geltman PL, Grant-Knight W, Mehta SD, et al. The "Lost Boys of Sudan": Functional and behavioral health of unaccompanied refugee minors resettled in the United States. Archives of Pediatric and Adolescent Medicine 2005; 159: 585-591.
[f] Montgomery E, Foldspang A. Seeking asylum in Denmark: Refugee children's mental health and exposure to violence. European Journal of Public Health 2005; 15: 233-237.
[g] Freitag S, Brahler E, Schmidt S, Glaesmer H. The impact of forced displacement in World War II on mental health disorders and health-related quality of life in late life: A German population-based study. International Psychogeriatrics 2013; 25: 310-319.
[h] Alemi Q, James S, Cruz R, et al. Psychological distress in Afghan refugees: A mixed-method systematic review. Journal of Immigrant and Minority Health 2014; 16: 1247-1261.
[i] Elhabiby MM, Radwan DN, Okasha TA, El-Desouky ED. Psychiatric disorders among a sample of internally displaced persons in South Darfur. International Journal of Social Psychiatry 2015; 61: 358-362.
[j] Slewa-Younan S, Uribe Guarjardo MG, Heriseanu A, Hasan T. A systematic review of post-traumatic stress disorder and depression among Iraqi refugees located in western countries. Journal of Immigrant and Minority Health 2015; 17: 1231-1239.

risks to their health and safety. Their fears are not unfounded. The United States has forcibly returned Guatemalan and El Salvadoran asylum-seekers to their countries of origin, where some have been killed by death squads.[1] Lebanon has threatened to force thousands of Syrian refugees back to Syria. And many Afghan refugees in Pakistan have been forced to return to Afghanistan.[15]

Even many years after resettlement, refugees have high rates of mental disorders. For example, 20 years after a civil war in Guatemala, many Guatemalan refugees in Mexico had psychiatric disorders, often associated with human rights violations.[16] More than 20 years after their resettlement in the United States, more than half of Cambodian refugees had trauma-related PTSD or major depression.[17] Tibetan nuns and lay students, who had been arrested and tortured in Tibet and were living in exile as refugees in India, had increased anxiety.[18]

Women

Women are at increased risk of mental disorders during war and its aftermath. For example, civilian women in Bosnia and Herzegovina exposed to traumatic war and postwar events had a 28% prevalence of PTSD, compared to 4.4% among women not directly exposed, and a high prevalence of anxiety, hostility, paranoid ideation, depression, and other psychological symptoms.[19] Female victims of sexual violence have often suffered from high rates of PTSD, depression, social phobia, and other mental disorders.[20] Other major causes of mental disorders in women include injuries from use of indiscriminate weapons, communicable diseases, severe injuries and deaths of loved ones, disruption of family structure, and social disintegration (Figure 8-1).

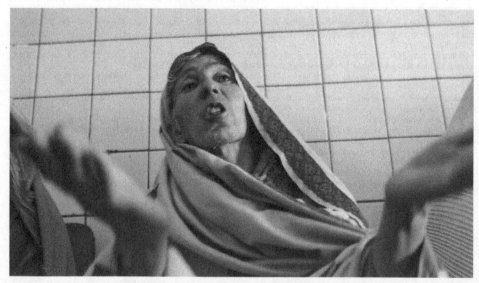

FIGURE 8-1 A 45-year-old woman who had two sons killed during war and a daughter injured by a bomb at their home cries during a therapy session in 2003 at the Kabul Mental Health Hospital in Kabul, Afghanistan. (AP Photo/Silvia Izquierdo.)

The mental disorders among Syrian women are illustrative. Among married Syrian refugee women living in Jordan—almost all of whom had experienced war-related traumas—about one-third had PTSD, often accompanied by reduced intimacy.[21] Syrian women in a refugee camp in Greece experienced a high prevalence of anxiety, depression, and somatization.[22]

Wives of veterans with PTSD may be at increased risk of developing PTSD. A study in Croatia of 56 veterans' wives with PTSD found that 57% of them had six or more symptoms of secondary traumatic stress and 39% met the diagnostic criteria for secondary traumatic stress.[23]

Children

Children in war zones generally have high rates of mental disorders, including PTSD, depression, fear, anxiety, sleep problems, difficulty concentrating, and psychosomatic symptoms. Often detachment from their families and communities is a major contributing factor. Societal instability and the undermining of civil society have a great detrimental impact on children. These disorders among children often have long-term adverse consequences on performance in school and at work, on ability to form and maintain relationships, and on family life, coping skills, and overall health and well-being.[24-31]

Children displaced by war often have distressing experiences, such as physical assault, deprivation of food and water, imprisonment, hearing nearby gunshots and explosions, and witnessing torture and murder. They may worry that they or family members will be injured or killed.[32]

Children may commit acts of violence, sometimes after joining gangs. Risk factors include displacement from their homes; serious injury to or death of parents, other relatives, friends, or neighbors; military deployment of parents; witnessing violent acts; and witnessing or experiencing domestic violence within their families.[33] Fathers returning home from war with a "battlefield mentality" sometimes attack their spouses and children. (See Chapter 12.)

In the Middle East, a study found that the number of children's war-related traumatic experiences was associated with their subsequent prevalence of mental, behavioral, and emotional problems. The prevalence of PTSD in children and adolescents was estimated to be 5% to 8% in Israel, 23% to 70% in Palestine, and 10% to 30% in Iraq. Contributing factors included level and type of exposure, socioeconomic adversity, and inadequate social support. The number of their war-related traumatic exposures was associated with PTSD, depression, anxiety, functional impairment, behavioral problems, risk-taking behavior, and emotional disorders. Also associated with PTSD were a history of being tear-gassed or shelled, witnessing a friend's beating, being close to a terrorist attack, losing one's home, suffering violent acts, and experiencing bereavement.[34]

Depression occurs frequently in children affected by war, adversely affecting their sense of purpose in life, impairing educational achievement, and increasing the probability of physical and mental disorders, including suicide. Although depression is a treatable illness, many cases are not diagnosed because of lack of facilities and personnel and the difficulty of providing mental healthcare during war and its aftermath.[35]

During war, children may develop profound psychological disorders after witnessing traumatic events. Young children exposed to war often develop anxiety as well as low frustration tolerance, excessive thumb-sucking, changes in eating habits, demanding behavior, attention-seeking, aggressiveness, and temper tantrums. They may develop prolonged periods of crying. And they may develop over-dependency.[36]

Mental disorders have been prevalent in children during war and its aftermath:

- In South Africa, Sierra Leone, the Gambia, and Rwanda, children's exposure to community violence and war-related violence was consistently associated with PTSD, depression, and aggression.[37]
- In Bosnia and Herzegovina, 7 years after the war, foster children had higher rates of PTSD and depression.[38]
- During the Iraq War, 37% of children in Mosul had mental disorders, including PTSD, bedwetting, separation anxiety disorder, phobias, stuttering, refusal to attend school, learning disorders, and conduct disorders.[39]
- In the Gaza Strip, young children who had been exposed to day raids and shelling of their homes by tanks had higher rates of behavioral and emotional problems.[40]
- Colombian children displaced by war had, in the previous 12 months, twice the prevalence of posttraumatic stress and triple the prevalence of anxiety disorder.[41]
- In war-affected southern Thailand, almost half of students had direct exposure to a war-related event, which doubled their probability of developing mental disorders.[42]

There has only been limited research on substance abuse among children adversely affected by war. One example, however, is a study of Syrian refugee youth in Jordan that found that current smoking was associated with loss of family members.[43]

ADDRESSING MENTAL DISORDERS

Overview

Addressing mental disorders is a major challenge during war and its aftermath, given the major traumas experienced by war-affected populations and limited resources. In war-affected low-income countries, formal mental health services may be inadequate, but families and communities often support individual and group mental health through personal interactions and cultural and religious practices.

There are a number of measures that can support mental health of civilians during war and its aftermath. While providing direct assistance, health professionals and humanitarian aid workers should respect and support existing frameworks and approaches for mental health. Community health workers can be trained to better address mental health needs. Programs that are integrating displaced people into communities, reuniting families, and providing educational and employment opportunities can help address mental health needs. Truth and reconciliation commissions may play a helpful role (Chapter 15).

Improving Mental Health Assessment Tools

Existing tools to assess the mental health of conflict-affected populations are inadequate. Self-report tools, which have been widely used in conflict settings, do not accurately estimate the prevalence of mental disorders. Many of these tools, which have been developed for use in Western cultures, are not culturally appropriate. A standard assessment tool that can be adapted to various conflict settings needs to be developed.[44]

Developing Multifaceted Approaches

Measures to address mental health needs of children are illustrative of the multifaceted approaches that are necessary. Preventive interventions and treatments for children traumatized by war include strengthening community and family support, providing mental healthcare, and giving children emotional support.[45] Immediate and mid-term interventions also include promoting connectiveness, hope, a sense of safety, and a sense of self and community efficacy.[46] Focused psychosocial interventions can be effective in reducing PTSD and functional impairment and in increasing hope, coping, and social support.[47] Interventions need to be systematically and independently evaluated.

Ideally, all phases of emergency and reconstruction assistance should include psychosocial considerations and prioritize prevention of further mental trauma. Programs can support healing processes and reestablish normalcy by establishing daily routines of family and community life and by providing children with opportunities for expression and structured activities.[48] Ongoing risk factors in children's families, such as harsh parenting, distress of parents, and intimate partner violence among parents, need to be addressed.[49]

Addressing Mental Health Needs of Displaced Children

After displacement, children who had been internally displaced and their families may need much time to achieve stability. Protection and support of these children and their families include protection from attacks, harassment, intimidation, and persecution; compensation for reconstructing damaged or destroyed homes; and assistance with reintegration, including psychosocial support and access to education, healthcare, and social protections.[50]

Governments, UN agencies, and humanitarian relief organizations assist unaccompanied children with housing, education, food and nutrition, water and sanitation, and healthcare. They also reunify displaced children with their families and help to reintegrate them into communities. They also protect them from physical and sexual assaults, harassment and intimation, and persecution.[51]

Refugee children, especially if unaccompanied, should be provided documentation on the identity of their parents and their place of birth. Because family tracing is difficult during war, unaccompanied children should not be available for adoption unless all family tracing efforts have been exhausted.[48]

Governments, UN agencies, and relief organizations need to improve programs to disarm, demobilize, and reintegrate child soldiers into their families and communities. Interventions are most effective if they account for both war-related and post-conflict factors.

By accepting and forgiving child soldiers, communities can increase the likelihood of their being successfully reintegrated and becoming self-sufficient. Effective psychosocial interventions include mental healthcare, traditional rituals of cleansing and healing, and provision of training and employment opportunities.[52] (See Chapter 4.)

Sustainable Improvement in Mental Healthcare

Armed conflict can sometimes provide opportunities for creating sustainable improvement in mental healthcare. These opportunities can arise because the news media and governments may give increased attention to the mental health status and needs of war-affected civilians.

The World Health Organization has reviewed, in retrospect, 10 emergency situations, most of which were related to armed conflict, to determine what could be learned for improving mental healthcare after armed conflict and other emergency situations. It made the following observations that may be applicable in similar situations:

1. An early commitment for long-term mental health reform was important.
2. Reforms that were achieved addressed a wide range of mental health problems.
3. The government's central role was respected, even when certain functions were temporarily assigned to nongovernmental organizations.
4. Local mental health professionals played key roles in promoting and shaping mental health reform.
5. Coordination among diverse agencies was critically important.
6. Review and revision of national policies and plans was a critical component in mental health reform.
7. A key strategy was decentralizing mental health resources and promoting community-based care.
8. Health workers who were reorganized, trained, and provided with ongoing supervision were more capable of managing mental health problems.
9. Demonstration projects offered proof of concept and created opportunities for long-term funding.
10. Individuals and groups who were engaged in the process became effective advocates for broader mental health reform.[53]

SUMMARY POINTS

- War-related mental disorders among civilians are prevalent, but have generally been neglected.
- PTSD, depression, anxiety, and substance use disorders frequently occur.
- Women, children, and displaced people are at especially high risk.
- Improving mental health requires a multifaceted approach that includes respect for local cultures and concepts of mental health.

- Methods to assess and respond to mental disorders among war-affected civilians need to be improved.

REFERENCES

1. Charlson F, van Ommeren M, Flaxman A, et al. New WHO prevalence estimates of mental disorders in conflict settings: A systematic review and meta-analysis. Lancet 2019: 394: 240-248.
2. Hassan G, Ventevogel P, Jefee-Bahloul H, et al. Mental health and psychosocial wellbeing of Syrians affected by armed conflict. Epidemiology and Psychiatric Sciences 2016; 25: 129-141.
3. de Jong JTVM, Komproe IH, Van Ommeren M. Common mental disorders in postconflict settings. Lancet 2003; 361: 2128-2130.
4. Morina N, Stam K, Pollet TV, Priebe S. Prevalence of depression and posttraumatic stress disorder in adult civilian survivors of war who stay in war-afflicted regions: A systematic review and meta-analysis of epidemiological studies. Journal of Affective Disorders 2018: 239: 328-338.
5. American Psychiatric Association. Diagnostic and Statistical Manual or Mental Disorders (5th edition) (DSM-5). Washington, DC: American Psychiatric Publishing, 2013.
6. Mirković M, Djurić S, Trajković G, et al. Predictors of depression problems of adults who live in the security endangered territory. Srpski Arhiv za Celokupno Lekarstvo 2015; 143: 584-589.
7. Ezard N. Substance use among populations displaced by conflict: A literature review. Disasters 2012; 36: 533-557.
8. Roberts B, Ezard N. Why are we not doing more for alcohol use disorder among conflict-affected populations? Addiction 2015; 110: 889-890.
9. Bogic M, Njoku A, Priebe S. Long-term mental health of war-refugees: A systematic literature review. BMC International Health and Human Rights 2015; 15: 20. doi: 10.1186/s12914-015-0064-9.
10. Bustamante LHU, Cerqueira RO, Leclerc E, Brietzke E. Stress, trauma, and posttraumatic stress disorder in migrants: A comprehensive review. Brazilian Journal of Psychiatry 2017; 40: 220-225.
11. Buhmann CB. Traumatized refugees: Morbidity, treatment and predictors of outcome. Danish Medical Journal 2014; 61: B4871.
12. Weaver H, Roberts B. Drinking and displacement: A systematic review of the influence of forced displacement on harmful alcohol use. Substance Use & Misuse 2010; 45: 2340-2355.
13. Bogic M, Njoku A, Priebe S. Long-term mental health of war-refugees: A systematic literature review. BMC International Health and Human Rights 2015; 15: 29.
14. Pavli A, Maltezou H. Health problems of newly arrived migrants and refugees in Europe. Journal of Travel Medicine 2017; 24: 1-8. doi: 10.1093/jtm/tax016.
15. Human Rights Watch. Pakistan coercion, UN complicity: The mass forced return of Afghan refugees. February 13, 2017. Available at: https://www.hrw.org/report/2017/02/13/pakistan-coercion-un-com plicity/mass-forced-return-afghan-refugees. Accessed on February 4, 2021.
16. Sabin M, Cardozo BL, Nackerud L, et al. Factors associated with poor mental health among Guatemalan refugees living in Mexico 20 years after civil conflict. Journal of the American Medical Association 2003; 290: 635-642.
17. Marshall GN, Shell TL, Elliott MN, et al. Mental health of Cambodian refugees 2 decades after resettlement in the United States. Journal of the American Medical Association 2005; 294: 571-579.
18. Holtz TH. Refugee trauma versus torture trauma: A retrospective controlled cohort study of Tibetan refugees. Journal of Nervous & Mental Disease 1998; 186: 24-34.
19. Klarić M, Klarić B, Stevanović A, et al. Psychological consequences of war trauma and postwar social stressors in women in Bosnia and Herzegovina. Croatian Medical Journal 2007; 48: 167-176.
20. Lončar M, Medved V, Jovanović N, Hotujac L. Psychological consequences of rape on women in 1991–1995 war in Croatia and Bosnia and Herzegovina. Croatian Medical Journal 2006; 47: 67-75.
21. Rizkalla N, Segal SP. War can harm intimacy: Consequences for refugees who escaped Syria. Journal of Global Health 2019; 9: 020407. doi: 10.7189/jogh.09.020407.

22. Braun-Lewensohn O, Abu-Kaf S, Al-Said K. Women in refugee camps: Which coping resources help them to adapt? International Journal of Environmental Research and Public Health 2019; 16: 3990. doi: 10.3390/ijerph16203990.

23. Frančišković T, Stevanović A, Jelušić I, et al. Secondary traumatization of wives of war veterans with posttraumatic stress disorder. Croatian Medical Journal 2007; 48: 177-184.

24. UNICEF USA. UNICEF: More than 1 in 10 children living in countries and areas affected by armed conflict. Available at: https://www.unicefusa.org/press/releases/unicef-more-1-10-children-living-countries-and-areas-affected-armed-conflict/21551. Accessed on April 7, 2020.

25. Kadir A, Shenoda S, Goldhagen J, Pitterman S. The effects of armed conflict on children. Pediatrics 2018; 142: e20182586. doi: https://doi.org/10.1542/peds.2018-2586.

26. Attanayake V, McKay R, Joffres M, et al. Prevalence of mental disorders among children exposed to war: A systematic review of 7,920 children. Medicine, Conflict and Survival 2009; 25: 4-19.

27. Slone M, Mann S. Effects of war, terrorism and armed conflict on young children: A systematic review. Child Psychiatry and Human Development 2016; 47: 950-965.

28. Hasanović M, Sinanović O, Selimvašić Z, et al. Psychological disturbances of war-traumatized children from different foster and family settings in Bosnia and Herzegovina. Croatian Medical Journal 2006; 47: 85-94.

29. Pine DS, Castillo J, Masten A. Trauma, proximity, and developmental psychopathology: The effects of war and terrorism on children. Neuropsychopharmacology 2005; 30: 1781-1792.

30. Panter-Brick C, Eggerman M, Gonzalez V, et al. Violence, suffering, and mental health in Afghanistan: A school-based survey. Lancet 2009; 374: 807-816.

31. Waugh MJ, Robbins I, Davies S, Feigenbaum J. The long-term impact of war experiences and evacuation on people who were children during World War Two. Aging & Mental Health 2007; 11: 168-174.

32. Drury J, Williams R. Children and young people who are refugees, internally displaced persons or survivors or perpetrators of war, mass violence and terrorism. Current Opinion in Psychiatry 2012; 25: 277-284.

33. Lustig SL, Kia-Keating M, Knight WG, et al. Review of child and adolescent refugee mental health. Journal of the American Academy of Child and Adolescent Psychiatry 2004; 43: 24-36.

34. Dimitry L. A systematic review on the mental health of children and adolescents in areas of armed conflict in the Middle East. Child: Care, Health and Development 2012; 38: 153-161. doi: 10.1111/j.1365-2214.2011.01246.x.

35. Kar N. Depression in youth exposed to disasters, terrorism and political violence. Current Psychiatry Reports 2019; 21: 73. doi: 10.1007/s11920-019-1061-9.

36. Slone M, Mann S. Effects of war, terrorism and armed conflict on young children: A systematic review. Child Psychiatry and Human Development 2016; 47: 950-965. doi: 10.1007/s10578-016-0626-7.

37. Foster H, Brooks-Gunn J. Children's exposure to community and war violence and mental health in four African countries. Social Science & Medicine 2015; 146: 292-299.

38. Hasanović M, Sinanović O, Selimvašić Z, et al. Psychological disturbances of war-traumatized children from different foster and family settings in Bosnia and Herzegovina. Croatian Medical Journal 2006; 47: 85-94.

39. Al-Jawadi AA, Abdul-Rhman S. Prevalence of childhood and early adolescence mental disorders among children attending primary healthcare centers in Mosul, Iraq: A cross-sectional study. BMC Public Health 2007; 7: 274.

40. Thabet AA, Karim K, Vostanis P. Trauma exposure in preschool children in a war zone. British Journal of Psychiatry 2006; 188: 154-158.

41. Gómez-Restrepo C, Cruz-Ramirez V, Medine-Rico M, Rincón CJ. Mental health in displaced children by armed conflict—National Mental Health Survey Colombia 2015. Acta Espanolas de Psiquiatria 2018; 46: 51-57.

42. Jayuphan J, Sangthong R, Hayeevani N, et al. Mental health problems from direct vs indirect exposure to violent events among children born and growing up in a conflict zone of southern Thailand. Social Psychiatry and Psychiatric Epidemiology 2019; 55: 57-62.

43. Kheirallah KA, Cobb CO, Alsulaiman JW, et al. Trauma exposure, mental health, and tobacco use among vulnerable Syrian refugee youth in Jordan. Journal of Public Health 2019; 42: e343-e351. doi: 10.1093/pubmed/sdz128.

44. Moore A, van Loenhout JAF, de Almeida MM, et al. Measuring mental health burden in humanitarian settings: A critical review of assessment tools. Global Health Action 2020; 13: 1783957. doi: 10.1080/16549716.2020.1783957.

45. Jordans MJD, Pigott H, Tol WA. Interventions for children affected by armed conflict: A systematic review of mental health and psychosocial support in low- and middle-income countries. Current Psychiatry Report 2016; 18: 9. doi: 10.1007/s11920-015-0648-z.

46. Betancourt TS, Meyers-Ohki SE, Charrow AP, Tol WA. Interventions for children affected by war: An ecological perspective on psychosocial support and mental health care. Harvard Review of Psychiatry 2013; 21: 70-91.

47. Purgato M, Gross AL, Betancourt T, et al. Focused psychosocial interventions for children in low-resource humanitarian settings: A systematic review and individual participant data meta-analysis. Lancet Global Health 2018; 6: e390-e400.

48. Keren M, Abdallah G, Tyano S. WAIMH position paper: Infants' rights in wartime. Infant Mental Health Journal 2019; 40: 763-767.

49. Miller KE, Jordans MJD. Determinants of children's mental health in war-torn settings: Translating research into action. Current Psychiatry Reports 2016; 18: 58. doi: 10.1007/s11920-016-0692-3.

50. United Nations Children's Fund. Lost at Home: The Risks and Challenges for Internally Displaced Children and the Urgent Actions Needed to Protect Them. New York: UNICEF, 2020.

51. United Nations, Office of the Special Representative of the Secretary-General for Children and Armed Conflict. Working Paper No. 1: The Six Grave Violations Against Children During Armed Conflict: The Legal Foundation, 2013. Available at: https://childrenandarmedconflict.un.org/publications/WorkingPaper-1_SixGraveViolationsLegalFoundation.pdf. Accessed on May 2, 2020.

52. Betancourt TS, Borisova II, Williams TP, et al. Sierra Leone's former child soldiers: A follow-up study of psychosocial adjustment and community reintegration. Child Development 2010; 81: 1077-1095.

53. World Health Organization. Building Back Better: Sustainable Mental Health Care After Emergencies. Geneva: WHO, 2013. Available at: https://www.who.int/mental_health/emergencies/building_back_better/en/. Accessed on June 3, 2021.

Profile 8:
Zaher Sahloul, M.D.
Responding to Refugees' Health Needs

Zaher Sahloul, a pulmonary medicine and critical care physician in Chicago, always yearned to return to his native Syria to share his medical expertise and train others in critical care medicine. In 1998, he joined the Syrian American Medical Society (SAMS), a nonprofit, apolitical professional association, and, several times over the next few years, returned to Syria to train local physicians and to volunteer at clinics for underserved people.

When the Arab Spring began in early 2011, he and many other Syrians became very hopeful that this movement would bring about political and social change in Syria for which they had waited so long. He went to Turkey to assess the health status of some of the 20,000 Syrian refugees who were living in camps there. Then, as president of SAMS, he and three other Syrian American physicians organized the first SAMS mission to Turkey to provide care for the refugees.

The number of Syrian refugees in Turkey and subsequently in Iraq, Jordan, and Lebanon grew quickly. Dr. Sahloul established hubs in neighboring countries, staffed largely with Syrian physicians to serve the many Syrians who were seeking refuge there. In order to help Syrians within the country's borders, he established networks of physicians and nurses inside Syria to staff clinics, build field hospitals, and recruit other health workers.

Dr. Sahloul and his colleagues also provided training in Turkey and Jordan for Syrian physicians, who crossed the border to take courses in surgery, disaster medicine, treatment of people exposed to chemical weapons, and the use of portable ultrasound equipment—a valuable tool in settings without advanced imaging techniques. They established satellite Internet communication with physicians inside Syria to provide further training and guidance with specific patients. Because many hospitals in Syria were without electricity during the war, they arranged for generators and diesel fuel to operate them. In 2016, during the siege of

From Horror to Hope. Barry S. Levy, Oxford University Press. © Oxford University Press 2022.
DOI: 10.1093/oso/9780197558645.003.0016

Aleppo, he led a medical mission to Syria, which included work in an underground hospital to highlight the plight of civilians during bombing.

Meanwhile, Dr. Sahloul did extensive fundraising and gained the support of the International Medical Corps and the International Rescue Committee. Between 2012 and 2015, his program grew from one full-time employee and an annual budget of $100,000 to a program with 160 staff members, 1,800 healthcare providers inside Syria, and an annual budget of $100 million. Within 5 years from the beginning of the crisis, the program served more than five million Syrian patients. When many Syrian refugees arrived in Greece, he set up mobile clinics there and recruited physicians to staff them.

In 2017, Dr. Sahloul co-founded MedGlobal to reduce healthcare inequity by building resilience in disaster regions, low-income countries, and fragile states. MedGlobal provides health services in Yemen, Syria, the Gaza Strip, Lebanon, Bangladesh, and elsewhere. In 2020, it served 1.8 million people in 11 countries. Throughout this entire period, Dr. Sahloul continued to practice in Chicago with 15 other physicians, who supported his work and covered for him when he was away.

Dr. Sahloul has published many medical journal articles and op-eds in the U.S. and global media on the impact of war on health and on the importance of medical neutrality. He was awarded the 2020 Gandhi Peace Award for his humanitarian work in Syria. When asked why he has done—and continues doing—this work, sometimes risking his life and taking a cut in his income, he responds:

> I have gained much more than I have given. I believe that I am not only helping people in dire need and training other physicians to meet this need, but also giving voice to the voiceless and, in doing so, having a major influence on decision-makers in the U.S. government and at the United Nations. As a result, I clearly see how a physician serving people affected by war can advocate on their behalf to improve their health and well-being.

Dr. Sahloul is President and Co-Founder of MedGlobal and an Associate Clinical Professor at the University of Illinois at Chicago.

9

Adverse Impacts on Reproductive Health

History, despite its wrenching pain, cannot be unlived, but if faced with
courage, need not be lived again.
MAYA ANGELOU

INTRODUCTION

During war, reproductive health issues have received inadequate attention by humanitarian
aid organizations, the academic research community, and other sectors of society. As a result, many of the impacts of war on reproductive health have not been fully recognized,
adequately studied, or otherwise addressed. Compared to other categories of morbidity and
mortality addressed in this book, reproductive health issues have received far less adequate
attention and therefore there are fewer published reports of research concerning the impact
of war on reproductive health.

INADEQUATE CARE

During war, women face increased risks of death during pregnancy and childbirth, largely
because of inadequate antenatal, intrapartum, and postpartum care. Inadequate care partly
results from attacks on healthcare facilities, looting of medical supplies, and injuring, kidnap-
ping, and killing healthcare workers and forcing them to flee (Chapter 2). It also results from
poverty, inadequate education and low literacy, and limited access to services.[1,2] Inadequate
support for women's rights is an important contributing factor.

Antenatal care (ANC), which aims for the best health conditions for mother and infant
during pregnancy, includes risk identification, prevention and management of pregnancy-
related disorders or concurrent diseases, and health education and health promotion. The
World Health Organization (WHO) has produced extensive ANC recommendations, including nutritional interventions, maternal and fetal assessment, and preventive measures.
It has also produced health system measures to improve the utilization and quality of ANC.

From Horror to Hope. Barry S. Levy, Oxford University Press. © Oxford University Press 2022.
DOI: 10.1093/oso/9780197558645.003.0017

WHO recommends a minimum of eight ANC contacts during pregnancy to reduce perinatal mortality and improve women's experience of care.[3]

Compared to the WHO recommendations, ANC has been woefully inadequate in the vast majority of war settings. For example, a study in Afghanistan conducted between 2010 and 2015, found that, among the 68% of women who gave birth at home, 47% received no ANC and, among women who delivered in a public clinic or public hospital, 75% received inadequate ANC.[4] A study in Kenya, based on data from 2010, found that ANC was of lower quality if it was provided within 6.2 miles (10 km) of a conflict event (in a high-conflict month). Other risk factors for low-quality ANC included poverty, low educational level, and long distance between residence and ANC clinic.[5]

When ANC is not received or is inadequate, the risks of abnormal pregnancy outcome increase. For example, a study in Sarajevo during the Bosnian War found that when ANC services were reduced, spontaneous abortions (miscarriages) increased by 64%, perinatal mortality (fetal deaths in addition to infant deaths in the first 7 days of life) increased by 70%, and mean birthweight decreased by 19%.[6]

COMPLICATIONS OF PREGANCY AND ADVERSE BIRTH OUTCOMES

Pregnancy-related disorders include preeclampsia and complications of labor and delivery, such as hemorrhage and maternal death. Adverse birth outcomes include spontaneous abortions (miscarriages), premature births, stillbirths, low-birthweight infants, birth defects, and neonatal morbidity and mortality. During war, pregnancy-related disorders and adverse birth outcomes often increase. For example, during the Second Lebanon War, pregnant women reported an increased number of interruptions in maternity care and experienced more complications of pregnancy. Displacement was associated with a tripling of the rate of complications (39% during displacement, compared to 13% before displacement).[7]

Maternal Mortality

Maternal mortality can be extremely high in conflict-affected countries, especially those suffering from inadequate maternal healthcare prior to conflict. A 2007 study found that, in 21 countries in sub-Saharan Africa that had experienced recent conflict, the maternal mortality ratio (MMR) was 1,000 per 100,000 live births, compared to 690 per 100,000 live births in countries without recent conflict.[8]

In 2017, the MMR for Uganda was 375 deaths per 100,000 live births. (For comparison, the MMR in 2017 for South Africa was 119 and the MMR for the United States was 19 per 100,000 live births.) In Uganda, the MMR was especially high in rural areas and among women with less education and lower socioeconomic status. Contributing factors included the increased incidence of sexual violence and rape during armed conflict, inadequate quality and accessibility of maternal health services, lack of medications, inadequate training of staff, and inequities in provision of care.[9]

Surveys in 35 African countries from 1990 to 2016 found that conflict within 31 miles (50 km) significantly increased the overall mortality rate of women by 112 deaths per 100,000 person-years. Of these deaths, 10% occurred during pregnancy or childbirth. In high-intensity conflicts, the mortality rate of women tripled.[10]

A micro-level study investigated maternal mortality among more than 1.3 million sisters of more than 530,000 women of reproductive age in 30 countries in sub-Saharan Africa. It found that the presence of recent organized violence events within 50 km (31 miles) of respondents was associated with an increased risk of maternal death among the sisters. Specifically, the study found that each additional logged conflict event increased maternal mortality by about 10% and, among women 20 to 35 years of age, by about 14%.[11]

According to a 2005 study, in areas affected by the armed conflict in Chiapas, Mexico, where 87% of births occurred at home, the MMR was increased more than 10-fold: 607 maternal deaths per 100,000 live births, compared to 54 per 100,000 in Mexico as a whole. Women frequently died because they could not access emergency obstetric care. The rates of fetal deaths and deaths of infants during their first 7 days of life were also increased.[12]

A study in Afghanistan found that between 2003 and 2015, the percentage of births with a skilled birth attendant increased from 14% to 51%, and the percentage of births in a facility increased from 13% to 48%.[4] However, a study in 2016 found considerable gaps in the quality of recordkeeping; the cause of death was not recorded in almost half of maternal deaths. When causes of maternal deaths were recorded, the most frequent causes were preventable or treatable conditions, including hypertensive disorders of pregnancy, obstetric hemorrhage, and unanticipated complications of clinical management.[13]

Maternal mortality has adverse consequences for infant and child survival. A longitudinal analysis of the consequences of maternal mortality from 1987 to 2011 in Butajira, Ethiopia, which experienced two wars during this period, found that children whose mothers died within 42 days of their birth faced a *46-fold greater risk* of dying within 1 month compared to infants whose mothers survived.[14]

Premature Delivery and Stillbirth

Premature delivery and stillbirth can be increased during war and its aftermath. For example, at a hospital in the Democratic Republic of the Congo, premature deliveries, the most frequent adverse pregnancy outcome, increased from 6.3% in 1996, before the Second Congo War, to 11.5% in 2001, during the war. The occurrence of stillbirths increased from 3.5% to 7.2% of pregnancies during this period.[15]

Low Birthweight

Several studies have found associations between armed conflict and both reduced mean birthweight and an increased percentage of infants born with low birthweight:

- A study of 53 "developing countries" that experienced conflict between 1990 and 2018 found that intrauterine exposure to armed conflict in the first trimester decreased birthweight by 2.8% and increased the occurrence of low birthweight by 3.2%. It also found that infants born to poor and low-educated mothers were especially vulnerable to the adverse consequences of armed conflict.[16]

- A study found that exposure to the Second Lebanon War in early and mid pregnancy was associated with lower birthweight and an increased probability of low birthweight. There was a 13-gram decrease in birthweight associated with exposure to war in the first trimester and a 16-gram decrease associated with exposure in the second trimester.[17]
- A study in Libya in 2011 found an increased percentage of low-birthweight infants during armed conflict (10.1%) compared with several months before armed conflict (8.5%), and an increased percentage of preterm births during the conflict (3.6%) compared with several months before (2.5%).[18]

Neonatal Mortality

Armed conflict is also associated with increases in neonatal mortality (deaths during the first 28 days of life). Among the 15 countries with the highest rates of neonatal mortality in 2015, all but one were experiencing chronic conflict or political instability—accounting for 42% of all neonatal deaths worldwide.[19]

Birth Defects

There is some, but limited, evidence that children born to female veterans have an increased occurrence of birth defects (congenital anomalies). Female veterans who had served in the Vietnam War or the Gulf War self-reported increased rates of birth defects in their children.[20] Among female Vietnam War veterans, the risk of having children with "moderate-to-severe" birth defects was increased by 46%.[21] Women deployed in the U.S. military in the Gulf War reported a 180% increase, and men reported a 78% increase, in the rate of moderate-to-severe birth defects among their liveborn children.[22]

The U.S. military exposed almost five million Vietnamese people to Agent Orange, which adversely affected their health. A systematic review and meta-analysis of 22 studies found a significant association between Agent Orange exposure and congenital malformations, with a summary relative risk of 1.95. It also found a dose–response relationship between exposure to Agent Orange and congenital malformations. Some of the studies were based on self-reports of congenital malformations and some were based on medical examinations.[23] However, the U.S. government has not supported any systematic study of adverse pregnancy outcomes among Vietnamese civilians exposed to Agent Orange. (For more on Agent Orange, see Chapters 10, 12, and 13.)

During wars in Kuwait, Iraq, Lebanon, and Egypt, depleted uranium (DU) contaminated air, water, soil, and food. However, it has been difficult to determine if DU exposure during these wars caused adverse health effects.[24] Animal studies have shown that DU might cause congenital malformations, and epidemiological studies have demonstrated increased risk of congenital malformations in children of DU-exposed parents.[25] In Basra, Iraq, the incidence of congenital malformations increased after the Gulf War—from 2.5 per 1,000 births in 1991–1994 to 4.6 per 1,000 in 1995–1998—and the occurrence of chromosomal aberrations and congenital heart disease also increased.[26] (For more on DU, see Chapters 10, 12, and 13.)

Women exposed to other heavy metals might be at higher risk of giving birth to children with birth defects. A study in Gaza found a progressive increase in birth defects since 2006, when there were repeated military attacks that deposited heavy metals in the environment. Between 2011 and 2016, there was an increase in the rate of birth defects (from 1.1% to 1.8% of all births) and in the rate of preterm infants (from 1.1% to 7.9%). Adverse birth outcomes from 2016 until 2019 were associated with mothers' exposure to military attacks in 2014 and/or to hot spots of heavy metal contamination. The content of the following metals was consistently high in mothers' hair between 2014 and 2018–2019: barium, arsenic, cobalt, cadmium, chromium, vanadium, and uranium.[27]

ACCESS TO CONTRACEPTION AND ABORTION SERVICES

There is a complex interaction of several factors that influence availability and use of reproductive health services. These factors include intensity of conflict, the status of preexisting health services, and the type and quality of humanitarian intervention. These factors and their interaction were illustrated in a study in conflict-affected northern Uganda between 1988 and 2011 that found contraceptive use and institutional deliveries in this area of conflict were both lower than in the rest of the country.[9] In Afghanistan between 2003 and 2018, those provinces with minimal intensity of conflict had greater gains in contraceptive use.[28]

Cost of contraception and lack of awareness of family planning services can be barriers to use of contraception. For example, a study of Syrian refugee women in Lebanon found that cost was a major barrier to use of contraception and some Syrian refugee women were not aware of free services for sexual and reproductive health.[29]

Access to and availability of reproductive health services, such as for contraception and abortion care, is often inadequate or absent for displaced populations. Uganda, which has hosted 1.4 million refugees and conflict-affected people, is an illustrative example. Although Uganda's policies have encouraged self-sufficiency and local integration for refugees, abortion has been legally restricted and, as a result, displaced women and girls have had persistent unmet sexual and reproductive health needs. A study of Congolese refugees in Uganda found that, because of legal restrictions, they were unable to obtain lawful abortions and were therefore engaging in unsafe abortion practices. Conflicting and ambiguous laws and policies as well as their fear of legal consequences also reduced their access to safe abortions and post-abortion care.[30]

Although protection of abortion services under international humanitarian law has been increasingly recognized by the United Nations, the European Union, and other international and national organizations, abortion services have not been comprehensively or uniformly provided during armed conflict. In fact, women and girls who become pregnant due to rape during armed conflict infrequently have access to abortion services. Reasons for this gap include funding restrictions and misinterpretation of protections that are included in international humanitarian law. If safe abortion services are not available, women may receive unsafe abortions and suffer resultant complications, including death. International humanitarian law ensures that victims of armed conflict receive necessary medical care, including the option of abortion services. The denial of abortion services causes mental and physical suffering that can constitute torture and other cruel, inhuman, and degrading treatment in certain contexts.[31]

IMPROVING MATERNAL AND REPRODUCTIVE HEALTH SERVICES

The vast majority of maternal deaths and other complications of pregnancy can be prevented by improving the availability, accessibility, and quality of maternal healthcare. Substantial reductions in maternal morbidity and mortality can be achieved by the provision of ANC and ensuring the presence of a trained birth attendant at time of labor and delivery. Providing maternal health services with trained midwives can substantially reduce maternal morbidity and mortality and improve pregnancy outcomes (Figure 9-1).

Four years after the civil war in Liberia ended in 2003, the government rebuilt the healthcare system. It developed and implemented cost-effective interventions to improve maternal health. It identified and responded to high-priority needs. And it made education of women and girls a high priority. Measures of maternal healthcare utilization, including

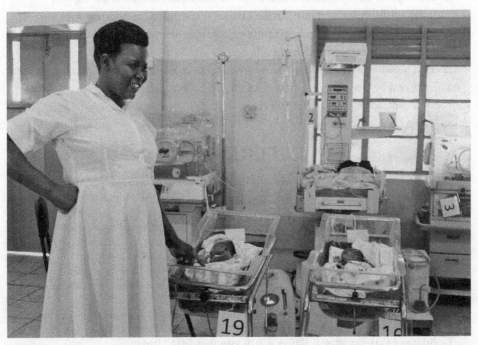

FIGURE 9-1 Midwife stands in ward for premature infants at Juba Teaching Hospital in Juba, South Sudan, in 2019. Despite a civil war that killed almost 400,000 people, maternal and infant health improved as a result of a concerted effort by the government and its partners to dramatically increase the number of trained midwives. (AP Photo/Sam Mednick.)

numbers of prenatal care visits and facility-based delivery of infants, steadily increased between 2007 and 2016, and both the MMR and the infant mortality rate steadily decreased.[32]

Humanitarian protocols, laws, and other policies need to protect the sexual and reproductive rights of women and respond to their needs. Policies need to ensure access to maternal health services, contraception, and abortion services.

Abortion services are protected under international humanitarian and human rights laws. However, during war, humanitarian aid organizations have often not provided sexual and reproductive health services because they have deferred to national law, have had restrictions on their funding, and have failed to consider abortion as part of healthcare. The Global Justice Center, a nongovernmental organization that develops legal strategies to define, establish, and protect human rights and gender equity, has proposed use of international humanitarian law to ensure comprehensive care for women and girls adversely affected by war.[33]

In 2013, the UN Security Council and the UN Committee on Elimination of Discrimination Against Women reaffirmed the rights of women living in conflict settings to comprehensive reproductive health services. Security Council Resolution 2122 called on UN member states to ensure that all sexual and reproductive healthcare options are given to women affected by conflict, especially to women impregnated by rape.[34]

SUMMARY POINTS

- Adverse impacts on reproductive health receive inadequate attention during war.
- Antenatal, intrapartum, and postpartum care are often inadequate during war.
- The rates of maternal deaths, premature births, low-birthweight infants, and neonatal deaths are often increased during war.
- Maternal health can be improved by increasing access to and improving quality of antenatal care and by ensuring the presence of trained birth assistants.
- Access to contraception and abortion services needs to be ensured.

REFERENCES

1. Gopalan SS, Das A, Howard N. Maternal and neonatal service usage and determinants in fragile and conflict-affected situations: A systematic review of Asia and the Middle-East. BMC Women's Health 2017; 17: 20. doi: 10.1176/s12905-017-0379-x.
2. Che Chi P, Bulage P, Urdal H, Sundby J. Perceptions of the effects of armed conflict on maternal and reproductive health services and outcomes in Burundi and northern Uganda: A qualitative study. BMC International Health and Human Rights 2015; 15: 7. doi: 10.1186/s12914-015-0045-z.
3. World Health Organization. WHO Recommendations on Antenatal Care for a Positive Pregnancy Experience. Geneva: World Health Organization, 2016. Available at: https://www.who.int/publications/i/item/9789241549912. Accessed on May 4, 2021.
4. Kim C, Erim D, Natiq K, et al. Combination of interventions needed to improve maternal healthcare utilization: A multinomial analysis of the inequity in place of childbirth in Afghanistan. Frontiers in Global Women's Health 2020; 1: 571055. doi: 10.3389/fgwh.2020.571055.
5. Chukwuma A, Wong KLM, Ekhator-Mobayode UE. Disrupted service delivery? The impact of conflict on antenatal care quality in Kenya. Frontiers in Global Women's Health 2021; 2: 599731. doi: 10.3389/fgwh.2021.599731.

6. Centers for Disease Control and Prevention. Status of public health—Bosnia and Herzegovina, August–September 1993. Morbidity and Mortality Weekly Report 1993; 42: 979-982.

7. Kabakian-Khasholian T, Shayboub R, El-Kak F. Seeking maternal care at times of conflict: The case of Lebanon. Health Care for Women International 2013; 34: 352-362.

8. O'Hare BAM, Southall DP. First do no harm: The impact of recent armed conflict on maternal and child health in sub-Saharan Africa. Journal of the Royal Society of Medicine 2007; 100: 564-570.

9. Namasivayam A, González PA, Delgado RC, Che Chi P. The effect of armed conflict on the utilization of maternal health services in Uganda: A population-based study. PLoS Currents 2017; 9. doi: 10.1371/currents.dis.557b987d6519d8c7c96f2006ed3c271a.

10. Wagner Z, Heft-Neal S, Wise PH, et al. Women and children living in areas of armed conflict in Africa: A geospatial analysis of mortality and orphanhood. Lancet Global Health 2019; 7: e1622-e1631.

11. Kotsadam A, Östby G. Armed conflict and maternal mortality: A micro-level analysis of sub-Saharan Africa, 1989–2013. Social Science & Medicine 2019; 239: 112526. https://doi.org/10.1016/j.socscimed.2019.112526.

12. Brentlinger PE, Javier Sánchez-Pérez H, Arana Cedeño M, et al. Pregnancy outcomes, site of delivery, and community schisms in regions affected by the armed conflict in Chiapas, Mexico. Social Science and Medicine 2005; 61: 1001-1014.

13. Maruf F, Tappis H, Stekelenburg J, van den Akker T. Quality of maternal death documentation in Afghanistan: A retrospective health facility record review. Frontiers in Global Women's Health 2021; 2: 610578. doi: 10.3389/fgwh.2021.610578.

14. Moucheraud C, Worku A, Molla M, et al. Consequences of maternal mortality on infant and child survival: A 25-year longitudinal analysis in Butajira, Ethiopia (1987–2011). Reproductive Health 2015; 12: S4.

15. Ahuka OL, Chabikuli N, Ogunbanjo GA. The effects of armed conflict on pregnancy outcomes in the Congo. International Journal of Gynecology and Obstetrics 2004; 84: 91-92.

16. Le K, Nguyen M. Armed conflict and birth weight. Economics and Human Biology 2020; 39: 100921. https://dx.doi.org/10.1016/j.ehb.2020.100921.

17. Torche F, Shwed U. The hidden costs of war: Exposure to armed conflict and birth outcomes. Sociological Science 2015; 2: 558-581.

18. Bodalal Z, Agnaeber K, Nagelkerke N, et al. Pregnancy outcomes in Benghazi, Libya, before and during the armed conflict in 2011. Eastern Mediterranean Health Journal 2014; 20: 175-180.

19. Wise PH, Darmstadt GL. Confronting stillbirths and newborn deaths in areas of conflict and political instability: A neglected global imperative. Paediatrics and International Child Health 2015; 35: 220-226.

20. Rivera JC, Johnson AE. Female veterans of Operations Enduring and Iraqi Freedom: Status and future directions. Military Medicine 2014; 179: 133-136.

21. Kang HK, Mahan CM, Lee KY, et al. Pregnancy outcomes among U.S. women Vietnam veterans. American Journal of Industrial Medicine 2000; 38: 447-454.

22. Kang H, Magee C, Mahan C, et al. Pregnancy outcomes among U.S. Gulf War veterans: A population-based survey of 30,000 veterans. Annals of Epidemiology 2001; 11: 504-511.

23. Ngo AD, Taylor R, Roberts CL, Nguyen TV. Association between Agent Orange and birth defects: Systematic review and meta-analysis. International Journal of Epidemiology 2006; 35: 1220-1230.

24. Bešić L, Muhović I, Mrkulić F, et al. Meta-analysis of depleted uranium levels in the Middle East region. Journal of Environmental Radioactivity 2018; 192: 67-74.

25. Hindin R, Brugge D, Panikkar B. Teratogenicity of depleted uranium aerosols: A review from an epidemiological perspective. Environmental Health: A Global Accessed on Science Source 2005; 4: 17. doi:10.1186/1476-069X-4-17.

26. Al-Sadoon I, Hassan GG, Yacoub AA-H. Depleted uranium and health of people in Basrah: Epidemiological evidence. Hassan Medical Journal of Basrah University 1999; 17. Available at: https://nointervention.com/archive/Iraq/ABC/DU/Iraq_incidence/DU-1-INCIDENCE.htm. Accessed on August 3, 2020.

27. Manduca P, Al Baraquni N, Parodi S. Long-term risks to neonatal health from exposure to war: 9 years long survey of reproductive health and contamination by weapon-delivered heavy metals in Gaza, Palestine. International Journal of Environmental Research and Public Health 2020; 17: 2538. doi: 10.3390/ijerph17072538.

28. Akseer N, Rizvi A, Bhatti Z, et al. Association of exposure to civil conflict with maternal resilience and maternal and child health and health system performance in Afghanistan. JAMA Network Open 2019; 2: e1914819. doi: 10.1001/jamanetworkopen.2019.14819.

29. Cherri Z, Gil Cuesta J, Rodriguez-Llanes JM, Guha-Sapir D. Early marriage and barriers to contraception among Syrian refugee women in Lebanon: A qualitative study. International Journal of Environmental Research and Public Health 2017; 14: 836. doi: 10.3390/ijerph14080836.

30. Nara R, Banura A, Foster AM. Exploring Congolese refugees' experiences with abortion care in Uganda: A multi-methods qualitative study. Sexual and Reproductive Health Matters 2019; 27: 262-271. doi: 10.1080/26410397.2019.1681091.

31. Global Justice Center. Shifting Good Policy to Practice: Armed Conflict, Humanitarian Aid, and Reproductive Rights. June 19, 2019. Available at: https://globaljusticecenter.net/blog/19-publications/1139-shifting-good-policy-to-practice-armed-conflict-humanitarian-aid-and-reproductive-rights. Accessed on April 15, 2021.

32. Yaya S, Uthman OA, Bishwajit G, Ekholuenetale M. Maternal health care service utilization in post-war Liberia: Analysis of nationally representative cross-sectional household surveys. BMC Public Health 2019; 19: Article 28. https://bmcpublichealth.biomedcentral.com/articles/10.1186/s12889-018-6365-x.

33. Radhakrishnan A, Sarver E, Shubin G. Protecting safe abortion in humanitarian settings: Overcoming legal and policy barriers (Commentary). Reproductive Health Matters 2017; 25: 40-47. doi: 10.1080/09688080.2017.1400361.

34. UN Security Council. Resolution 2122 (2013), adopted by the Security Council at its 7044th meeting, on 18 October 2013. Available at: https://undocs.org/en/S/RES/2122(2013). Accessed on May 12, 2020.

Profile 9:
Rohini Haar, M.D., M.P.H.
Documenting Human Rights Violations

As Rohini Haar, an emergency medicine physician who has worked extensively on war-related and human rights issues in many low- and middle-income countries, will tell you, there is no standard career path for doing this work. But finding inspiring mentors and finding—and creating—opportunities to participate are critically important.

As an undergraduate, she worked on a refugee water and sanitation project in Ethiopia for several months. As a medical student, she visited Morocco, where she trained local physicians and nurses on human rights issues, including how to identify evidence of torture, and visited India, where she saw physicians in overwhelmed public hospitals having to make difficult choices about whom to treat. During her residency in emergency medicine, Dr. Haar spent a month in Senegal, visiting health centers and interviewing health workers. And after completing her residency, she worked in Guyana, where she assessed care in clinics, and in Ghana, where she trained mid-level health workers in emergency medicine.

Over the next several years, Dr. Haar completed a master of public health program, while working in emergency medicine and raising a family. After completing her education and training, she became an Adjunct Professor at the University of California at Berkeley School of Public Health, where she has taught graduate and undergraduate students, and performed research focusing on the impact of human rights violations on the health and protection of health workers and health services during war. She has studied the immediate and long-term consequences of attacks on healthcare in the Syrian Civil War and other armed conflicts. She has done research in Colombia, documenting human rights violations during civil war and unrest. She investigated the health effects of torture among health workers in Sudan and of war crimes among Rohingya refugees in Bangladesh.

From Horror to Hope. Barry S. Levy, Oxford University Press. © Oxford University Press 2022.
DOI: 10.1093/oso/9780197558645.003.0018

Dr. Haar has recognized that the impact of war on civilian populations extends long after fighting has ceased. She has seen that availability of military-style weapons occurs not only in war zones in low-income countries, but also among police forces in the United States. And she has documented the use of lacrimogenic chemical weapons (tear gas) used against peaceful protesters in the United States.

Looking back, she recognizes the important influences of her mentors. Her father shared his deep concern about social injustice. A medical school professor opened her eyes to violations of human rights. Mentors on refugees and protection of civilians during war have provided valuable guidance. She now collaborates with some of her former mentors on small-scale studies on health and human rights in war-torn countries and on large-scale projects, such as developing guidelines for investigating torture and other violations of international humanitarian law.

Dr. Haar has learned that, to do this work as a physician, you do not need to leave clinical medicine. And, with four children under the age of 10, she has realized that you can also raise a family while doing this work. She has taken her oldest children to low-income countries to enable them to see what she does and to get a glimpse of life in underserved communities.

When asked what has been most important in sustaining her in this work, she responds, "The human connections with my collaborators and the people I serve. The intellectual challenges. The unwavering support of my husband. And my passion for this work."

Dr. Haar is an Adjunct Professor of Epidemiology at the School of Public Health, University of California at Berkeley, and a Medical Advisor to Physicians for Human Rights.

10

Noncommunicable Diseases

War does not determine who is right—only who is left.
BERTRAND RUSSELL

INTRODUCTION

Noncommunicable diseases include cancer, coronary artery disease, diabetes mellitus, chronic respiratory disease, and other chronic disorders. Mortality rates for these diseases are often high when healthcare has been disrupted by war, displacement, and damage to civilian infrastructure.[1,2]

Noncommunicable diseases may increase in a war-affected population even years after the war has ended. For example, studies have found:

- Women exposed to the Dutch Famine (1944–1945) during childhood and young adulthood had an increased risk of type 2 diabetes, with a "dose–response" relationship.[3]
- Women exposed in utero or during early childhood to the Korean War had an increased risk for abdominal obesity, elevated serum triglyceride level, and metabolic syndrome as adults.[4]
- Individuals affected by fetal or infant undernutrition in the Biafran Famine (1968–1970) during the Nigerian Civil War had an increased risk of hypertension and impaired glucose tolerance (prediabetes or diabetes) during adulthood.[5]

These findings are consistent with the Barker Hypothesis, proposed by British epidemiologist David Barker in 1990, in which he hypothesized that adverse nutrition in utero and in early life was causally related to hypertension, coronary heart disease, and non–insulin-dependent diabetes in later life.[6,7]

ACCESS TO HEALTHCARE

Complications of noncommunicable diseases occur more frequently during war and its aftermath, often because civilians have reduced access to healthcare facilities and

From Horror to Hope. Barry S. Levy, Oxford University Press. © Oxford University Press 2022.
DOI: 10.1093/oso/9780197558645.003.0019

essential medications.[8] Displaced people generally have great difficulty accessing health-care for noncommunicable diseases.[9] Examples include (a) acute myocardial infarction and stroke occurring in patients with inadequately treated hypertension, and (b) chronic renal disease developing in patients with poorly controlled diabetes.

Because access to cancer treatment may be limited during war, cancer patients may seek treatment in other nearby countries. For example, in recent years, some Iraqi cancer patients have traveled to Lebanon, Jordan, and elsewhere for cancer treatment because Iraqi oncology specialists fled, hospitals were destroyed, and medical facilities lacked equipment to diagnose cancer, perform radiation therapy, and reliably provide chemotherapy. Patients often relied on the sale of possessions, including their homes, and vast networks to raise money for treatment.[10,11]

Individuals with end-stage renal disease (ESRD), who require regular dialysis or kidney transplantation, suffer during war. For example, in Yemen, before the start of the civil war in 2015, a network of 28 dialysis centers provided treatment for about 4,400 ESRD patients. After the war began and import restrictions were implemented, the network had to reduce its services. Many smaller dialysis centers closed or reduced their hours of operation. Some ESRD patients moved to Sana'a, where dialysis centers were overwhelmed and had to reduce the number and duration of dialysis sessions. Therefore, patients who were able to continue dialysis suffered from lethargy, disorientation, pain, and anxiety. And those who could not access dialysis died.[12]

Even when civilians have access to healthcare in war settings, the quality of care may be inadequate. Often, common noncommunicable diseases are not diagnosed or overlooked. For example, a study in conflict-affected northern Uganda found that hypertension was common, but unexpectedly accounted for only a small fraction of diagnoses. In one district, hypertension accounted for only 0.83% of all diagnoses in outpatient populations.[13] In contrast, the *actual* prevalence of hypertension in Uganda as a whole was between 21% and 34%.[14]

CANCER

Civilians are potentially exposed during war and its aftermath to ionizing radiation and car-cinogenic chemicals. But there is only limited reliable evidence on the occurrence of war-related cancer among civilians. The most complete cancer studies related to war are based on a cohort of survivors of the atomic bomb attacks on Hiroshima and Nagasaki.

Cancer in Atomic Bomb Survivors

Atomic bomb survivors of Hiroshima and Nagasaki have been studied by the Atomic Bomb Casualty Commission and its successor organization, the Radiation Effects Research Foundation. Among survivors, risk for acute myelogenous leukemia, acute lymphocytic leukemia, and chronic myelogenous leukemia increased markedly about 2 years after the bombings and peaked about 7 to 8 years after, especially in people exposed at young ages. Survivors have also been at increased risk of myelodysplastic syndrome and cancers of the bladder, female breast, lung, brain, ovary, thyroid, colon, esophagus, stomach, and liver as well as non-melanoma skin cancer.[15] The risk of these radiation-induced malignancies has persisted for six decades.[16]

Survivors have also been at increased risk of nonmalignant diseases, such as hemor-rhagic stroke (including subarachnoid hemorrhage), nonmalignant thyroid nodules, and cataracts. Survivors exposed before age 40 have been at increased risk for hypertension and myocardial infarction.

There have been relatively few studies on psychological effects among atomic bomb survivors; a questionnaire survey of survivors 17 to 20 years after the bombings found in-creased prevalence of anxiety symptoms and somatization.[17] Another survey among sur-vivors of the Nagasaki bombing found, in 1997, severe apathy, disordered relationships, and anhedonia (inability to feel pleasure) among these survivors—52 years after the bombing.[18]

Children who had been exposed in utero to the atomic bomb explosions had impaired physical and mental development. Those exposed between 8 and 15 gestational weeks suf-fered a high frequency of severe mental retardation, often accompanied by small head size and decreased intelligence quotient (IQ). Those exposed in utero to radiation of 1 Gy or higher were several centimeters shorter during their teenage years than counterparts without exposure to this level of radiation. Those exposed in utero during the second trimester of pregnancy had increased prevalence of systolic hypertension.[15]

Cancer in People Exposed to Nuclear Weapons Tests

Participating military personnel and many people residing downwind of atmospheric nu-clear tests received large doses of radiation from radioactive fallout. Hundreds of thousands of them likely developed cancer.[19,20] Atmospheric nuclear tests at the Nevada Test Site caused between 11,300 and 212,000 additional cases of thyroid cancer in the United States.[21] A cancer mortality study of U.S. military veterans exposed to at least 5 rem of radiation during atmospheric nuclear weapons tests found increased mortality for all causes combined and more than a threefold increased risk for all lymphohematopoietic cancers combined (leu-kemia, lymphoma, and multiple myeloma).[22] A study performed on more than 8,500 Navy veterans who had participated in an atmospheric nuclear test in 1958 found that they had a 42% increase in cancer mortality overall and more than a sixfold increase in deaths from liver cancer.[23] A case–control study of leukemia in a population exposed to atmospheric nu-clear tests between 1952 and 1958 found a weak association between bone marrow dose of radiation and all types of leukemia, with the greatest excess risk in those who received high doses when they were age 20 or younger at the time of exposure.[24] A study in Kazakhstan near the Semipalatinsk nuclear test site found an increased incidence of thyroid cancer and Hashimoto's (autoimmune) thyroiditis.[25] (See Chapter 13.)

Cancer and Other Diseases in Nuclear Weapons Industry Workers

Workers in the nuclear weapons industry have faced substantial health risks as a result of ex-posures to beryllium, ionizing radiation, and hazards unique to this industry. A cohort mor-tality study of workers at a nuclear materials production plant in Tennessee found increased death rates for lung cancer, brain cancer, several lymphohematopoietic malignancies, and can-cers of the pancreas, prostate, kidney, and female breast.[26] Another study found that workers in the nuclear weapons industry had more than a sixfold increase in chronic beryllium disease.[27] The U.S. government has acknowledged that nuclear weapons workers have been exposed to ionizing radiation and chemicals that have caused cancer and early death among these workers at 14 nuclear weapons plants.[28] The U.S. Department of Energy has established an occupational illness compensation program for workers in the nuclear weapons industry.[29]

Other Cancer Studies of War-Affected Populations

Between 1993 and 2007, a study found that the leukemia rate in children under age 15 in Basra, Iraq, more than doubled from 2.6 per 100,000 in 1993 to 6.9 per 100,000 in 2007. The greatest rate increase was in children under age 6. Of the 97 total cases of childhood leukemia, 82% were acute lymphoblastic leukemia and 13% were acute myeloid leukemia. It was difficult to determine the cause of this increase. The Basra region was exposed to chemical weapons agents, pyrophoric depleted uranium, and benzene as well as ongoing undifferentiated water and air pollution.[30]

Another study in Iraq found that the incidence of breast cancer, lung cancer, leukemia, and lymphoma almost doubled to tripled since the start of the Gulf War. Between 1991 and 2003, about 1,200 tons of ammunition, much of it contaminated with depleted uranium, had been dropped on Iraq, contaminating more than 350 sites.[31]

A study of more than 100,000 migrants to Sweden from the former Yugoslavia during the Balkan Wars and more than 147,000 migrants to Sweden from 24 other European countries during the same period (1991–2001) found that being a migrant from the Balkan Wars was associated with a 16% increased probability of being diagnosed with cancer and a 27% increased probability of dying from cancer.[32]

Many studies of cancer in war-affected populations have been of poor quality. A systematic review of the impact of armed conflict on cancer among civilians in low- and middle-income countries found that two-thirds of the 20 studies reviewed were of low methodological quality and that their findings were often conflicting. The main limitations in many studies were ecological design and the failure to account for sudden demographic changes after forced migration. There was also limited adjustment for confounding variables. During war, the ability to collect reliable cancer incidence and mortality data from registries, hospitals, and camps for displaced persons is often inadequate because information systems are destroyed, relevant data are not collected, and information collection is not standardized. In addition, reported data may be inaccurate due to limited diagnostic facilities, reduced access to cancer care, and the availability of only a few pathologists to confirm diagnoses.[33]

In contrast to the deficiencies of cancer studies performed on civilians exposed to war, systematic studies have been performed on U.S. military veterans. Most notably, studies have been performed on veterans who served in the Vietnam War regarding their wartime exposures to Agent Orange, which was contaminated with dioxin, a known carcinogen (Figure 10-1). These studies demonstrated "sufficient evidence" of an association between Agent Orange and soft tissue sarcoma, non-Hodgkin lymphoma, chronic lymphocytic leukemia, and Hodgkin lymphoma. (See Chapters 12 and 13.) However, few, if any, systematic studies have been performed on Vietnamese civilians who were also exposed to Agent Orange.

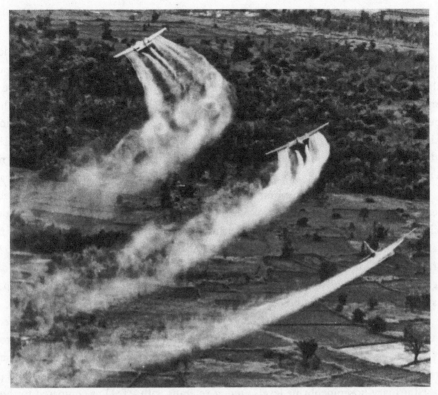

FIGURE 10-1 U.S. Air Force planes spray Agent Orange during Operation Ranch Hand in 1966 in South Vietnam. (AP Photo.)

CARDIOVASCULAR DISEASE

War is associated with an increased incidence of cardiovascular disease (CVD) as well as CVD risk factors, including smoking, hypertension, and hyperlipidemia.[34] A study of CVD mortality in 134 countries during the 1960–2000 period found that armed conflict increased CVD mortality rates in both men and women, with a greater increase in women. It found that, in the year after occurrence of armed conflict with 25 or more battle-related deaths, women had a 14% increase and men a 12% increase in CVD mortality rates. Reasons for these increases appeared to include damage to civilian infrastructure (including healthcare), damage to the economy, and overall destruction of society. Other factors included stress, breakdowns in supply chains for medicines and other necessary supplies, flight of health-care personnel, and insufficient attention to treatable CVD risk factors, such as hypertension and hyperlipidemia.[35] The study of more than 100,000 migrants to Sweden from the former Yugoslavia cited on page 172 found that being a migrant from the Balkan Wars was associated with a 39% increased probability of being diagnosed with CVD and a 45% increased probability of dying from CVD.[32]

Elderly Holocaust survivors had a higher prevalence of ischemic heart disease than counterparts not exposed to the Holocaust. Possible causative and contributing factors were physical and mental torture, poor hygiene, malnutrition, and lack of preventive and medical health services during the Holocaust.[36]

A study found that women who had a cumulative exposure to five or more human-loss or property-loss events related to the Lebanese Civil War, which lasted more than 15 years, had more than a fourfold increase in CVD mortality, and men who had exposure to five or more war-related loss events had more than a doubling of CVD mortality. Women who had experienced human traumas had a 237% increase in CVD mortality risk. Men displaced during the war had a 68% higher risk for CVD mortality, and women a 50% higher risk.[37] This study illustrated the need for governments and humanitarian aid organizations to focus not only on short-term emergency needs, but also on the long-term health consequences of war.

As noted earlier, undernutrition early in life can increase risks for noncommunicable diseases during adulthood. A study of adults who had been exposed to food deprivation as children, adolescents, or young adults during the 1940–1945 German occupation of the Channel Islands found that postnatal exposure to the occupation was associated with a 152% increase in CVD in adulthood.[38] A study of older Colombian adults who experienced displacement and poor nutrition early in life showed that they had an increased risk of hypertension and diabetes during adulthood.[39] (See Chapter 7.)

Posttraumatic stress disorder (PTSD) exerts a number of potentially adverse effects on the cardiovascular system. Multiple studies have shown that patients suffering from PTSD have increased resting heart rate as well as increased heart rate and blood pressure in response to traumatic stimuli (slides, sounds, and scripts). Some studies have found increased urinary norepinephrine levels among veterans with PTSD as compared to those without PTSD. Hyperactivity of the sympathoadrenal axis might contribute to CVD via effects of catecholamines on the heart, the blood vessels, and the function of platelets.[40] (See Chapter 8.)

DISORDERS DUE TO TOXIC EXPOSURES

During war and its aftermath, children have been exposed to lead, other heavy metals, and other hazardous chemicals. Lead exposure can cause cognitive impairment, other neurobehavioral abnormalities, and other health problems. A study of deciduous teeth in children from Basra, Iraq, found that dentine lead levels were highest in children who had been born with congenital anomalies (birth defects).[41] A study of weapon-related heavy metals in hair samples of Palestinian mothers in the first trimester of pregnancy during the Gaza War found that higher levels of chromium and uranium were associated with abnormal early emotional development in their children.[42]

ADDRESSING
NONCOMMUNICABLE DISEASES

During war and its aftermath, the diagnosis, treatment, and prevention of noncommunicable diseases needs to be improved. Efforts need to focus on the use of community health workers and sustainable systems. Important elements of a comprehensive program to address noncommunicable diseases include the following:

- Training of health professionals and allied workers
- Patient education and improvement in health literacy
- Coordinated efforts to discourage cigarette smoking and to promote smoking cessation
- Systems to ensure provision of essential medications for treating hypertension, diabetes, coronary artery disease, and other prevalent noncommunicable diseases
- Systems to ensure continuity of care.

International aid programs need to give increased priority to noncommunicable diseases, especially for programs serving middle-aged and older adults. These programs need to focus not only on diagnosis and treatment of noncommunicable diseases, but also on identification of risk factors for these diseases and other preventive measures. These aid programs need to transition into locally sustainable efforts that are integrated into primary healthcare.

In addition, there is a need to improve the number and quality of epidemiological studies investigating associations between exposure to war and development of cancer. The quality of studies could be improved by making better use of hospital-based registries and other sources of data that are routinely collected. There needs to be better consideration of and adjustment for confounders. And there needs to be more research on how screening programs and increased access to healthcare may affect the reported incidence of cancer after war. Research also needs to investigate the impact of inequities in access to diagnostic, treatment, and preventive services for cancer. Finally, future research on cancer etiology should focus, to the extent possible, on cohort and case–control studies, rather than ecological studies.[33] (See Chapter 14.)

SUMMARY POINTS

- War and famine early in life may increase the incidence of hypertension, hyperlipidemia, and diabetes in adulthood.
- Disruption of healthcare and public health services during war and its aftermath causes increased morbidity and mortality due to noncommunicable diseases.
- Civilians may be exposed to carcinogens and radioactive materials during war and its aftermath, increasing their risk of various forms of cancer.
- The incidence of cardiovascular disorders may also increase due to war-related exposures and decreased access to healthcare.
- During war and its aftermath, noncommunicable diseases generally do not receive adequate attention from humanitarian aid organizations and UN agencies.

REFERENCES

1. Toole MJ, Waldman RJ. The public health aspects of complex emergencies and refugee situations. Annual Review of Public Health 1997; 19: 283-312.

2. El Saghir NS, Pérez de Celis ES, Fares JE, Sullivan R. Cancer care for refugees and displaced populations: Middle East conflicts and global natural disasters. American Society of Clinical Oncology Educational Book 2018; 38: 433-440.

3. van Abeelen AFM, Elias SG, Bossuyt PMM, et al. Famine exposure in the young and the risk of type 2 diabetes in adulthood. Diabetes 2012; 61: 2255-2260.

4. Han C, Hong Y-C. Fetal and childhood malnutrition during the Korean War and metabolic syndrome in adulthood. Nutrition 2019; 62: 186-193.

5. Hult M, Tornhammar P, Ueda P, et al. Hypertension, diabetes and overweight: Looming legacies of the Biafran famine. PloS ONE 2010; 5: e13582. doi: 10.1371/journal.pone.0013582.

6. "Barker Hypothesis" in Dictionary of Public Health. Oxford Reference. Available at: https://www.oxfordre ference.com/view/10.1093/oi/authority.20110803095447459#:~:text=A%20hypothesis%20proposed%20 in%201990,dependent%20diabetes%2C%20in%20middle%20age. Accessed on March 31, 2021.

7. Edwards M. "The Barker Hypothesis" in V Preedy, VB Patel (eds.). The Handbook of Famine, Starvation, and Nutrient Deprivation. Cham, Switzerland: Springer. https://doi.org/10.1007/978-3-319-40007-5_ 71-1, pp. 1–21.

8. Kerridge BT, Khan MR, Sapkota A. Terrorism, civil war, one-sided violence and global burden of disease. Medicine, Conflict and Survival 2012; 28: 199-218.

9. Greene-Cramer B, Summers A, Lopes-Cardozo B, et al. Noncommunicable disease burden among conflict-affected adults in Ukraine: A cross-sectional study of prevalence, risk factors, and effect of conflict on severity of disease and access to care. PLoS ONE 2020; 15: e0231899. doi: 10.1371/journal. pone.0231899.

10. Skelton M, Alameddine R, Saifi O, et al. High-cost cancer treatment across borders in conflict zones: Experience of Iraqi patients in Lebanon. JCO Global Oncology 2020; 6: 59-66. doi: 10.1200/jgo.19.00281.

11. Skelton M. "Iraqi's Cancer Itineraries: War, Medical Travel, and Therapeutic Geographies" in C Lutz, A Mazzarino (eds.). War and Health: The Medical Consequences of the Wars in Iraq and Afghanistan. New York: New York University Press, 2019, pp. 152-171.

12. Pérache AH, van Leeuwen C, Fall C. The politics of exclusion: Fighting for patients with kidney failure in Yemen's war. Journal of Public Health 2019; 42: e311-e315.

13. Whyte SR, Park S-J, Odong G, et al. The visibility of non-communicable diseases in northern Uganda. African Health Sciences 2015; 15: 82-89.

14. Schwartz JI, Guwatudde D, Nugent R, Kiiza CM. Looking at non-communicable diseases in Uganda through a local lens: An analysis using locally derived data. Globalization and Health 2014; 10: 77.

15. Ozasa K, Cullings HM, Ohishi W, et al. Epidemiological studies of atomic bomb radiation at the Radiation Effects Research Foundation. International Journal of Radiation Biology 2019; 95: 879-881. doi: 10.1080/09553002.2019.1569778.

16. Tsushima H, Iwanaga M, Miyazaki Y. Late effect of atomic bomb radiation on myeloid disorders: Leukemia and myelodysplastic syndromes. International Journal of Hematology 2012; 95: 232-238. doi: 10.1007/s12185-012-1002-4.

17. Yamada M, Izumi S. Psychiatric sequelae in atomic bomb survivors in Hiroshima and Nagasaki two decades after the explosions. Social Psychiatry and Psychiatric Epidemiology 2002; 37: 409-415.

18. Ohta Y, Mine M, Wakasugi M, et al. Psychological effect of the Nagasaki atomic bombing on survivors after half a century. Psychiatry and Clinical Neurosciences 2000; 54: 97-103.

19. International Physicians for the Prevention of Nuclear War, and Institute for Energy and Environmental Research. Radioactive Heaven and Earth: The Health and Environmental Effects of Nuclear Weapons Testing in, on and Above the Earth. New York: Apex Press, 1991.

20. Prăvălie R. Nuclear weapons test and environmental consequences: A global perspective. AMBIO 2014; 43: 729-744.

21. Institute of Medicine and National Research Council. Exposure of the American People to Iodine-131 from Nevada Nuclear-Bomb Tests: Review of the National Cancer Institute Report and Public Health Implications. Washington, DC: National Academy Press, 1999. Available at: https://www.ncbi.nlm.nih. gov/books/NBK100842/pdf/Bookshelf_NBK100842.pdf. Accessed on November 27, 2020.

22. Dalager NA, Kang HK, Mahan CM. Cancer mortality among the highest-exposed US atmospheric nuclear test participants. Journal of Occupational and Environmental Medicine 2000; 42: 798-805.

23. Watanabe KK, Kang HK, Dalager NA. Cancer mortality risk among military participants of a 1958 atmospheric nuclear weapons test. American Journal of Public Health 1995; 85: 523-527.
24. Stevens W, Thomas DC, Lyon JL, et al. Leukemia in Utah and radioactive fallout from the Nevada test site: A case-control study. Journal of the American Medical Association 1990; 264: 585-591.
25. Zhumadilov Z, Gusev BI, Takada J, et al. Thyroid abnormality trend over time in northeastern regions of Kazakhstan, adjacent to the Semipalatinsk nuclear test site: A case review of pathological findings for 7271 patients. Journal of Radiation Research 2000; 41: 35-44.
26. Loomis DP, Wolf SH. Mortality of workers at a nuclear materials production plant at Oak Ridge, Tennessee, 1947–1990. American Journal of Industrial Medicine 1996; 29: 131-141.
27. Van Dyck MV, Martyny JW, Mroz MM, et al. Exposure and genetics increase risk of beryllium sensitization and chronic beryllium disease in the nuclear weapons industry. Occupational and Environmental Medicine 2011; 68: 842-848.
28. Wald ML. U.S. acknowledges radiation killed weapons workers. New York Times, January 29, 2000. Available at: https://www.nytimes.com/2000/01/29/us/us-acknowledges-radiation-killed-weapons-workers.html. Accessed on August 25, 2020.
29. Office of Workers' Compensation Programs, United States Department of Labor, Division of Energy Employees Occupational Illness Compensation (DEEOIC): Executive Order 13179: Providing Compensation to American's Nuclear Weapons Workers, December 7, 2000. Available at: https://www.dol.gov/owcp/energy/regs/compliance/law/eo13179.htm. Accessed on August 25, 2020.
30. Hagopian A, Lafta R, Hassan J, et al. Trends in childhood leukemia in Basrah, Iraq, 1993–2007. American Journal of Public Health 2010; 100: 1081-1087.
31. Fathi RA, Matti LY, Al-Salih HS, Godbold D. Environmental pollution by depleted uranium in Iraq with special reference to Mosul and possible effects on cancer and birth defect rates. Medicine, Conflict and Survival 2013; 29: 7-25.
32. Thordardottir EB, Yin L, Hauksdottir A, et al. Mortality and major disease risk among migrants of the 1991–2001 Balkan wars to Sweden: A register-based cohort study. PLoS Medicine 2020; 17: e1003392.
33. Jawad M, Millett C, Sullivan R, et al. The impact of armed conflict on cancer among civilian populations in low- and middle-income countries: A systematic review. eCancer 2020; 14: 1039. doi: https://doi.org/10.3332/ecancer.2020.1039.
34. World Bank. Fragility, Conflict & Violence. Available at: https://www.worldbank.org/en/topic/fragility conflictviolence/overview. Accessed on May 18, 2021.
35. Poole D. Indirect health consequences of war. International Journal of Sociology 2012; 42: 90-107.
36. Kagansky N, Knobler H, Stein-Babich M, et al. Holocaust survival and the long-term risk of cardiovascular disease in the elderly. Israel Medical Association Journal 2018; 21: 241-245.
37. Sibai AM, Fletcher A, Armenian HK. Variations in the impact of long-term wartime stressors on mortality among the middle-aged and older population in Beirut, Lebanon, 1983–1993. American Journal of Epidemiology 2001; 154: 128-137.
38. Head RF, Gilthrope MS, Byrom A, Ellison GTH. Cardiovascular disease in a cohort exposed to the 1940–45 Channel Islands occupation. BMC Public Health 2008; 8: 303. doi: 10.1186/1471-2458-8-303.
39. McEniry M, Samper-Ternent R, Flórez CE, Cano-Gutierrez C. Early life displacement due to armed conflict and violence, early nutrition, and older adult hypertension, diabetes, and obesity in the middle-income country of Colombia. Journal of Aging and Health 2019; 31: 1479-1502.
40. Bedi US, Arora R. Cardiovascular manifestations of posttraumatic stress disorder. Journal of the National Medical Association 2007; 99: 642-649.
41. Savabieasfahani M, Sadik Ali S, Bacho R, et al. Prenatal metal exposure in the Middle East: Imprint of war in deciduous teeth of children. Environmental Monitoring and Assessment 2016; 188: 505. doi: 10.1007/s10661-016-5491-0.
42. Vänskä M, Diab SY, Perko K, et al. Toxic environment of war: Maternal prenatal heavy metal load predicts infant emotional development. Infant Behavior and Development 2019; 55: 1-9.

Profile 10:
Sheri Fink, M.D., Ph.D.
Reporting on the
Complexities of War

War and humanitarian assistance during war raise complex medical and ethical issues. They defy simple narratives. And journalists have the challenging task of objectively documenting and describing war in its many complexities—searching for the historical truth. Few people are more capable for performing this task than Sheri Fink, physician, former humanitarian aid worker, book author, and, since 2014, a Correspondent with the *New York Times*.

After graduating from the University of Michigan as a psychology major, Sheri enrolled at Stanford Medical School. While working toward her M.D. degree and her Ph.D. in neuroscience, she organized a course on the lessons for medicine from the Holocaust. Then she and other students learned about and protested the genocide in Bosnia-Herzegovina. In 1997, she attended a conference on "Medicine, War, and Peace" in Bosnia and became intensely interested in the medical and ethical issues that physicians there had faced during the war. She was so interested that she took a year off before graduating from medical school and went to Bosnia to study the roles of physicians during the war and the challenges that they had faced. There she listened to physicians, nurses, and humanitarian aid workers describe their experiences. Often they had been torn between their responsibilities to serve their patients and their personal struggles to survive.

Her 1-year study turned into a 5-year project in which she meticulously gathered information about the small number of physicians who provided medical care to 50,000 Bosnians under siege in Srebrenica from 1992 to 1995. She interviewed survivors and found and reviewed numerous publications, documents, videotapes, films, and other materials. She reconstructed a narrative about the physicians, their colleagues, and patients in her book *War Hospital: A True Story of Surgery and Survival*, which was published in 2003 and received outstanding reviews.

From Horror to Hope. Barry S. Levy, Oxford University Press. © Oxford University Press 2022.
DOI: 10.1093/oso/9780197558645.003.0020

After one of her trips to Bosnia, Dr. Fink provided humanitarian aid to Kosovar refugees at the Kosovo-Macedonian border, where 100,000 who were seeking refuge in Macedonia were trapped in a "no man's land." She served as a triage physician there with the International Medical Corps in a makeshift tent between borders as refugees brought family members and others needing medical attention: men, women, and children suffering from injuries, seizures, dehydration, and exacerbations of chronic mental health problems. Given a dearth of equipment, supplies, and personnel, the staff faced ethical dilemmas about whom to treat.

While gathering information for her book, Dr. Fink worked in other war-affected countries. With Physicians for Human Rights, she worked in Macedonia, interviewing refugees about the human rights abuses that they had witnessed and they and their household members had directly experienced. With the International Medical Corps, she worked in Iraq shortly after the war began in 2003, delivering basic supplies to hospitals that had been looted, and she also worked in Mozambique, Tajikistan, and Ingushetia in Russia.

By the late 2000s, Dr. Fink chose to work full time as a journalist. Soon after she was hired by ProPublica in 2008, she performed a retrospective investigation of the impact of Hurricane Katrina on the doctors, nurses, and patients at a public hospital in New Orleans. She wrote a Pulitzer Prize–winning article about that situation and subsequently her next book, *Five Days at Memorial*, which received other awards.

In 2014, she joined the staff of the *New York Times*, where she has covered a wide range of issues from the psychological effects of "enhanced interrogation" at Guantanamo to the COVID-19 pandemic. She was among a small group of *Times* correspondents who covered the Ebola outbreak in West Africa, for which she shared another Pulitzer Prize (in International Reporting). And she continues to have the challenging task of objectively documenting and describing issues in their many complexities—searching for the historical truth.

Dr. Fink is a Correspondent with the New York Times.

11

Vulnerable Populations

There is no flag large enough to cover the shame of killing innocent people.
HOWARD ZINN

INTRODUCTION

This chapter summarizes the health impacts of war on (a) women, children, and displaced people, as described in Chapters 6 through 10, and (b) people with disabilities, older people, and Indigenous Peoples, not previously described in this book. Many individuals belong to two or more of these vulnerable groups. This chapter also describes UN conventions concerning women, children, refugees, and people with disabilities.

What causes these populations to be especially vulnerable to the health impacts of war? The causes vary by war and population affected. Women may be malnourished because a military force is restricting their access to food. Children may develop diarrheal disease because a water treatment plant has been bombed. Older people may suffer because they have been separated from their families during mass displacement. And populations are often vulnerable because they lack political power and because those with political power do not adequately protect or provide for them—or have persecuted, oppressed, or directly attacked them.

WOMEN

A substantial and increasing percentage of women worldwide—10% in 2017—have been living dangerously close to armed conflict or have been displaced by armed conflict.[1,2] As described in Chapters 6 through 9, during war and its aftermath, women are at especially increased risk for physical and sexual assaults, malnutrition, mental disorders, and adverse impacts on reproductive health. Rape and other forms of gender-based violence have profound adverse effects on women's health and well-being.[3,4] Inadequate or absent antenatal, intrapartum, and postpartum care increases the risk of maternal mortality and other complications of pregnancy.[5,6] And, as a result of war, many women become widows—often before

From Horror to Hope. Barry S. Levy, Oxford University Press. © Oxford University Press 2022.
DOI: 10.1093/oso/9780197558645.003.0021

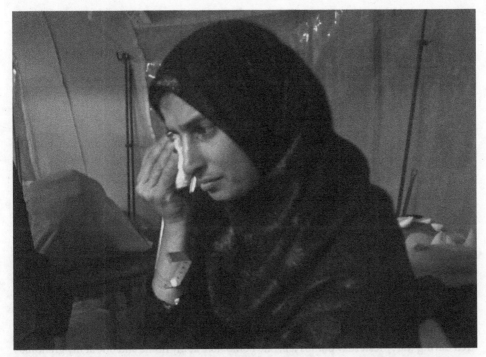

FIGURE 11-1 An Iraqi woman wipes tears from her eyes as she recuperates from injuries to her legs at a U.S. Army combat surgical hospital in Iraq in April 2003. Her husband died when he was caught in a crossfire between Iraqi and U.S. forces. (AP Photo/Julie Jacobson.)

age 30—and must shoulder alone the burdens of family and household responsibilities, frequently with limited psychosocial and financial support (Figure 11-1).[7-9]

Convention on the Elimination of All Forms of Discrimination against Women (CEDAW)

In 1979 the UN General Assembly adopted the CEDAW, an international bill of rights for women and an agenda for action. Its action plan requires states parties to eventually achieve full compliance concerning women's civil rights, reproductive rights, and rights equal to those of men concerning education and employment.[10] (Although the United States has signed the Convention, it is one of the few countries that has not ratified it.)

In order to ensure that states parties comply with their CEDAW obligations before, during, and after armed conflict, the UN Committee on the Elimination of Discrimination against Women has recommended that states parties:

- Prevent, investigate, and punish all forms of gender-based violence, especially sexual violence, and implement a policy of zero tolerance
- Prohibit all forms of gender-based violence, such as by legislation, policies, and protocols
- Ensure women's and girls' access to justice, such as by adopting gender-sensitive investigative procedures to address sexual and gender-based violence, adopting codes of conduct

and protocols for police and military personnel, and building the capacity of the judiciary to ensure its independence, impartiality, and integrity

- Ensure that victims of gender-based violence have access to comprehensive medical treatment, mental healthcare, and psychosocial support
- Establish early warning systems and adopt gender-specific security measures to prevent escalation of gender-based violence and other violations of women's rights.[11]

The UN Security Council has adopted a series of resolutions that focus on issues of women's human rights and gender equality before, during, and after armed conflict. Resolution 1325, adopted in 2000, emphasized the importance of women's equal and full participation as active agents in peace and security. Between 2000 and 2013, the Security Council adopted six additional resolutions concerning women, peace, and security. For example, Security Council Resolution 1820, adopted in 2008, recognized sexual violence during conflict as a tactic of war and that sexual violence can constitute a war crime.[12]

CHILDREN

The words of a 7-year-old girl in Aleppo, Syria, capture the fear and terror perceived by children during war: "Yesterday bombs fell, one bomb here at my home and one at my grandma's house. People are dying like flies here. I don't know what is next. The bombs are just like falling rain."[13]

More than 10% of children worldwide live in areas affected by war. Children, especially those under age 5, are at increased risk of malnutrition, injury, lifelong disability, or death from indiscriminate weapons, such as antipersonnel landmines and cluster munitions (Chapters 4 and 6).

Young children are at increased risk of malnutrition because of breakdowns in the food supply and separation from caregivers. They are at increased risk of communicable diseases, especially diarrheal diseases, acute respiratory infections, malaria, and measles.[14,15] They are far less likely to be immunized against childhood diseases and to receive other preventive measures. And, because of malnutrition, they may be at increased risk of cardiovascular and other disorders later in life (Chapter 7).[16]

Trade sanctions and embargoes that restrict imports of food and medicine disproportionately affect children. For example, after the Gulf War began in mid-1990, the mortality rate for Iraqi children under age 5 more than tripled due to the war and trade sanctions, which limited import of food and medicines for the next 7 years.[17] An analysis based on a logistic regression model indicated a minimum of 100,000 and a more likely estimate of 227,000 excess deaths among young children in Iraq from August 1991 through March 1998; about one-fourth of these deaths were mainly associated with the Gulf War, most of which were primarily associated with sanctions.[18]

Children are at increased risk of mental disorders because of physical and sexual assault, mistreatment and abuse, displacement, and separation from parents (Chapter 8). Children in war zones face an increased risk of one or both of their parents dying—almost 9% in one study in Africa.[19] They may be forced to become child soldiers (Chapter 6).[20] Exposure to carcinogens may increase children's risks for cancer later in life. And during war children lose opportunities for education and social development.

Convention on the Rights of the Child (CRC)

The CRC, which entered into force in 1990, is intended to promote and protect the well-being of all children.[21] Together with the Sustainable Development Goals and the work of the World Health Organization and UNICEF, the CRC provides frameworks for protecting children, including during war and its aftermath.[22] It affirms children's political, economic, social, and cultural rights, including rights to health, protection from abuse, and freedom of expression. It also addresses rights related to education, healthcare, juvenile justice, and disabilities.[21] Nevertheless, these and other children's rights are frequently violated during war.[23]

The CRC has 196 states parties. The United States, which has signed the CRC, is the only country that has not ratified it. However, the United States has ratified two optional protocols to the CRC, one on child soldiers (see below) and the other on the sale of children, child prostitution, and child pornography.[24]

The CRC obligates states parties to ensure that children younger than 15 do not directly participate in combat.[21] One of its optional protocols proclaims: "States Parties shall take all feasible measures to ensure that persons who have not attained the age of 15 years do not take a direct part in hostilities."[25] The International Criminal Court has outlawed as a war crime the conscription of children under age 15. But the CRC does not prevent children from ages 15 to 18 from voluntarily participating in combat as soldiers.

DISPLACED PEOPLE

During war, people are frequently uprooted from their homes (made homeless), sometimes suddenly and violently, and often permanently. Worldwide, 48.0 million people are internally displaced due to war and violence and 26.4 million are refugees, with many never returning to their home countries. Most displaced people are women, children, and older people, for whom displacement acts as a multiplier of their war-related health risks. (See Chapter 2.)

Internally displaced persons, who during war are often desperately challenged to meet their basic needs, are generally far worse off than refugees (Figure 11-2). They may be repeatedly displaced during the course of war. They often have little or no access to healthcare or public health services, which adversely affects their health. From a perspective of protecting public health and providing humanitarian assistance, it is often difficult to obtain both numerator data (incidence or prevalence of disease among internally displaced persons) and denominator data (the size and characteristics of the population at risk).

Displaced Women

A review of 31 studies of the health of internally displaced women in Africa found that violence, mental health, sexual and reproductive health, and malaria were health issues that were most frequently studied. It reported that prolonged displacement during protracted conflict

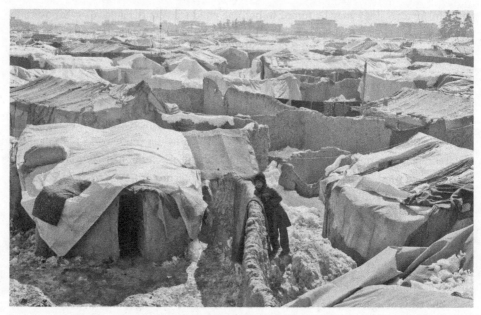

FIGURE 11-2 An internally displaced boy from Helmand Province stands in a refugee camp in Kabul, Afghanistan, in 2012. (AP Photo/Musadeq Sadeq.)

has often led to community apathy about violence against internally displaced women, with domestic violence becoming normalized. It found that several factors affected the mental health of these women, including excessive responsibilities for caregiving, inadequate financial and family support, sustained experiences of violence, family dysfunction, and chronic alcoholism of men. It reported that access to reproductive health services was associated with relevant knowledge, geographical proximity to services, consent of spouse, and affordability of services. And it found that a few studies indicated that, although malaria prevalence was high among these women, they often did not understand how it is transmitted and did not implement recommended preventive measures.[26]

Displaced Children

"This is not a place for children," says Ramez, 10, of his new home, a juvenile detention center-turned-shelter in Syria. Between late 2019 and mid-2020, an escalation in violence affecting the southern rural province of Idlib had forced nearly 300,000 Syrians to find safety elsewhere in the country. Women and children made up an estimated 80% of these internally displaced persons. Ramez's family was one of 45 families that had taken shelter in the juvenile detention center, where they lived in the most basic conditions. Shourouk, a 10-year-old girl living at the center, said, "This is such a gloomy place. I cannot sleep well." Other families had settled in schools, mosques, and makeshift tented settlements.[27]

In 2017, 16% of children worldwide were living dangerously close to armed conflict or had been displaced by armed conflict. Between 2000 and 2017, the number of children who had not been displaced but were living within 31 miles (50 km) of armed conflict increased 47%, from 250 million to 368 million.[2] By 2019, there were more than 31 million

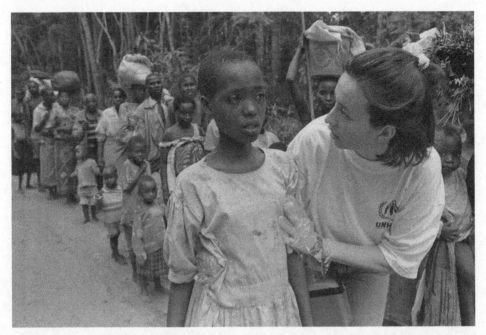

FIGURE 11-3 A field worker with UNHCR: The UN Refugee Agency helps a young Rwandan Hutu girl find her parents while evacuating refugees from the Biaro refugee camp in Zaire (now the Democratic Republic of the Congo) in 1997. UN and humanitarian aid agencies were trying to reunite thousands of unaccompanied children with their parents before repatriation to Rwanda. (AP Photo/John Moore.)

children who had been forcibly displaced because of violence and conflict—in direct violation of the CRC. Most of these children were in Africa and the Middle East; three countries—Syria, the Democratic Republic of the Congo, and Yemen—accounted for about one-third of them.[28]

Displaced children are often separated from their parents, who may have been seriously injured or killed, and these children may be caring for younger siblings (Figure 11-3). Unaccompanied children are at especially increased risk of physical and sexual assault and abuse, malnutrition, communicable diseases, and mental disorders.[27,28] (See Chapters 6, 7, and 8.)

Convention Relating to the Status of Refugees

This convention, also known as the 1951 Refugee Convention, defined refugees and asserted the rights of people who are granted asylum and the responsibilities of the countries that grant it. But it only applied to people displaced, mainly in Europe, due to events before 1951. The 1967 Protocol Relating to the Status of Refugees and UN General Assembly Resolution 2198 removed the restrictions of the Convention and committed states parties to treating refugees according to recognized legal and humanitarian standards, including protecting their legal status and not sending them to places where they might be persecuted.[29] Various international agreements protect the right of refugees to make a free and informed choice about returning to their countries of origin and not to be subjected to pressure to leave their countries of asylum.

PERSONS WITH DISABILITIES

More than one billion people live with physical, sensory, intellectual, or mental health impairments that adversely affect their daily lives. About one-fourth of all families worldwide include one or more people with a significant disability. The issues faced by persons with disabilities include not only their specific impairments, but also social stigma, decreased access to resources, and poverty.[30]

People with disabilities are disproportionately vulnerable because of poverty, social disadvantage, and structural exclusion—not because of any natural vulnerability. Those who are displaced are at increased vulnerability because of loss of their social and family network as well as decreased access to medical care; they therefore do not receive the specialized attention that they need. Often, people with war-related disabilities receive more attention than people who had disabilities before war began.[31]

People with disabilities have often been targeted during war. They are vulnerable because they are sometimes clustered in psychiatric hospitals, orphanages, and other institutions, which may tempt combatants to attack them or use them as human shields.[32] In Nazi Germany, at least 90,000 people with disabilities were killed. In armed conflict in Sierra Leone, people with disabilities were deliberately shot by soldiers. In Rwanda in 1994, almost all of 700 patients at a psychiatric hospital who had mental health problems or learning difficulties were killed. In addition, people with disabilities are injured or killed by indiscriminate attacks that impact the civilian population.[33]

People with different types of disabilities face different challenges during war and its aftermath (Figure 11-4). For example, people with blindness or hearing impairment face

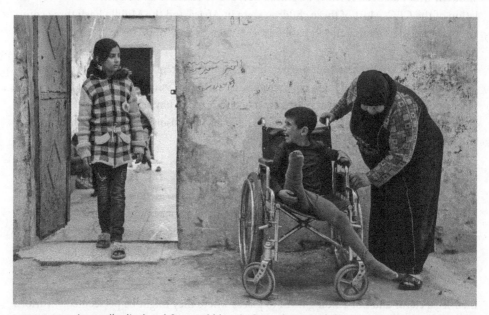

FIGURE 11-4 Internally displaced 9-year-old boy in Syria shown with his grandmother and sister. He lost his right foot and his memory in an air raid during their displacement to the town of Ma'arrat Misrin in 2020. His grandmother was caring for her 16 orphaned grandchildren after losing six of her own children during the Syrian Civil War. (AP Photo/Anas Alkharboutli.)

difficulties receiving emergency communications. People with blindness or mobility issues have difficulty navigating steep or slippery footpaths in order to access latrines and food distribution sites, and may have difficulty during evacuations. People with intellectual disabilities face increased risks of injury and death because of targeted attacks on them and because of their disabilities, their being abandoned and neglected, and difficulties accessing healthcare and other services.[33] And war damages or threatens healthcare and other support systems for all people with disabilities.

People with disabilities experience social stigma, which may reduce their social interaction and exclude them from participating in many activities. Those with intellectual or psychological impairments are especially stigmatized, and may not seek assistance from mental health professionals in order to avoid additional stigma.[34] And people with disabilities who are exposed to war are at high risk of developing posttraumatic stress symptoms.[35]

In low-income countries, many people with disabilities have rarely, if ever, seen a physician and many of them do not know what caused their disability. If they do not receive adequate healthcare, they are at increased risk of developing exacerbations or complications of their disabilities.[36]

During war, persons with disabilities have faced violent attacks, forced displacement, and ongoing neglect. Some persons with disabilities are unable to flee from attacks. Those left behind are at increased risk of assault, abuse, malnutrition, communicable disease—and death. A 45-year-old woman in South Sudan said: "When the fighting broke out, we fled to the UN compound and we left my mother and brother-in-law behind because they couldn't walk, and we couldn't carry them."[37] They later died in a fire. Some people with disabilities eventually reach camps for displaced persons, but even then they often find it difficult to access food, healthcare, and safe and secure living conditions.[37]

Children with disabilities face additional challenges. If they are stigmatized, they may not attend school. They may find it difficult and frightening to flee danger during war. In many countries, they are unlikely to receive rehabilitation services. Children who have lost an arm or a leg in a landmine explosion may need several prostheses as they grow. But many never receive even one prosthesis.[38]

Convention on the Rights of Persons With Disabilities

This convention, which entered into force in 2008, reaffirms the human rights and fundamental freedoms of all persons with disabilities, and calls for their full participation and equal access to resources. It also includes a specific provision pertaining to humanitarian emergencies, including armed conflict.[39] As of June 2021, the Convention had been ratified by 182 countries. The United States has signed but not ratified it, even though the Americans with Disabilities Act of 1990 contains more stringent protections than the Convention. Because it did not ratify the Convention, the United States can play only a limited role at international meetings where states parties discuss best practices and share advances in implementation.[40]

The 2016 Charter on Inclusion of Persons with Disabilities in Humanitarian Action, which has been endorsed by 32 countries (including the United States) and many civil society organizations, commits participating countries to strive to ensure that services and humanitarian assistance are equally available and accessible to all persons with disabilities.[41]

In 2019, the UN Security Council adopted Resolution 2475, in which it called upon UN member states and parties to armed conflict to protect persons with disabilities during armed conflict and ensure that they have access to justice, basic services, and unimpeded humanitarian assistance. It emphasized the need for countries to end impunity for criminal acts against persons with disabilities and other civilians and ensure that, in additional to access to justice, they have effective remedies and appropriate reparation.[42]

OLDER PEOPLE

During war and its aftermath, older people are at increased risk of injury, illness, and death because of vulnerability to physical attacks, psychosocial stress, and reduced access to food, safe water, and healthcare. Even in dangerous situations, many older people choose to remain in their homes rather than to leave and face the unknown. During protracted wars, when civilian infrastructure has been damaged or destroyed and there is less security and socioeconomic stability, many older people who stay behind die. Even when they have been able to get to camps for displaced persons, they are often overlooked and marginalized. And sometimes humanitarian aid organizations neglect older people, mistakenly assuming that they will be cared for by their families.[43]

Older people often find themselves alone. They may suffer from physical or cognitive impairments. They may have no financial support. They may be subject to abuse, such as looting, destruction of their property, and physical and sexual violence, especially if they belong to a minority group or live in a remote location.[44]

Older people are at increased risk of posttraumatic stress disorder (PTSD), depression, and poor psychological quality of life. They have difficulty accessing healthcare, often because they do not have money for treatment or transport. They frequently have limited knowledge about healthcare and available programs for financial or other assistance.[45]

War-related experiences during young adulthood may increase the risk of mental disorders later in life. For example, child survivors of the Second World War who had been placed in internment camps and had experienced violence under Japanese occupation in the Dutch East Indies had more trauma-related experiences and more mental disorders in later life as compared with age-matched control subjects who had lived through the German occupation in The Netherlands during the war.[46] Recent onset of PTSD symptoms in older Vietnamese people has been associated with a history during the Vietnam War of having killed or severely injured others, having witnessed war atrocities or the death of their children, or having been separated from their spouses.[47]

INDIGENOUS PEOPLES

For centuries, Indigenous Peoples have been targeted during war—and at other times—by national governments or other military forces. They have been killed and disabled. They have been forcibly displaced from their homelands. They have been marginalized. They have suffered the physical, psychological, and social consequences not only of war, but also of social injustice. And their cultures have been damaged or destroyed.[48]

For Indigenous Peoples, land exists for material and spiritual benefit collectively and must be preserved for future generations. They perceive that they have the authority to assert their rights to their lands and resources, cultural heritage, and religious practices, and that they must protect their institutions and their culture.[49,50]

During colonization of the "New World," colonizers committed acts of extreme racism against Indigenous Peoples with massacres, forced relocations, and death by starvation and disease. This subjugation of Indigenous Peoples was legally sanctioned by *doctrines of discovery*, which enabled countries to claim "unoccupied lands" or lands belonging to "heathens" or "pagans." In many parts of the world, these doctrines led to situations in which Indigenous Peoples were forced to become dependent nations or "wards of the State"—situations in which the government could revoke their ownership of land at any time.[51]

Killing of Indigenous Peoples drastically reduced their numbers or totally eliminated them. During the 15th century, before the arrival of Columbus, the population of North America was estimated to have been 10 to 12 million people. By the 1890s, the population of Indigenous Peoples in North America had been reduced to about 300,000. Even today, in parts of Latin America where Indigenous Peoples represent most of the population, they are marginalized, disadvantaged, and separated from their land.[51] And they have also been marginalized, disadvantaged, and separated from their land in the United States and many other countries where Indigenous Peoples today are minorities.

Indigenous Peoples have been harmed not only by war, but also by the preparation for war, such as in the development and testing of nuclear weapons. For example, Navajos in the southwestern United States have been intensely engaged in the mining of uranium, a toxic

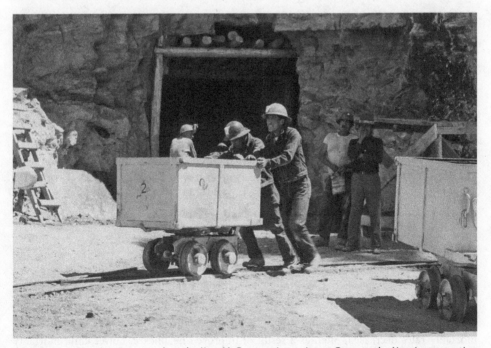

FIGURE 11-5 Navajo miners work at the Kerr McGee uranium mine at Cove on the Navajo reservation in Arizona in 1953. (AP Photo.)

and radioactive heavy metal used to produce nuclear weapons and fuel nuclear power plants (Figure 11-5). Although it was known for decades that uranium miners were at increased risk of lung cancer and possibly other diseases because of their occupational exposures, Navajo miners were not given adequate protection; even when protective measures were provided, adoption was slow and incomplete. As a result, many Navajo miners developed occupational lung cancer.[52] As another example, Indigenous Peoples in the Marshall Islands were exposed to atmospheric tests of nuclear weapons and their environment was heavily contaminated with radioactive fallout (Chapter 5).

ADDRESSING THE NEEDS OF VULNERABLE POPULATIONS

While the specific needs of war-affected vulnerable people differ, the health and well-being of all vulnerable people should be protected by:

- Provision of safe food, water, and shelter
- Facilities for sanitation and hygiene
- Access to healthcare and public health services
- Measures to prevent violence and ensure their safety and security
- Support for individual and community mental health
- Respect, protection, and fulfillment of their human rights
- Access to justice.

Specific measures for preventing morbidity and mortality are described in previous chapters.

Responding to the Needs of Women

Chapters 6 through 9 have addressed specific measures to reduce risks that women face during war and its aftermath, including physical and sexual assaults and reproductive health threats. With regard to gender-based violence, specific measures have been discussed in Chapter 6 and earlier in this chapter. With regard to reproductive health threats faced by women, preventive measures focus on improving the availability, accessibility, and quality of maternal healthcare; increasing availability of contraception and family planning services; and ensuring the right to reproductive choice and access to abortion services (Chapter 9). More broadly, women's rights need to be respected, protected, and fulfilled so that women attain political and socioeconomic power equal to that of men.

Responding to the Needs of Children

Multiple interventions are necessary to protect and to respond to the needs of children during war and its aftermath. (See Profile 11.) Achieving and maintaining peace may be the most important intervention. A study of peace agreements in 73 countries that had been engaged in war from 1989 to 2012 found that after war ended neonatal, infant, and under-5 mortality rates decreased, often as a result of improved healthcare. Lower child mortality rates after war were also associated with higher per-capita gross domestic product, higher levels of democracy, and higher primary school enrollment.[53]

In her 2001 book *The Impact of War on Children*, Graça Machel, an international advocate for women's and children's rights and former First Lady of South Africa, issued an urgent call to action to protect the rights of children, including:

- Ending impunity for crimes committed against children
- Monitoring and reporting on violations of children's rights during conflicts
- Improving the collection and analysis of data concerning children during war
- Supporting civil society to protect children
- Mobilizing international resources for war-affected children.[54]

Her call to action remains relevant today.

Responding to the Needs of Displaced People

Basic elements of addressing the health needs of displaced persons during the emergency phase of a war include assessment of health status; provision of medical care; prevention and control of communicable diseases; and programs for food distribution and nutrition, protection and security, water supply and sanitation, and public health surveillance.[55] (See Profile 8.)

In post-conflict situations, it is often challenging to create a transition from an emergency humanitarian aid response to a situation in which only local health workers and facilities provide healthcare and public health services. During an emergency, huge infusions of external assistance and health workers can undermine local health services by creating two parallel systems of care with different levels of expertise and resources. Sudden departure of emergency workers after a war has ended may leave local residents with inadequate follow-up and unrealistic expectations for local health services.[56]

In order to provide healthcare to displaced populations, physicians and others often need to work in challenging environments without sufficient resources. They need to adapt, sometimes very quickly, to rapidly changing situations and security threats. In host countries, they need to develop and maintain trusting relationships with refugees; screen for and treat diseases while considering the sociocultural contexts of refugees' lives; educate refugees about the host country's healthcare system, including patients' rights and health insurance programs; and identify and address discrimination. They also need to bridge language barriers and understand refugees' beliefs about health and illness in order to obtain accurate case histories, explain consent for medical procedures, and ensure that refugees understand treatment options.[57-59]

Health professionals and other humanitarian aid workers face a number of ethical dilemmas. For example, after witnessing violations of human rights or international humanitarian law, they may need to choose between keeping silent in order to have continued access to an endangered population in need and speaking out about these violations.[56]

Improving Humanitarian Assistance

There is a need to make humanitarian assistance more systematic, evidence-based, and tailored to the setting and the needs of the affected population.[60] The BRANCH Consortium Steering Committee has proposed a framework that prioritizes interventions based on the needs of those affected, potential interventions and feasibility of implementing them, and the potential risks for those providing assistance. The framework consists of three levels of assistance:

- In conflict settings where violence is acute and ongoing, providing a small set of lifesaving interventions
- In insecure areas where the threat of violence may be imminent but people are not being exposed to active conflict, considering a wider range of interventions
- In stable situations where displaced people are settled in camps or integrated in communities in host countries, providing a comprehensive package of interventions, while targeting those who have the greatest needs.[61]

The Assessment Capacities Project (ACAPS) assesses the severity of various aspects of humanitarian crises in order to support evidence-based decision-making. It compares the scale and severity of various crises worldwide, including assessing and analyzing humanitarian needs for specific population groups in specific settings and access for humanitarian aid in these settings. It also assesses physical and security constraints, such as ongoing violence, the presence of landmines and improvised explosive devices, and constraints in the physical environment. And it communicates its findings to humanitarian aid organizations, governments, and other entities. ACAPS also develops potential scenarios on how situations may evolve and create humanitarian needs.[62] (See section on SMART Methodology in Chapter 14.)

The Sphere Association has developed universal minimum standards for humanitarian responses, which have been used extensively by governments, donors, businesses, and military forces. *The Sphere Handbook* includes the ethical, legal, and practical bases for these standards and a humanitarian charter, which reviews international humanitarian law, human rights, and refugee law. It also provides guidance on communicable diseases, child health, sexual and reproductive health, injury and trauma care, mental health, noncommunicable diseases, and palliative care.[63]

Governments and humanitarian organizations can improve long-term healthcare for war-affected civilians, such as by radically expanding the range of mass-delivered interventions for various diseases, offering these interventions in integrated mass campaigns, and expanding use of negotiated ceasefires to implement these campaigns. They can address chronic communicable diseases, such as tuberculosis and HIV/AIDS, and noncommunicable diseases more systematically, such as by registering prevalent cases that can be treated locally, developing simplified home-based care guidelines, and developing and evaluating new methods of treatment. And they can help ensure that healthcare is accessible and affordable for war-affected civilians, such as by integrating services into existing national health services.[64]

The ever-changing nature of armed conflict presents ongoing challenges for protecting civilians and providing humanitarian assistance. These challenges, which include systematic use of sexual violence, frequent deployment of explosive devices in populated areas, and the increasingly complex political context of armed conflict, often make it difficult for humanitarian aid organizations to gain access to populations in need and ensure safety and security for humanitarian aid workers. COVID-19 and other emerging infectious diseases represent additional problems. The changing nature of combatants in intrastate wars, including fighters from militias, guerrilla groups, and military forces from other countries, presents further challenges. Governmental and UN agencies and nongovernmental organizations providing humanitarian assistance need to adapt to these challenges.[65]

SUMMARY POINTS

- Populations are vulnerable for many reasons, including lack of political power.
- Each vulnerable population has specific needs during war and its aftermath.
- Inadequate healthcare and public health services during war increase health risks for vulnerable populations.
- UN conventions support the protection of some vulnerable populations.
- In addition to addressing immediate needs of vulnerable populations, aid organizations must also facilitate development of sustainable local efforts to meet the long-term needs of these populations.

REFERENCES

1. Clark H. A commitment to support the world's most vulnerable women, children, and adolescents (Comment). Lancet 2021; 397: P450-P452. doi: 10.1016/S0140-6736(21)00137-9.
2. Bendavid E. The effects of armed conflict on the health of women and children. Lancet 2021; 397: P522-532. doi: 10.1016/S0140-6736(21)00131-8.
3. United Nations. Conflict related sexual violence: Report of the United Nations Secretary-General. March 29, 2019. Available at: https://www.un.org/sexualviolenceinconflict/wp-content/uploads/2019/04/report/s-2019-280/Annual-report-2018.pdf. Accessed on April 23, 2020.
4. Lamb C. Our Bodies Their Battlefield: What War Does to Women. London: William Collins, An Imprint of HarperCollins Publishers, 2020.
5. Torche F, Shwed U. The hidden costs of war: Exposure to armed conflict and birth outcomes. Sociological Science 2015; 2: 558-581.
6. Wagner Z, Heft-Neal S, Wise PH, et al. Women and children living in areas of armed conflict in Africa: A geospatial analysis of mortality and orphanhood. Lancet Global Health 2019; 7: e1622-e1631.
7. Changoiwala P. The hidden struggle of India's war widows. Women's Advancement Deeply, June 22, 2018. Available at: https://www.newsdeeply.com/womensadvancement/articles/2018/06/22/the-hidden-struggles-of-indias-war-widows. Accessed on May 9, 2020.
8. Basnet S, Kandel P, Lamichane P. Depression and anxiety among war-widows of Nepal: A post-civil war cross-sectional study. Psychology, Health & Medicine 2018; 23: 141-153.
9. Witting AB, Lambert J, Wickrama T. War and disaster in Sri Lanka: Implication for widows' family adjustment and perception of self-efficacy in caring for one's family. International Journal of Psychology 2019; 54: 126-134.

10. UN Women. Convention on the Elimination of All Forms of Discrimination against Women. Available at: https://www.un.org/womenwatch/daw/cedaw/. Accessed April 14, 2021.

11. Committee on the Elimination of Discrimination against Women. General Recommendation No. 30 on Women in Conflict Prevention, Conflict and Post-conflict Situations (Advance Unedited Version). United Nations. October 18, 2013. Available at: https://www.ohchr.org/documents/hrbodies/cedaw/gcomments/cedaw.c.cg.30.pdf. Accessed on April 14, 2021.

12. UN Women. Guidebook on CEDAW General Recommendation No. 30 and the UN Security Council Resolutions on Women, Peace and Security, New York, 2015. Available at: http://peacewomen.org/sites/default/files/CEDAW-Guide-REV2_UNW.pdf. Accessed on April 14, 2021.

13. The Syria war as seen through a child's eyes. ITV News, October 4, 2016. Available at: youtube.com/watch?tv=bC0tUgvKsus. Accessed on September 15, 2020.

14. Guha-Sapir D, van Panhuis WG. Conflict-related mortality: An analysis of 37 datasets. Disasters 2004; 28: 418-428.

15. Albertyn R, Bickler SW, van As AB, et al. The effects of war on children in Africa. Pediatric Surgery International 2003; 19: 227-232.

16. Head RF, Gilthrope MS, Byrom A, Ellison GTH. Cardiovascular disease in a cohort exposed to the 1940–45 Channel Islands occupation. BMC Public Health 2008; 8: 303. doi: 10.1186/1471-2458-8-303.

17. Ascherio A, Chase R, Coté T, et al. Effect of the Gulf War on infant and child mortality in Iraq. New England Journal of Medicine. 1992; 327: 931-936.

18. Garfield R. Morbidity and mortality among Iraqi children from 1990 through 1998: Assessing the impact of the Gulf War and economic sanctions. Unpublished paper. Available at: https://reliefweb.int/sites/reliefweb.int/files/resources/A2E2603E5DC88A4685256825005F211D-garfie17.pdf. Accessed on July 12, 2021.

19. Wagner Z, Heft-Neal S, Wise PH, et al. Women and children living in areas of armed conflict in Africa: A geospatial analysis of mortality and orphanhood. Lancet 2019; 7: e1622-e1631.

20. Song SJ, de Jong J. Child soldiers: Children associated with fighting forces. Child and Adolescent Psychiatric Clinics of North America 2015; 24: 765-775.

21. Office of the High Commissioner, United Nations Human Rights. Convention on the Rights of the Child, November 20, 1989. Available at: https://www.ohchr.org/en/professionalinterest/pages/crc.aspx. Accessed on January 5, 2021.

22. Uchitel J, Alden E, Bhutta ZA, et al. The rights of children for optimal development and nurturing care. Pediatrics 2019; 144: e20190487. doi: https://doi.org/10.1542/peds.2019-0487.

23. United Nations, Office of the Special Representative of the Secretary-General for Children and Armed Conflict. Working Paper No. 1: The Six Grave Violations Against Children During Armed Conflict: The Legal Foundation, 2013. Available at: https://childrenandarmedconflict.un.org/publications/WorkingPaper-1_SixGraveViolationsLegalFoundation.pdf. Accessed on May 2, 2020.

24. Human Rights Watch. United States ratification of international human rights treaties. July 24, 2009. Available at: https://www.hrw.org/news/2009/07/24/united-states-ratification-international-human-rights-treaties. Accessed on April 1, 2021.

25. Office of the United Nations High Commissioner for Human Rights. Optional Protocol to the Convention on the Rights of the Child on the Involvement of Children in Armed Conflict. Available at: https://www.ohchr.org/en/professionalinterest/pages/opaccrc.aspx. Accessed on April 22, 2020.

26. Amodu OC, Richter MS, Salami BO. A scoping review of the health of conflict-induced internally displaced women in Africa. International Journal of Environmental Research and Public Health. 2020; 17: 1280. doi:10.3390/ijerph17041280.

27. United Nations Children's Fund. Lost at Home: The Risks and Challenges for Internally Displaced Children and the Urgent Actions Needed to Protect Them. New York: UNICEF, 2020. Available at: https://www.unicef.org/media/70131/file/Lost-at-home-risks-and-challenges-for-IDP-children-2020.pdf. Accessed on August 26, 2020.

28. Salami B, Iwuagwu S, Amodu O, et al. The health of internally displaced children in sub-Saharan Africa: A scoping review. BMJ Global Health 2020; 5: e002584. doi: 10.1136/bmjgh-2020-002584.

29. UNHCR: The UN Refugee Agency. Convention and Protocol Relating to the Status of Refugees, December 2010. Available at: https://www.unhcr.org/protect/PROTECTION/3b66c2aa10.pdf. Accessed on September 1, 2020.

30. Groce NE. "People with Disabilities" in BS Levy (ed.). Social Injustice and Public Health (3rd edition). New York: Oxford University Press, 2019, pp. 155-174.

31. Portero IB, Bolaños Enriquez TG. Persons with disabilities and the Colombian armed conflict. Disability & Society 2018; 33: 487-491.

32. Devanda C, Barriga SR, Quinn PG, Lord JE. Protecting civilians with disabilities in conflicts. NATO Review. December 1, 2017. Available at: https://www.nato.int/docu/review/articles/2017/12/01/protecting-civilians-with-disabilities-in-conflicts/index.html. Accessed at May 4, 2021.

33. Rohwerder B. Intellectual disabilities, violent conflict and humanitarian assistance: Advocacy of the forgotten. Disability & Society 2013; 28: 770-783.

34. Stough LM, Ducy EM, Kang D. Addressing the needs of children with disabilities experiencing disaster or terrorism. Current Psychiatry Reports 2017; 19: 24. doi: 10.1007/s11920-017-0776-8.

35. Shpigelman C, Gelkopf M. The impact of exposure to war and terror on individuals with disabilities. Psychological Trauma: Theory, Research, Practice and Policy 2019; 11: 189-196.

36. Human Rights Watch. South Sudan: People with disabilities, older people face danger. May 31, 2017. Available at: https://www.hrw.org/news/2017/05/31/south-sudan-people-disabilities-older-people-face-danger. Accessed on September 22, 2020.

37. Human Rights Watch. UN: War's impact on people with disabilities. December 2, 2018. Available at: https://www.hrw.org/news/2018/12/03/un-wars-impact-people-disabilities. Accessed on September 22, 2020.

38. Taipale V. "Children and war" in I Taipale (ed.). War or Health?: A Reader. Dhaka, Bangladesh: University Press, 2001, pp. 249-258.

39. United Nations. Convention on the Rights of Persons with Disabilities (CRPD). 2006. Available at: https://www.un.org/development/desa/disabilities/convention-on-the-rights-of-persons-with-disabilities.html. Accessed on September 22, 2020.

40. Jones R. U.S. Failure to Ratify the Convention on the Rights of Persons with Disabilities. April 19, 2013. Available at: https://www.awid.org/news-and-analysis/us-failure-ratify-convention-rights-persons-disabilities#:~:text=FRIDAY%20FILE%20%2D%20In%20December%202012,Persons%20with%20Disabilities%20(CRPD).&text=This%20resulted%20in%20the%20treaty,ratification%20under%20the%20U.S.%20constitution. Accessed on March 31, 2021.

41. United Nations. Charter on Inclusion of Persons with Disabilities in Humanitarian Action, 2016. Available at: http://humanitariandisabilitycharter.org/. Accessed on September 22, 2020.

42. United Nations Security Council. Resolution 2475 [On Protection of Persons with Disabilities in Armed Conflict], June 20, 2019. Available at: https://digitallibrary.un.org/record/3810259?ln=en. Accessed on May 4, 2021.

43. Global Action on Aging. In wars and disasters, old people get left behind (Reuters). September 29, 2009. Available at: http://globalag.igc.org/armedconflict/countryreports/general/warsolderleft.htm. Accessed on September 21, 2020.

44. Global Action on Aging. Older persons caught in armed conflict and other emergency situations. Available at: http://globalag.igc.org/armedconflict/index.htm. Accessed on September 21, 2020.

45. Massey E, Smith J, Roberts B. Health needs of older populations affected by humanitarian crises in low- and middle-income countries: A systematic review. Conflict and Health 2017; 11: 29. doi: 10.1186/s13031-017-01330-x.

46. Mooren TTM, Kleber JR. The significance of experiences of war and migration in older age: Long-term consequences in child survivors from the Dutch East Indies. International Psychogeriatrics 2013; 25: 1783-1794.

47. Korinek K, Loebach P, Teerawichitchainan B. Physical and mental health consequences of war-related stressors among older adults: An analysis of posttraumatic stress disorder and arthritis in Northern Vietnamese war survivors. Journal of Gerontology: Social Sciences 2017; 72: 1090-1102.

48. Hitchcock RK. The impacts of conservation and militarization on indigenous peoples. Human Nature 2019; 30: 217-241.

49. Lutz EL. Indigenous peoples and violent conflict: Preconceptions, appearances, and realities. Cultural Survival Quarterly Magazine, March 2005. Available at: https://www.culturalsurvival.org/publications/

cultural-survival-quarterly/indigenous-peoples-and-violent-conflict-preconceptions. Accessed on September 23, 2020.

50. Commission on Human Rights, United Nations Economic and Social Council. Human Rights of Indigenous Peoples: Study on treaties, agreements and other constructive arrangements between States and indigenous populations. Final report by Miguel Alfonso Martínez, Special Rapporteur, June 22, 1999. Available at: https://digitallibrary.un.org/record/276353?ln=en#record-files-collapse-header. Accessed on September 23, 2020.

51. World Conference Against Racism. "Doctrines of Dispossession": Racism Against Indigenous Peoples. World Conference Against Racism, Racial Discrimination, Xenophobia and Related Intolerance. Durban, South Africa, August 31–September 7, 2001. Available at: https://www.un.org/WCAR/e-kit/indigenous.htm. Accessed on September 23, 2020.

52. Brugge D, Goble R. The history of uranium mining and the Navajo people. American Journal of Public Health 2002; 92: 1410-1419.

53. Joshi M. Comprehensive peace agreement implementation and reduction in neonatal, infant and under-5 mortality rates in post-armed conflict states, 1989-2012. BMC International Health and Human Rights 2015; 15: 27. doi: 10.1186/s12914-015-0066-7.

54. Machel G. The Impact of War on Children. New York: Palgrave, 2001.

55. Médecins Sans Frontières. 11 Humanitarian Priorities in Refugee Camps: Video tutorials produced as a result of MSF Refugee Evaluations in 2012. Available at: https://evaluation.msf.org/11-humanitarian-priorities-refugee-camps. Accessed on March 11, 2021.

56. Leaning J, Guha-Sapir D. Natural disasters, armed conflict, and public health. New England Journal of Medicine 2013; 369: 1836-1842.

57. Robertshaw L, Dhesi S, Jones LL. Challenges and facilitators for health professionals providing primary healthcare for refugees and asylum seekers in high-income countries: A systematic review and thematic synthesis of qualitative research. BMJ Open 2017; 7: e015981. doi: 10.1136/bmjopen-2017-015981.

58. Mangrio E, Sjögren Forss K. Refugees' experiences of healthcare in the host country: A scoping review. BMC Health Services Research 2017; 17: 814. doi: 10.1186/s12913-017-2731-0.

59. Wylie L, Van Meyel R, Harder H, et al. Assessing trauma in a transcultural context: Challenges in mental health care with immigrants and refugees. Public Health Reviews 2018; 39: 22. doi: 10.1186/s40985-018-0102-y.

60. Singh NS, Ataullahjan A, Ndiaye K, et al. Delivering health interventions to women, children, and adolescents in conflict settings: What have we learned from ten country case studies? Lancet 2021; 397: 533-542. doi: 10.1016/S0140- 6736(21)00132-X.

61. Gaffey MF, Waldman RJ, Blanchet K, et al. Delivering health and nutrition interventions for women and children in different conflict contexts: A framework for decision making on what, when, and how. Lancet 2021; 397: 543-554.

62. Assessment Capacities Project (ACAPS). Available at: www.acaps.org. Accessed on June 7, 2021.

63. Sphere Association. The Sphere Handbook: Humanitarian Charter and Minimum Standards in Humanitarian Response (4th edition). Geneva, Switzerland: Sphere Association, 2018.

64. Spiegel EB, Checchi F, Colombo S, Paik E. Health-care needs of people affected by conflict: Future trends and changing frameworks. Lancet 2010; 375: 341-345.

65. Wise PH, Shiel A, Southard N, et al. The political and security dimensions of the humanitarian health response to violent conflict. Lancet 2021; 397: 511-521. doi: 10.1016.S0140-6736(21)00130-6.

Profile 11:
Samantha Nutt, M.D., M.Sc.
Protecting Children

In medical school, Samantha Nutt developed a strong commitment to women's health as a way of supporting women's rights. But she was frustrated with the medical paradigm, which focuses on treating disease rather than on promoting health. So she went on to complete her family practice certification and her specialization in public health, with a focus on global health.

In the mid-1990s, she was recruited by UNICEF to evaluate the impact of war and violence in Somalia, where only a few nongovernmental organizations were still providing humanitarian assistance and armed groups were attacking civilians with impunity. There, as part of a three-person team, she assessed public health needs, especially those of women, and made recommendations to the UN Security Council on priorities for future public health responses.

Soon after, she participated in humanitarian aid missions to Burundi, Iraq, and Liberia. In all of this humanitarian work, she recognized that the existing framework for emergency humanitarian assistance failed to disrupt cycles of violence, hunger, and dependency in these countries. She envisioned the need for a different approach, based on local civil-society organizations, local resilience, and local sustainable solutions.

In 2000, in partnership with her husband, Eric Hoskins, and others, she established War Child Canada (and later War Child USA), an organization based on developing long-term partnerships with local leaders to build capacity to address health, nutrition, and related problems. At first—and many times since—she traveled to several war-torn countries, met with local leaders, and actively listened to their needs and what they saw as solutions. As a result of many conversations, the organization evolved to provide grants to grassroots projects in three areas: education for women and children, access to justice for victims of sexual and gender-based violence, and economic development and food security.

From Horror to Hope. Barry S. Levy, Oxford University Press. © Oxford University Press 2022.
DOI: 10.1093/oso/9780197558645.003.0022

Over the past two decades, this grassroots approach has demonstrated its effectiveness, which has given War Child Canada credibility and has helped to elicit financial support. It now has an annual budget of approximately $20 million and 400 full-time and part-time staff members. It works in partnership with local communities and local civil-society organizations. Throughout the world, 99% of its staff members are local to the communities and the countries that they serve. Some of its national partners are now independently funded, but some still need an additional capacity boost that its teams provide.

During 2019, the organization served 600,000 children in eight regions of the world. In the Democratic Republic of the Congo, one of its programs focuses on catch-up learning for children displaced by conflict; it has served a half million children, who now do better on national examinations than comparable children attending school. In Afghanistan and Uganda, War Child Canada provides legal defense for children who have been sexually exploited and for girls and women who refuse to succumb to family pressures to marry at a very young age. In Sudan and South Sudan, it provides food security, peacebuilding initiatives, and economic development by providing vocational training for women.

Looking back, Dr. Nutt recognizes that building a new organization in a different paradigm took determination, willful persistence, tenacity, resilience, and personal and financial sacrifice. She observes, "Giving up was never an option."

Why does Dr. Nutt continue to do this work? "It is extremely gratifying to be part of something much bigger than yourself, to fight so that others can have the rights and opportunities everyone deserves," she replies. "The work is deeply rewarding—intellectually, psychologically, and emotionally. It addresses issues that really matter."

Dr. Nutt is Founder and President of War Child Canada/USA and a Staff Physician at Women's College Hospital, Toronto.

PART IV

Other Impacts and Their Documentation

12

Health Impacts on Military Personnel and Veterans

Older men declare war. But it is youth that must fight and die.
HERBERT HOOVER

INTRODUCTION

This chapter focuses mainly on morbidity and mortality of U.S. military personnel. But it does not reflect the higher morbidity and mortality rates of military forces in low- and middle-income countries, who have had far less access than U.S. service members to protective equipment, emergency evacuation, and quality medical care.

MORTALITY

It was reported in 1991 that military forces worldwide in the first nine decades of the 20th century incurred 458,000 deaths annually, on average—a number *more than 36 times greater* than in the three previous centuries. And their annual average mortality rate of 183 per one million military personnel was *more than 11 times greater* than in the three previous centuries.[1]

Compared to the U.S. Civil War, the First World War, the Korean War, and the Vietnam War, the Second World War had, by far, the highest *total number of deaths of all military forces*—more than 5.5 million per year of warfare. Considering these five wars as well as the American Revolution, the highest *rates* of *U.S. service members* killed and wounded occurred during the Civil War (Table 12-1).

Before the First World War, more U.S. troops died from diseases than battles. For example, during the Spanish-American War, U.S. troops had more than five times more disease deaths than battle deaths. In contrast, during the First World War, U.S. troops had almost three times as many battle deaths than disease deaths (before the influenza pandemic). And during the Second World War, U.S. troops in Europe incurred about 100 times more battle deaths than disease deaths. The significant decrease in the percentage

From Horror to Hope. Barry S. Levy, Oxford University Press. © Oxford University Press 2022.
DOI: 10.1093/oso/9780197558645.003.0023

TABLE 12-1 Battle Deaths and Nonmortal Woundings Among U.S. Service Members, Selected Wars

War	Total U.S. Service Members	Battle Deaths		Nonmortal Woundings	
		Number	Rate[a]	Number	Rate[a]
American Revolution	217,000[b]	4,435	2,044	6,188	2,852
Civil War	3,263,363	214,938	6,586	281,881[c]	8,638
First World War	4,734,991	53,402	1,128	204,002	4,308
Second World War	16,112,566	291,557	1,810	670,846	4,163
Korean War	1,789,000[d]	33,739	1,886	103,284	5,773
Vietnam War	3,403,000[e]	47,434	1,394	153,303	4,505
Gulf War	694,550[f]	148	21	467	67
Iraq War	141,450[g]	3,479	306[h]	31,993	2,837[h]
Afghanistan War	30,400[i]	1,844	280[j]	20,131	2,584[j]

[a] Per 100,000 service members.
[b] Exact number is unknown; this number is the median of the estimated range of 184,000 to 250,000.
[c] Union troops only; for Confederate troops, this number is not known.
[d] Total U.S. service members in theater of war.
[e] Total U.S. service members deployed to Southeast Asia.
[f] Total U.S. service members deployed to the Persian Gulf.
[g] Median annual number, fiscal years 2003–2010. Range: 88,300–157,800.
[h] Average annual rate, fiscal years 2003–2010.
[i] Median annual number, 2001–2014. Range: 2,500–90,000.
[j] Average annual rate, 2001–2014.
(Sources: For the first seven wars listed: Department of Veterans Affairs. America's Wars. Washington, DC: Department of Veterans Affairs, November 2020. Available at: https://www.va.gov/opa/publications/factsheets/fs_americas_wars.pdf. Accessed on February 3, 2021. For the Iraq War: Gollob S, O'Hanlon ME. Iraq Index. Foreign Policy at Brookings, August 2020. Available at: https://www.brookings.edu/wp-content/uploads/2020/08/FP_20200825_iraq_index.pdf. Accessed on August 24, 2021; and U.S. Department of Defense, Defense Casualty Analysis System. U.S. Military Casualties—Operation Iraqi Freedom [OIF] Casualty Summary by Month and Service. Available at: https://dcas.dmdc.osd.mil/dcas/pages/report_oif_month.xhtml. Accessed on August 24, 2021. For the Afghanistan War: Gollob S, O'Hanlon ME. Afghanistan Index. Foreign Policy at Brookings, August 2020. Available at: https://www.brookings.edu/wp-content/uploads/2020/08/FP_20200825_afganistan_index.pdf. Accessed on August 24, 2021; and U.S. Department of Defense, Defense Casualty Analysis System. U.S. Military Casualties—Operation Enduring Freedom [OEF] Casualty Summary by Month and Service. Available at: https://dcas.dmdc.osd.mil/dcas/pages/report_oef_month.xhtml. Accessed on August 24, 2021.)

of deaths from disease during war resulted mainly from vastly improved medical care and public health measures.[1] An exception to this trend occurred among Australian troops who fought in the Second World War in tropical areas of Asia, where malaria and other communicable diseases were highly prevalent; they had 16 times more disease deaths than battle deaths.[1]

Over the course of decades, there have been three other major trends in deaths among U.S. military personnel during war:

- The case-fatality rate for combat wounds markedly decreased—from 14.1% in the Civil War, to 4.5% in the Second World War, and 3.6% in the Vietnam War.
- The proportion of all deaths during war due to nonintentional (accidental) injuries markedly increased from 3% during the Civil War, to 16% during the Second World War, and 46% in the Gulf War.[1]

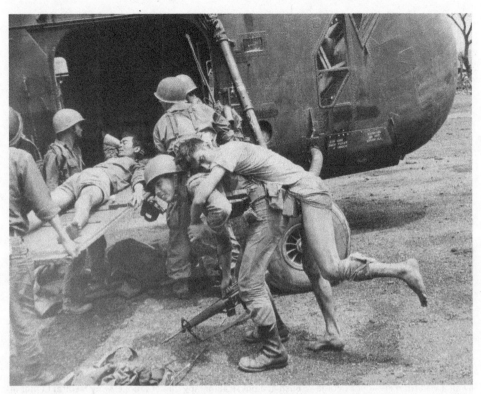

FIGURE 12-1 An exhausted and wounded South Vietnamese paratrooper is dragged by a comrade to a rescue helicopter in Thuan Loi, South Vietnam, in 1965. (AP Photo/Horst Faas.)

- Starting with the Vietnam War, many wounded soldiers survived because of rapid evacuation from war zones and highly specialized and coordinated treatment (Figure 12-1).

INJURIES AND MUSCULOSKELETAL DISORDERS

During war, injuries generally occur more frequently than illnesses. Among *combat* injuries suffered by U.S. military personnel deployed to Iraq and Afghanistan, 82% were caused by explosive blasts and 14% from gunshots. Fractures accounted for 40% of musculoskeletal combat wounds and 6% of musculoskeletal combat wounds required amputations (Figure 12-2).[2] *Non-combat* injuries among deployed U.S. military personnel occurred at more than three times the rate of combat injuries.[3]

Costs for treating veterans of the Iraq and Afghanistan wars have been extremely high for two major reasons. First, many injured veterans survived injuries that would have killed soldiers in previous wars. Second, attacks with improvised explosive devices caused polytraumatic injuries—brain injury, severe facial trauma, blindness, and multiple limb injuries—that have required long periods of treatment and rehabilitation.[4]

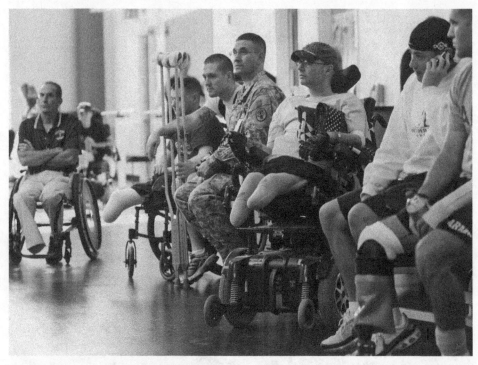

FIGURE 12-2 American veterans with disabilities, several of whom had suffered limb amputations, await a visit from President George W. Bush at a physical therapy unit at Brooke Army Medical Center in San Antonio in 2007. (AP Photo/Gerald Hebert.)

Combat explosions during the Iraq War frequently caused multiple injuries—an average of 3.8 per explosion episode. The most frequent injury, affecting 11% of those injured, was mild traumatic brain injury (TBI, see page 209). Other frequent injuries included wounds of the legs and face and rupture of the tympanic membrane.[5]

Infections frequently occur as a result of combat-related injuries.[6] Infectious complications, especially skin and soft-tissue infections and osteomyelitis, have occurred in as many as 33% of wounded U.S. service members.[7] And chronic pain is a frequent complication of war-related injuries.[8]

Antimicrobial resistance has emerged as a major problem in treating infections in military personnel. During the Iraq War, a multiply resistant gram-negative bacterium, *Acinetobacter baumannii*, was detected in open wounds and fractures in U.S. soldiers. This organism spread to civilian populations in many other countries.[9] By 2014, it was among the six most important multidrug-resistant microorganisms in hospitals worldwide, most commonly causing ventilator-associated pneumonia and bloodstream infections, with high case-fatality rates.[10]

After deployment, combat-zone veterans have increased rates of fatal injuries. U.S. veterans who served in combat zones in the Vietnam War or the Gulf War had a 26% increase in injury-related deaths—many related to motor vehicle crashes. Possible causes and contributing factors to this increase have included posttraumatic stress, substance abuse, other war-related conditions, and reduced perception of risks on return to civilian society.[11]

Musculoskeletal disorders (MSDs)—injuries caused or aggravated by work tasks such as lifting, pushing, and pulling—frequently occur in military populations and often lead to long-term disability. For example, among Swedish soldiers serving in Afghanistan for 6-month deployments, 47% reported musculoskeletal complaints and injuries during deployment. The high occurrence of MSDs was partially due to the amount of weight carried—infantry soldiers wore equipment weighing 66 to 88 pounds, three or four times a week, up to 11 hours at a time.[12]

SEXUAL ASSAULTS

During deployment, women have faced many of the same health and safety risks as male military personnel. But, compared to men, they have been at increased risk of being sexually assaulted. Sexual assault of female veterans has been associated with a sixfold increase in reported posttraumatic stress disorder (PTSD) and a fourfold increase in reported depression.[13-15] (See Section on Gender-Based Violence in Chapter 6.)

Commanders in the U.S. military had long been responsible for prosecuting service members for sexual assaults. This policy constrained women who had been sexually assaulted in the military from reporting these assaults. In 2021, this policy, which had been part of the Uniform Code of Military Justice, was being changed to shift responsibility away from military commanders for prosecuting sexual assaults and related crimes. The Department of Defense was planning to create dedicated offices within each military service, with independent military lawyers taking over this role.[16]

MENTAL DISORDERS
PTSD and Depression

Over the past century, mental disorders have occurred frequently among soldiers. During the First World War, rates of hospital admission for "shell shock" increased during offensive military operations; among hospitalized soldiers, 21% "broke down" within 3 months of being deployed—and few directly returned to their combat units.[17] Among military veterans and nonmilitary war survivors of the Second World War—many of whom had experienced injuries, witnessed atrocities, or had been persecuted or placed in concentration camps—PTSD, depression, and suicidal thoughts were prevalent. During the decades after the war, these mental disorders were associated with higher mortality rates.[18]

During and after the Vietnam War, U.S. military personnel frequently suffered from mental disorders, including substance abuse. A study of Vietnam War veterans found that 19% had developed war-related PTSD and that, even 11 to 12 years after the war, 9% were suffering from PTSD.[19] Vietnam War–era veterans who fought in the war zone and probably had PTSD were more than twice as likely to have died than those without PTSD.[20] And 30 years after the war had ended, almost 75% of Vietnam War–era veterans reported at least one mental disorder, most frequently alcohol abuse and/or dependence (54%), nicotine dependence (48%), and PTSD (10%).[21]

A meta-analysis of studies on almost five million U.S. veterans of the Iraq and Afghanistan wars estimated that 23% had PTSD.[22] Risk factors for PTSD in veterans and military personnel included:

- *Pretrauma factors*, such as lower education, intelligence, military rank, and socioeconomic status; prior trauma; prior psychiatric history or symptoms; family psychiatric history; behavioral problems in childhood; and childhood abuse or adversity
- *Trauma characteristics*, including severity of trauma/combat exposure, perceived life threat, combat-related injury, peri-trauma distress or dissociation, and exposure to death, killing, or abusive violence
- *Posttrauma factors*, including lack of social support, negative homecoming experience, and exposure to additional life stressors.[23]

Depressive disorders also occur frequently among military personnel during and after deployment. A systematic review and meta-analysis found a 60% increase in depressive disorders as a result of military combat.[24] Another systematic review and meta-analysis found that Gulf War veterans had a 128% increased risk of depression.[25]

Mental Health of Women

In several countries, including France, Germany, New Zealand, Norway, Sweden, Canada, and the United States, an increasing number of women have served as military personnel—usually in non-combat roles, such as nursing, intelligence, logistics, and food preparation and service. U.S. female veterans of recent wars have had increased rates of mental disorders, including PTSD, depression, binge drinking, sleep disorders, and suicide.[26,27] Risk factors have included being attacked with improvised explosive devices, witnessing killing, handling human remains, and feeling helpless to defend or counterattack.

During post-deployment reintegration into society, female veterans have also suffered from psychosocial problems related to relationships, parenting, health issues, and homelessness. They have often faced gender-based barriers because their combat-related duties have been undervalued. And, after intense transformative experiences during military service, they have often returned to communities where gender relations and patriarchy are rigid.[28]

Mental Health of Prisoners of War

Prisoners of war (POWs) suffer from severe psychological trauma, which adversely affects their relationships. POWs, especially those who suffered severe trauma during captivity and those with PTSD symptoms, have often verbally and physically abused their partners after returning home.[29]

Some older veterans still suffer from having been POWs many years before. Former POWs from the Second World War and the Korean War have had an increased risk of PTSD.[30,31] POWs with PTSD have increased prevalence of cardiovascular disease and dementia.[31,32] And POWs from the Second World War and the Korean War age 75 and older have had an increased mortality rate due to heart disease.[33]

Suicide

From 1990 to 2007, annual suicide rates in the U.S. military were far below those in demographically similar civilian populations, possibly due to the *healthy soldier effect*—in which their morbidity and mortality rates have been lower than those of the general population because their selection by the military was partly based on their good health. These relatively low suicide rates may also have resulted from soldiers' perception of meaningful employment, military leadership, and high military morale. However, the suicide rates in the U.S. military increased after the start of the Iraq War in 2003; during that year, the suicide rate for soldiers deployed to Iraq was 18.3 per 100,000 compared to 11.9 per 100,000 among non-deployed soldiers. The suicide rate among active-duty members of the U.S. Army increased to 19.6 in 2008 and 29.2 in 2012—substantially higher than the suicide rate in the U.S. civilian population (12.1 per 100,000 in 2010).[34]

Among U.S. service members who committed suicide during the 2012–2015 period, 19% had three or more deployments, 38% had a failed or failing intimate partner relationship, and 25% had a disorder related to substance abuse or dependence.[35] Other potential contributing factors included killing or witnessing death in combat, dangers while patrolling civilian areas, PTSD, TBI, physical or sexual assault, chronic pain, separation from family, being ostracized, and feeling that one has let one's unit down.[36–38]

Suicide risk has also been strongly associated with *moral injury*—"perpetrating, failing to prevent, bearing witness to, or learning about acts that transgress deeply held moral beliefs."[39] Moral injury is characterized by a sense of meaninglessness, feelings of shame and grief, and remorse from having violated core moral beliefs. Military personnel who have been raised in a religious environment may be especially vulnerable to moral injury.[40]

Grief and Related Issues

Grief among veterans of wars is an important problem that has been largely overlooked. U.S. combat veterans of the Iraq and Afghanistan wars who had lost comrades due to combat or suicide have described prolonged mental and physical health consequences of grief, including adverse effects on family relationships.[41]

In transition to civilian life, military veterans experience loss of their military persona and nostalgia for military service.[42] Journalist Sebastian Junger has observed that what many veterans miss is "brotherhood"—"a mutual agreement in a group [such] that . . . you will put the safety of everyone in the group above your own."[43] Multiple deployments make this transition more challenging. Reflecting the challenges of this transition, military personnel have an increased risk of death within several years of discharge from active duty. U.S. Army Vietnam veterans had an increased mortality rate during the first 5 years after discharge from external causes of death, including unintentional poisoning and drugs.[44]

TABLE 12-2 Illustrative Examples of Communicable Diseases for Which Military Personnel Are at Increased Risk

Category	Illustrative Examples
Foodborne and waterborne diseases	Diarrheal diseases caused by bacteria and protozoa
	Hepatitis A and hepatitis E
	Typhoid and paratyphoid fever
	Brucellosis
Vector-borne diseases	Malaria
	Dengue fever
	Yellow fever
	Chikungunya viral infection
	Various rickettsial diseases
	West Nile fever
	Leishmaniasis
Infections associated with water contact	Schistosomiasis
	Leptospirosis
Sexually transmitted infections	Hepatitis B
	Gonorrhea
	Chlamydia infection
	HIV/AIDS
Airborne diseases	Tuberculosis
	Meningococcal meningitis
	COVID-19
	Influenza
Diseases transmitted by dust, soil, or animal contact	Lassa fever
	Rabies
	Q fever
	Anthrax
Other diseases transmitted person to person	Ebola virus disease
	Monkeypox

(Sources: Sanchez JL, Cooper MJ, Myers CA, et al. Respiratory infections in the U.S. military: Recent experience and control. Clinical Microbiology Reviews 2015; 28: 743-800; Murray CK, Yun HC, Markelz AE, et al. Operation United Assistance: Infectious disease threats to deployed military personnel. Military Medicine 2015; 180: 626-651.)

COMMUNICABLE DISEASES

Military personnel are at increased risk for a wide variety of communicable diseases (Table 12-2). Physicians sometimes fail to diagnose these diseases correctly because they are not familiar with them and because symptoms are often nonspecific.

Types of vector-borne illness threats to U.S. military personnel have evolved over time. Some diseases, such as yellow fever, have declined in incidence. Others, such as malaria and dengue fever, continue to occur frequently. Still others, such as those due to West Nile virus and chikungunya virus, have emerged.[45] The COVID-19 pandemic has presented new challenges for military service members.[46,47]

RESPIRATORY DISORDERS

U.S. military personnel deployed to Iraq and Afghanistan have been exposed to desert dust, burn pit emissions, diesel and jet-fuel exhaust, oil well fires (Figure 13-1 in Chapter 13), emissions from local industrial plants, and other air contaminants. Deployment-related respiratory disorders have included new-onset asthma and exacerbation of preexisting asthma. And they also have included chronic obstructive pulmonary disease (COPD), constrictive and respiratory bronchiolitis, allergic rhinitis, and other disorders.[48-54] Blast lung injury has occurred frequently and has often been fatal; most survivors have required ventilatory support.[55]

Open-air burn pits are areas on deployed military bases used for combustion of waste—chemicals, paint, cans, munitions, unexploded ordnance, and medical and human waste. Emissions from these burn pits often include particulate matter, dioxins, heavy metals, volatile organic compounds, and polycyclic aromatic hydrocarbons. Exposure to these air contaminants can cause asthma, bronchitis, COPD, constrictive bronchiolitis, and other chronic respiratory diseases.[56] Among U.S. military personnel deployed to Iraq and Afghanistan, there was a dose–response relationship between self-reported exposure to burn pit smoke and self-reported emphysema, chronic bronchitis, and COPD.[57]

TRAUMATIC BRAIN INJURY

Traumatic brain injury (TBI)—"a traumatically induced structural injury of the brain or physiologic disruption of normal brain function resulting from an external force"—has occurred among military personnel after they have been exposed to an explosion or other physically traumatic event. TBI can be caused by penetrating trauma or blunt force, including acceleration/deceleration forces that cause the brain to collide with the skull. More than 350,000 U.S. service members deployed to Iraq and Afghanistan were diagnosed with TBI between 2000 and 2016.[58]

The diagnosis of TBI is suggested by loss of consciousness, loss of memory of events immediately before or after the traumatic event, altered mental state, neurological deficits, and the presence of an intracranial lesion on imaging studies. Mild TBI is associated with nonspecific symptoms, such as headache, dizziness, nausea, and fatigue; cognitive symptoms, such as memory impairment, impulsiveness, and difficulty concentrating; and psychological symptoms, such as irritability, anxiety, and depression. Moderate to severe TBI can be associated with diminished sensation, impaired depth perception, seizures, tinnitus, dementia, aphasia, peripheral neuropathy, abnormal social behavior, abnormal executive functioning, and social detachment. The long-term consequences of TBI are not clear.[58-60]

ILLNESS DUE TO TOXIC EXPOSURES

Exposures to toxic chemicals can cause illness in military personnel. U.S. veterans of the Gulf War who had been exposed to chemical warfare agents, pesticides, prophylactic medications to protect against hazardous exposures, and emissions from hundreds of oil well fires returned home with multiple health problems. A substantial number developed *Gulf War Illness* (also known as *Gulf War Syndrome*), a multisystem illness characterized by fatigue, headaches, cognitive dysfunction, musculoskeletal pain, and respiratory, gastrointestinal, and skin symptoms.

A systematic review and meta-analysis of multisymptom illness in Gulf War veterans, based on seven studies of American, British, and Australian veterans, found that its prevalence ranged from 26% to 65% among them, in contrast to 12% to 37% in comparison groups.[61] Exposures to pesticides and/or pyridostigmine bromide, a prophylactic medication that was administered to protect against possible nerve gas attacks, likely caused Gulf War Illness and neurological dysfunction in Gulf War veterans. Exposures to sarin, cyclosarin, and oil well fires have also been associated with neurological disorders.[62,63]

During the Gulf War, U.S. military personnel were exposed to depleted uranium, a radioactive and toxic chemical that might cause birth defects (Chapter 9). Forty-two Gulf War veterans who had been wounded in "friendly fire" incidents involving depleted uranium and had then been monitored in a clinical surveillance program since 1993, underwent a comprehensive health assessment in 2017. After 24 years of surveillance, they had decreased bone density, increased blood estradiol concentrations, and slightly reduced kidney function. But no other abnormalities were identified.[64]

SENSORY IMPAIRMENT

Combat exposure to blasts can result in peripheral damage to the ears and eyes as well as central damage to the auditory and visual processing areas in the brain.[65] During the First World War and its aftermath, hearing impairment due to weapons fire occurred in soldiers who had exposures up to 185 dB (decibels) of sustained noise. (The permissible exposure limit of the Occupational Safety and Health Administration is 90 dB as an 8-hour time-weighted average.) An estimated 2.4% of British and Allied troops were disabled by hearing loss.[66] Among Iraq and Afghanistan war veterans, who had been exposed to blasts and explosions, ototoxic chemicals, and high levels of noise, 7.8% were diagnosed with hearing loss, 6.5% with tinnitus, and 6.2% with both disorders.[67]

NONCOMMUNICABLE DISEASES
Cardiovascular Disease

Hypertension and obesity have occurred at rates higher than expected in U.S. military personnel. Among service members, many of whom had been deployed to Iraq and Afghanistan, 6.9% developed hypertension between baseline assessment and follow-up approximately 3 years later. Among deployed service members, those reporting multiple combat exposures were 33% more likely to report hypertension than those who had no combat exposure.[68]

Among more than 50,000 U.S. service members wounded in Iraq and Afghanistan, severity of combat injury has been associated with subsequent development of hypertension and coronary artery disease (as well as diabetes mellitus and chronic kidney disease).[69] In addition, combat-related traumatic injury has been associated with an 80% increase in risk for death due to cardiovascular disease and, more specifically, a 57% increase in risk for death due to coronary heart disease, although the evidence for these findings has been weak.[70]

Cancer

Military personnel can be exposed to chemical carcinogens and ionizing radiation. The overall occurrence of cancer among military personnel as a result of these exposures has not been adequately studied. But the potential exists to study cancer morbidity and mortality, especially among military personnel of the United States and other high-income countries.

Occurrence of some malignancies has been increased among U.S. military personnel who had been exposed to Agent Orange, a mixture of chemicals that was contaminated with a potent carcinogen (tetrachlorodibenzo-*p*-dioxin, also known as TCDD and dioxin). Veterans who mixed and sprayed Agent Orange and other dioxin-contaminated herbicides in Vietnam from 1962 to 1971 have experienced increased incidence of several malignant and nonmalignant diseases (Figure 10-1 on page 173).[71]

A recent update on veterans who had been exposed to Agent Orange found "sufficient evidence" of an association between Agent Orange and soft-tissue sarcoma, non-Hodgkin lymphoma, chronic lymphocytic leukemia (CLL, a form of non-Hodgkin lymphoma), Hodgkin lymphoma, and chloracne. It also found "limited or suggestive evidence" of an association between Agent Orange exposure and (a) additional cancers, including laryngeal cancer, lung cancer, prostate cancer, bladder cancer, and multiple myeloma, and (b) nonmalignant diseases, including amyloid light-chain amyloidosis, early onset peripheral neuropathy, Parkinson disease, porphyria cutanea tarda, hypertension, ischemic heart disease, stroke, type 2 diabetes, and hypothyroidism.[72] Studies have also found evidence of increased mortality due to circulatory system disease and increased incidence of diabetes and high-grade prostate cancer among veterans exposed to Agent Orange and other herbicides during the Vietnam War.[73,74] (See Chapters 10 and 13.)

Several additional studies have found that military veterans have had increased morbidity or mortality due to cancer:

- U.S. veterans of the Gulf War who had been potentially exposed to the destruction of chemical munitions at Khamisiyah, Iraq, and to the smoke from oil well fires had increased brain cancer mortality.[75,76]
- Korean Vietnam veterans had a higher incidence of prostate cancer and other malignancies.[77]
- U.S. veterans deployed to the Persian Gulf during the Gulf War had an increased incidence of lung cancer.[78]

Many military personnel have been exposed to ionizing radiation, such as U.S. military participants in nuclear weapons tests. A study of more than 12,000 veterans who had been exposed to one or more of 30 atmospheric nuclear tests in 1957 at the Nevada Test Site found that the 3,020 veterans who had been exposed to the SMOKY test had an 89% increase in leukemia (excluding CLL).[79] A study of U.S. military personnel who received the highest gamma radiation doses while participating in atmospheric nuclear weapons tests found that they had more than a threefold increase in mortality from lymphopoietic cancers.[80] A study of U.S. Navy veterans who had participated in atmospheric nuclear tests in the Pacific in 1958 found that they had increased death rates, including more than a sixfold increase in liver cancer mortality.[81] But a study of more than 114,000 male military participants at eight above-ground nuclear weapons test series did not find any significant increase in mortality for non-CLL leukemia or several other malignancies, although their estimated mean doses of radiation to several organs were considered to be low.[82] (See Chapters 5 and 10.)

The U.S. Department of Veterans Affairs has recognized the following diseases as being associated with ionizing radiation exposure and for which veterans may be eligible for disability compensation and healthcare: cancers of the bile ducts, bone, brain, breast, colon, esophagus, gall bladder, liver, lung, pharynx, pancreas, ovary, salivary gland, small intestine, stomach, thyroid, and urinary tract as well as non-CLL leukemia, non-Hodgkin lymphoma, and multiple myeloma.[83]

Distribution of Tobacco Products to Military

The U.S. military has promoted tobacco use among service members. During the Second World War and the Korean War era, the U.S. military distributed cigarettes at no cost to overseas military personnel and provided tobacco products at a reduced cost on military bases within the United States. Although the United States stopped providing cigarettes to its overseas personnel as part of rations in 1975, tobacco products continued to be sold at subsidized prices on U.S. military bases until several years ago.[84,85]

PREVENTING MORBIDITY AND MORTALITY

Prevention of morbidity and mortality in military personnel focuses largely on preventing injuries and MSDs, communicable diseases, and mental disorders and substance abuse.

Preventing Injuries and MSDs

Strategies to prevent major injuries have included conditioning; footwear modification; bracing; physical fitness; leadership, supervision, and awareness; and reducing the volume of physical activity.[86] Medical surveillance programs can improve identification of problems needing specific attention.[87]

Preventing Communicable Diseases

Measures implemented to prevent communicable diseases are specific to the area of deployment. Prevention includes preparing for situations that may be encountered, such as treating communicable diseases in remote locations; educating service members on communicable disease threats endemic to the areas of deployment; implementing personal protective measures, such as avoiding disease-transmitting vectors and potentially contaminated water; providing recommended immunizations and malaria chemoprophylaxis, as indicated; and conducting ongoing surveillance.[88]

Preventing Mental Disorders and Substance Use

Much can be done to improve prevention of mental disorders and substance use. Military leaders can better recognize and understand risk factors for suicide and other mental disorders and can improve interventions at the individual and organizational level. Barriers that discourage service members from seeking care for mental disorders need to be reduced or eliminated.[89] And measures can be implemented to better address the impact of mental and substance use disorders on family members.

The Institute of Medicine, in 2014, conducted a systematic review of prevention strategies for behavioral and mental disorders in military personnel and their families. It found that most U.S. Department of Defense programs were not consistently based on evidence and that programs were not evaluated frequently or adequately. It recommended that the Department of Defense implement only evidence-based programs; develop, test, monitor, and evaluate new programs; and implement comprehensive evidence-based programs for psychological health for military personnel and their families.[90]

SUMMARY POINTS

- U.S. military personnel have lower rates of morbidity and mortality than do military forces in low- and middle-income countries.
- Survivors of war-related injuries often suffer infectious complications, long-term disabilities, and chronic pain.
- Military personnel are at high risk of PTSD, depression, substance use, and suicide.
- Depending on the nature and location of their deployments, military personnel can be at increased risk for a variety of communicable diseases.
- After deployment, military veterans face additional challenges to their physical and mental health, which can also impact their families.

REFERENCES

1. Garfield RM, Neugut AI. Epidemiologic analysis of warfare: A historical review. Journal of the American Medical Association 1991; 266: 688-692.
2. Belmont PJ Jr, McCriskin BJ, Hsiao MS, et al. The nature and incidence of musculoskeletal combat wounds in Iraq and Afghanistan (2005–2009). Journal of Orthopedic Trauma 2013; 27: e107-e113.
3. Belmont PJ, Owens BD, Schoenfeld AJ. Musculoskeletal injuries in Iraq and Afghanistan: Epidemiology and outcomes following a decade of war. Journal of the American Academy of Orthopedic Surgeons 2016; 24: 341-348.
4. Geiling J, Rosen JM, Edwards RD. Medical costs of war in 2035: Long-term care challenges for veterans of Iraq and Afghanistan. Military Medicine 2012; 177: 1235-1244.
5. Eskridge SL, Macera CA, Galarneau MR, et al. Injuries from combat explosions in Iraq. Injury 2012; 43: 1678-1682.
6. Murray CK, Hinkle MK, Yun HC. History of infections associated with combat-related injuries. Journal of Trauma 2008; Suppl 3: S221-S231.
7. McDonald JR, Liang SY, Li P, et al. Infectious complications after deployment trauma: Following wounded US military personnel into Veterans Affairs care. Clinical Infectious Diseases 2018; 67: 1205-1212.

8. George E, Elman I, Becerra L, et al. Pain in an era of armed conflicts: Prevention and treatment for warfighters and civilian casualties. Progress in Neurobiology 2016; 141: 25-44.

9. Dewachi O, Skelton M, Nguyen V-K, et al. Changing therapeutic geographies of the Iraqi and Syrian wars. Lancet 2014; 383: 449-457.

10. Antunes LCS, Visca P, Towner KJ. *Acinetobacter baumannii*: Evolution of a global pathogen. Pathogens and Disease 2014; 71: 292-301.

11. Knapik JJ, Marin RE, Grier TL, Jones BH. A systematic review of post-deployment injury-related mortality among military personnel deployed to conflict zones. BMC Public Health 2009; 9: 231. doi:10.1186/1471-2458- 9-231.

12. Halvarsson A, Hagman I, Tegem M, et al. Self-reported musculoskeletal complaints and injuries and exposure of physical workload in Swedish soldiers serving in Afghanistan. PLoS ONE 2018; 3(4): e0195548. doi: 10.1371/journal.pone.0195548.

13. Murphy F, Browne D, Mather S, et al. Women in the Persian Gulf War: Healthcare implications for active duty troops and veterans. Military Medicine 1997; 162: 656-660.

14. Doherty ME, Scannell-Desch E. Women's health and hygiene experiences during deployment to the Iraq and Afghanistan wars, 2003 through 2010. Journal of Midwifery and Women's Health 2012; 57: 172-177.

15. Pulverman CS, Creech SK, Mengeling MA, et al. Sexual assault in the military and increased odds of sexual pain among female veterans. Obstetrics & Gynecology 2019; 134: 63-71.

16. Lopez CT. Sexual assaults will no longer be prosecuted by commanders. DoD News, U.S. Department of Defense, July 2, 2021. Available at: https://www.defense.gov/News/News-Stories/Article/Article/2681848/sexual-assaults-will-no-longer-be-prosecuted-by-commanders/. Accessed on November 26, 2021.

17. Jones E, Thomas A, Ironside S. Shell shock: An outcome study of a First World War 'PIE' unit. Psychological Medicine 2007; 37: 215-223.

18. Bramsen I, Deeg DJ, van Der Ploeg E, Fransman S. Wartime stressors and mental health symptoms as predictors of late-life mortality in World War II survivors. Journal of Affective Disorders 2007; 103: 121-129.

19. Dohrenwend BP, Turner JB, Turse NA, et al. The psychological risk of Vietnam for U.S. veterans: A revisit with new data and methods. Science 2006; 313: 979-982.

20. Schlenger WE, Corry NH, Williams CS, et al. A prospective study of mortality and trauma-related risk factors among a nationally representative sample of Vietnam veterans. American Journal of Epidemiology 2015; 182: 980-990.

21. Eisen SA, Griffith KH, Xian H, et al. Lifetime and 12-month prevalence of psychiatric disorders in 8,169 male Vietnam War era veterans. Military Medicine 2004; 169: 896-902.

22. Fulton JJ, Calhoun PS, Wagner HR, et al. The prevalence of posttraumatic stress disorder in Operation Enduring Freedom/Operation Iraqi Freedom (OEF/OIF) veterans: A meta-analysis. Journal of Anxiety Disorders 2015; 31: 98-107.

23. Gates MA, Holowka DW, Vasterling JJ, et al. Posttraumatic stress disorder in veterans and military personnel: Epidemiology, screening, and case recognition. Psychological Services 2012; 9: 361-382.

24. Bonde MP, Utzon-Frank N, Bertelsen M, et al. Risk of depressive disorder following disasters and military deployment: Systematic review with meta-analysis. British Journal of Psychiatry 2016; 208: 330-336.

25. Blore JD, Sim MR, Forbes AB, et al. Depression in Gulf War veterans: A systematic review and meta-analysis. Psychological Medicine 2015; 45: 1565-1580.

26. Boyd MA, Bradshaw W, Robinson M. Mental health issues of women deployed to Iraq and Afghanistan. Archives of Psychiatric Nursing 2013; 27: 10-22.

27. Hoge CW, Clark JC, Castro CA. Commentary: Women in combat and the risk of post-traumatic stress disorder and depression. International Journal of Epidemiology 2007; 36: 327-329.

28. Rajivan AK, Senarathne R. Women in armed conflicts: Inclusion and exclusion (Asia-Pacific Human Development Report Background Papers Series, 2010/11). New York: United Nations Development Programme, 2011. Available at: https://www.undp.org/content/dam/rbap/docs/Research%20&%20Publications/human_development/RBAP-APHDR-TBP_2010_11.pdf. Accessed on September 7, 2020.

29. O'Donnell C, Cook JM, Thompson R, et al. Verbal and physical aggression in World War II former prisoners of war: Role of posttraumatic stress disorder and depression. Journal of Traumatic Stress 2006; 19: 859-866.

30. Port CL, Engdahl B, Frazier P. A longitudinal and retrospective study of PTSD among older prisoners of war. American Journal of Psychiatry 2001; 158: 1474-1479.

31. Kang HK, Bullman TA, Taylor JW. Risk of selected cardiovascular diseases and posttraumatic stress disorder among former World War II prisoners of war. Annals of Epidemiology 2006; 16: 381-386.

32. Meziab O, Kirby KA, Williams B, et al. Prisoner of war status, posttraumatic stress disorder, and dementia in older veterans. Alzheimer's & Dementia 2014; 10: S236-S241.

33. Page WF, Brass LM. Long-term heart disease and stroke mortality among former American prisoners of war of World War II and the Korean conflict: Results of a 50-year follow-up. Military Medicine 2001; 166: 803-808.

34. Reger MA, Tucker RP, Carter SP, Ammerman BA. Military deployment and suicide: A critical examination. Perspectives on Psychological Science 2018; 13: 688-699.

35. Pruitt LD, Smolenski DJ, Bush NE, et al. Suicide in the military: Understanding rates and risk factors across the United States Armed Forces. Military Medicine 2018; 184: 432-437.

36. Hyman J, Ireland R, Frost L, Cottrell L. Suicide incidence and risk factors in an active duty US military population. American Journal of Public Health 2012; 102: S138-S146.

37. Ursano RJ, Kessler RC, Stein MB, et al. Suicide attempts in the US Army during the wars in Afghanistan and Iraq, 2004 to 2009. JAMA Psychiatry 2015; 72: 917-926.

38. Nock MK, Deming CA, Fullerton CS, et al. Suicide among soldiers: A review of psychosocial risk and protective factors. Psychiatry 2013; 76: 97-125.

39. Litz BT, Stein N, Delaney E, et al. Moral injury and moral repair in war veterans: A preliminary model and intervention strategy. Clinical Psychological Review 2009; 29: 695-706.

40. Ames D, Erickson Z, Youssef NA, et al. Moral injury, religiosity, and suicide risk in U.S. veterans and active duty military with PTSD symptoms. Military Medicine 2018; 184: e271-e278.

41. Lubens P, Silver RC. U.S. combat veterans' responses to suicide and combat deaths: A mixed-methods study. Social Science & Medicine 2019; 236: 112341. doi: 10.1016/j.socscimed.2019.05.046.

42. Mobbs MC, Bonanno GA. Beyond war and PTSD: The crucial role of transition stress in the lives of military veterans. Clinical Psychology Review 2018; 59: 137-144.

43. Junger S. Why veterans miss war. TED Talk, May 23, 2014. Available at: https://www.ted.com/talks/sebastian_junger_why_veterans_miss_war?language=en. Accessed on July 6, 2021.

44. Catlin Boehmer TK, Flanders D, McGeehin MA, et al. Postservice mortality in Vietnam veterans: 30-year follow-up. Archives of Internal Medicine 2004; 164: 1908-1916.

45. Pages F, Faulde M, Orlandi-Pradines E, Parola P. The past and present threat of vector-borne diseases in deployed troops. Clinical Microbiology and Infection 2010; 16: 209-224.

46. Schmitt E, Cooper H. Navy secretary orders deeper inquiry into virus-stricken ship. New York Times, April 29, 2020.

47. Steinhauer J. Military and VA struggle with vaccination rates in their ranks. New York Times, July 1, 2021. Available at: https://www.nytimes.com/2021/07/01/us/politics/military-va-vaccines.html. Accessed on July 6, 2021.

48. Garshick E, Abraham JH, Baird CP, et al. Respiratory health after military service in Southwest Asia and Afghanistan. Annals of the American Thoracic Society 2019; 16: e1-e16.

49. Krefft SD, Rose CS, Nawaz S, Miller YE. Deployment-related lung disorders. Federal Practitioner 2015; 32: 32-38.

50. Falvo MJ, Osinubi OY, Sotolongo AM, Helmer DA. Airborne hazards exposure and respiratory health of Iraq and Afghanistan veterans. Epidemiologic Reviews 2015; 37: 116-130.

51. Barth SK, Dursa EK, Bossarte R, Schneiderman A. Lifetime prevalence of respiratory diseases and exposures among veterans of Operation Enduring Freedom and Operation Iraqi Freedom veterans: Results from the National Health Study for a new generation of U.S. veterans. Journal of Occupational and Environmental Medicine 2017; 58: 1175-1180.

52. Sanders JW, Putnam SD, Frankart C, et al. Impact of illness and non-combat injury during Operations Iraqi Freedom and Enduring Freedom (Afghanistan). American Journal of Tropical Medicine and Hygiene 2005; 73:713-719.

53. Soltis BW, Sanders JW, Putnam SD, et al. Self-reported incidence and morbidity of acute respiratory illness among deployed U.S. military in Iraq and Afghanistan. PLoS ONE 2009; 4: e6177. doi: http://dx.doi.org/10.1371/journal.pone.0006177.

54. Sanchez JL, Cooper MJ, Myers CA, et al. Respiratory infections in the U.S. military: Recent experience and control. Clinical Microbiology Reviews 2015; 28: 743-800.

55. Smith JE. The epidemiology of blast lung injury during recent military conflicts: A retrospective database review of cases presenting to deployed military hospitals, 2003–2009. Philosophical Transactions of the Royal Society 2011; 366: 291-294.

56. Coughlin SS, Szema A. Burn pits exposure and chronic respiratory illnesses among Iraq and Afghanistan veterans. Journal of Environment and Health Sciences 2019; 5: 13-14.

57. Liu J, Lezama N, Gasper J, et al. Burn pit emissions exposure and respiratory and cardiovascular conditions among airborne hazards and open burn pit registry participants. Journal of Occupational and Environmental Medicine 2016; 58: e249-e255.

58. Dixon KJ. Pathophysiology of traumatic brain injury. Physical Medicine and Rehabilitation Clinics of North America 2017; 28: 215-225.

59. Sayer NA. Traumatic brain injury and its neuropsychiatric sequelae in war veterans. Annual Review of Medicine 2012; 63: 405-419.

60. Swanson TM, Isaacson BM, Cyborski CM, et al. Traumatic brain injury, clinical overview, and policies in the US Military Health System since 2000. Public Health Reports 2017; 132: 251-259.

61. Gwini SM, Forbes AB, Sim MR, Kelsall HL. Multisymptom illness in Gulf War veterans: A systematic review and meta-analysis. Journal of Occupational and Environmental Medicine 2016; 58: 659-667.

62. White RF, Steele L, O'Callaghan JP, et al. Recent research on Gulf War Illness and other health problems in veterans of the 1991 Gulf War: Effects of toxicant exposures during deployment. Cortex 2016; 74: 449-475.

63. Kerr K. Gulf War Illness: An overview of events, most prevalent health outcomes, exposures, and clues as to pathogenesis. Reviews on Environmental Health 2015; 30: 273-286.

64. McDiarmid MA, Cloeren M, Gaitens JM, et al. Surveillance results and bone effects in the Gulf War depleted uranium-exposed cohort. Journal of Toxicology and Environmental Health, Part A 2018; 81: 1083-1097.

65. Saunders GH, Echt KV. Blast exposure and dual sensory impairment: An evidence review and integrated rehabilitation approach. Journal of Rehabilitation Research & Development 2012; 49: 1043-1058.

66. Conroy K, Malik V. Hearing loss in the trenches—A hidden morbidity of World War I. Journal of Laryngology and Otology 2018; 132: 952-955.

67. Swan AA, Nelson JT, Swiger B, et al. Prevalence of hearing loss and tinnitus in Iraq and Afghanistan veterans: A Chronic Effects of Neurotrauma Consortium study. Hearing Research 2017; 349: 4-12.

68. Granado NS, Smith TC, Swanson GM, et al. Newly reported hypertension after military combat deployment in a large population-based study. Hypertension 2009; 54: 966-973.

69. Stewart IJ, Sosnov JA, Howard JT, et al. Retrospective analysis of long-term outcomes after combat injury: A hidden cost of war. Circulation 2015; 132: 2126-2133.

70. Boos CJ, De Villiers N, Dyball D, et al. The relationship between military combat and cardiovascular risk: A systematic review and meta-analysis. International Journal of Vascular Medicine 2019; Article ID 9849465. https://doi.org/10.1155/2019/9849465.

71. Michalek JE, Pavuk M. Diabetes and cancer in veterans of Operation Ranch Hand after adjustment for calendar period, days of spraying, and time spent in Southeast Asia. Journal of Occupational and Environmental Medicine 2008; 50: 330-340.

72. Veterans and Agent Orange: Update 2014. Military Medicine 2017; 182: 1619-1620. doi: 10.7205/MILMED-D-17-00130.

73. Ketchum NS, Michalek JE. Postservice mortality of Air Force veterans occupationally exposed to herbicides during the Vietnam War: 20-year follow-up results. Military Medicine 2005; 170: 406-413.

74. Ansbaugh N, Shannon J, Mori M, et al. Agent Orange as a risk factor for high-grade prostate cancer. Cancer 2013; 119: 2399-2404. doi: 10.1002/cncr.27941.

75. Bullman TA, Mahan CM, Kang HK, Page WF. Mortality in US Army Gulf War veterans exposed to 1991 Khamisiyah chemical munitions destruction. American Journal of Public Health 2005; 95: 1382-1388.

76. Barth SK, Kang HK, Bullman A, Wallin MT. Neurological mortality among U.S. veterans of the Persian Gulf War: 13-year follow-up. American Journal of Industrial Medicine 2009; 52: 663-680.

77. Yi S-W. Cancer incidence in Korean Vietnam veterans during 1992–2003: The Korean Veterans Health Study. Journal of Preventive Medicine and Public Health 2013; 46: 309-318.

78. Young HA, Maillard JD, Levine PH, et al. Investigating the risk of cancer in 1990–1991 US Gulf War veterans with the use of state cancer registry data. Annals of Epidemiology 2010; 20: 265-272.

79. Caldwell GG, Zack MM, Mumma MT, et al. Mortality among military participants at the 1957 PLUMBBOB nuclear weapons test series and from leukemia among participants at the SMOKY test. Journal of Radiological Protection 2016; 36: 474-489.

80. Dalager NA, Kang HK, Mahan CM. Cancer mortality among the highest exposed US atmospheric nuclear test participants. Journal of Occupational and Environmental Medicine 2000; 42: 798-805.

81. Watanabe KK, Kang HK, Dalager NA. Cancer mortality risk among military participants of a 1958 atmospheric nuclear weapons test. American Journal of Public Health 1995; 85: 523-527.

82. Boice JD, Cohen SS, Mumma MT, et al. Mortality among U.S. military participants at eight aboveground nuclear weapons test series. International Journal of Radiation Biology 2020 [online before print]. https://doi.org/10.1080/09553002.2020.1787543.

83. U. S. Department of Veterans Affairs. Public Health: Diseases Associated with Ionizing Radiation Exposure. Available at: https://www.publichealth.va.gov/exposures/radiation/diseases.asp#presumptive. Accessed on June 4, 2021.

84. Bedard K, Deschênes O. The long-term impact of military service on health: Evidence from World War II and Korean War veterans. American Economic Review 2006; 96: 176-194.

85. Haddock CK, Jahnke SA, Poston WSC, Williams LN. Cigarette prices in military retail: A review and proposal for advancing military health policy. Military Medicine 2013; 178: 563-569.

86. Wardle SL, Greeves JP. Mitigating the risk of musculoskeletal injury: A systematic review of the most effective injury prevention strategies for military personnel. Journal of Science and Medicine in Sport 2017; 20: S3-S10.

87. Jones BH, Perrotta DM, Canham-Chervak ML, et al. Injuries in the military: A review and commentary focused on prevention. American Journal of Preventive Medicine 2000; 18: 71-84.

88. Murray CK, Horvath LL. An approach to prevention of infectious diseases during military deployments. Travel Medicine 2007; 44: 424-430.

89. Zamorski MA. Suicide prevention in military organizations. International Review of Psychiatry 2011; 23: 173-180.

90. Denning LA, Meisnere M, Warner KE (eds.). Preventing Psychological Disorders in Service Members and Their Families: An Assessment of Programs. Washington, DC: National Academies Press, 2014.

Profile 12:
Robert Gould, M.D., and Patrice Sutton, M.P.H.
Influencing Public Policy

When Robert (Bob) Gould and Patrice Sutton grew up in New York City, their families were on opposite sides of the political spectrum. But, by the mid-1980s, they had a shared passion for peace, health, and justice for all, which led them to the American Public Health Association (APHA) as a vehicle for advocacy.

Bob grew up in a politically engaged family in the midst of the civil rights and anti–Vietnam War movements. In medical school, he was inspired by Victor Sidel, Jack Geiger, and other physicians who demonstrated the inextricable links between health, peace, and social justice. Patrice grew up in a family where she developed a strong moral perspective on life and empathy for people who were less fortunate. Her work as a histologist came with heavy exposure to toxic chemicals and on-the-job learning about how workers and unions could bring pressure to make the workplace safer, inspiring her to seek a career in occupational and environmental health.

Bob and Patrice discovered that APHA policy statements are useful tools for supporting actions to protect the health of the public—to ban toxic chemicals, to condemn structural racism, to protect vulnerable populations, to address social injustice, to prevent war.

In 1984, Bob co-authored a policy statement opposing U.S. military intervention in Nicaragua, bringing a public health perspective to this contentious issue. The following year, he authored a position paper on the adverse health effects of militarism. APHA's adoption of both the policy statement and the position paper helped raise awareness of these issues within other organizations and mobilize political action.

In 1985, Patrice first attended the APHA Annual Meeting, when Gail Gordon founded the Peace Caucus in affiliation with APHA to highlight the health impacts of war. The following year, Peace Caucus members and the leadership of APHA organized a demonstration

From Horror to Hope. Barry S. Levy, Oxford University Press. © Oxford University Press 2022.
DOI: 10.1093/oso/9780197558645.003.0024

at the nuclear weapons test site in Nevada, in which more than 500 APHA members participated; 139 were arrested in acts of nonviolent civil disobedience. The demonstration drew the attention of the national news media and spurred additional protests at the test site to end testing of nuclear weapons.

The mobilization of public health professionals against nuclear weapons has served as a model for advocacy on many related fronts over the past 35 years by Patrice, Bob, and other Peace Caucus members. During this time, the Peace Caucus has organized hundreds of scientific-session presentations at APHA Annual Meetings, where speakers have documented the direct and indirect impacts of war on health and human rights.

Peace Caucus members have translated these findings and recommendations into policy statements, which have been adopted by APHA, including policies supporting bans of landmines and weapons of mass destruction, protection of civilians during war, opposition to specific wars, care for military veterans, and the primary prevention of war. These policies have educated APHA members and others about the impacts of war and the influence of militarism. They have also influenced other professional organizations, other nongovernmental organizations, and government agencies to address the health impacts of war. For example, APHA policies have helped promote efforts to abolish nuclear weapons and to condemn torture.

Looking back on their 35 years of work in helping to develop APHA policies on war-related issues, Bob and Patrice observe: "Health professionals can have a profound impact on the health of their patients and communities by leveraging the voice of their professional organizations in the primary prevention of war."

Dr. Gould is an Associate Adjunct Professor at the University of California San Francisco School of Medicine and President of San Francisco Bay Physicians for Social Responsibility. Ms. Sutton is a Collaborating Research Scientist in the Program on Reproductive Health and the Environment at the University of California San Francisco and Chair of the Environmental Health Committee, San Francisco Bay Physicians for Social Responsibility.

13

Impacts on the Environment

> We do not inherit the Earth from our ancestors; we borrow it from our children.
>
> WENDELL BERRY

INTRODUCTION

Military forces cause widespread damage to the environment during war and the preparation for war. Their use of explosive weapons destroys urban and rural infrastructure. Their use of fossil fuels releases air pollutants, including greenhouse gases. They contaminate sources of freshwater with hazardous chemicals. They damage farmland, causing displacement of populations. They damage animal habitats and ecosystems. They leave behind damaged military equipment, weapons, and ammunition as well as antipersonnel landmines and unexploded ordnance. And they divert human and financial resources away from environmental protection.[1,2]

Wars have always caused damage to the environment. As journalist Donovan Webster vividly described in his book *Aftermath: The Remnants of War*, environmental impacts of 20th-century wars remain in fields in France with unexploded shells from the First World War, at the nuclear weapons test site in Nevada, in mangrove forests in Vietnam contaminated with Agent Orange, and in Kuwait, where landmines from the Gulf War are still present.[3]

Wars cause environmental devastation, as illustrated by events during the Iraq War. Raw sewage was dumped into rivers because bombs had damaged sewage treatment facilities. Radioactive materials were released into the environment when a major nuclear research facility was destroyed. And land was contaminated with depleted uranium (DU), oil spills, and unexploded ordnance.[4,5]

AIR CONTAMINATION

Greenhouse gas emissions, chemical releases, and production and testing of nuclear weapons have accounted for much contamination of ambient air. So have open-air burn pits in war zones (Chapter 12).[6]

From Horror to Hope. Barry S. Levy, Oxford University Press. © Oxford University Press 2022.
DOI: 10.1093/oso/9780197558645.003.0025

Greenhouse Gas Emissions

The large amounts of fossil fuels used by military forces generate greenhouse gases, which cause climate change. The U.S. military, the largest institutional user of oil worldwide, consumes more than 100 million barrels annually to power vehicles, aircraft, ships, and other equipment. In 2017, it daily bought almost 270,000 barrels of oil and emitted more than 25,000 kilotons of carbon dioxide. Among the branches of the U.S. military, the U.S. Air Force has been by far the largest emitter of greenhouse gases.[7] (See the section "Freshwater Availability and Climate Change as Potential Causes of Armed Conflict" later in this chapter.)

Chemical Releases

During the Gulf War, retreating Iraqi troops ignited more than 600 oil well fires in Kuwait, contaminating the air with particulate matter, hydrogen sulfide, volatile organic compounds, and other chemicals—which threatened the health of civilians and military personnel (Figure 13-1).[8,9] A study of more than 1,500 Gulf War veterans found a dose–response relationship between self-reported exposure to smoke from these fires and both asthma and bronchitis.[10] But another study of Gulf War veterans did not find that they were at increased risk of hospitalization due to exposure to smoke from these fires.[11]

Air contaminants may have accounted for increased respiratory symptoms that occurred among U.S. military personnel deployed to Iraq and Afghanistan. A study of more than 46,000 of them found that they had a higher rate of newly reported respiratory symptoms (14%) than non-deployed military personnel (10%) and that duration of deployment was linearly associated with respiratory symptoms.[12] Other studies found that deployment was associated with prevalent and new-onset asthma.[13,14] (See Chapter 12.)

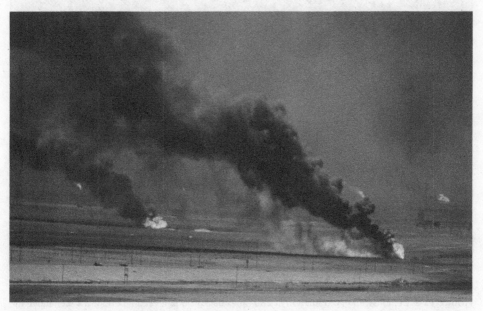

FIGURE 13-1 Burning oil wells in Kuwait, which were set on fire by retreating Iraqi troops shortly after the Gulf War in March 1991. (AP Photo.)

Nuclear Weapons Production

Workers at nuclear weapons production plants in Russia, the United States, and elsewhere as well as residents in nearby areas have been exposed to ionizing radiation and hazardous chemicals from these plants.

Starting in 1948, the Soviet Union produced material for nuclear weapons, including plutonium, at the Mayak nuclear weapons facility in southern Russia. For two decades, the facility exposed workers and area residents to ionizing radiation—much of it from long-acting strontium-90 and cesium-137. Planned disposals and unintentional releases of radioactive wastes contaminated the nearby Techa River, exposing residents of riverside villages downstream (Figure 13-2). Radioactive contamination of the environment also occurred from an explosion in a radioactive waste storage facility and from gaseous aerosol releases. Among a cohort of 30,000 nearby residents, 70 cases of leukemia occurred between 1953 and 2005; there was a dose–response relationship between radiation exposure and risk of leukemia.[15–17]

In the United States, nuclear weapons facilities, which mine, process, produce, and use radioactive and toxic materials, have contaminated the environment.[18] A production center in Fernald, Ohio, released 250 tons of uranium oxide into the air and contaminated surface water and groundwater with radioactive materials. The Hanford Reservation, a nuclear weapons facility in Washington State, released 200 billion gallons of contaminated water into groundwater and the Columbia River and released 1.2 million gallons of radioactive waste from underground tanks. The Oak Ridge Reservation, a facility in Tennessee, emitted thousands of pounds of uranium into the atmosphere and radioactive hazardous wastes into local

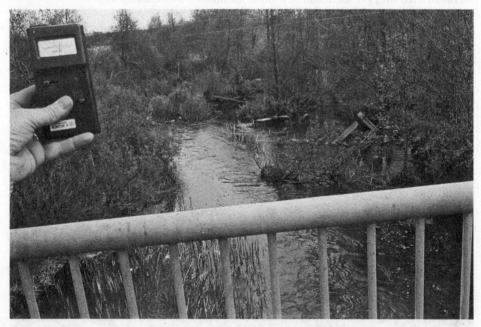

FIGURE 13-2 Demonstration of radiation at 280 times background level on a bridge 14 feet above the Techa River in Russia, not far from the Mayak (Chelyabinsk-40) nuclear weapons facility. (Photograph by Robert Del Tredici, the Atomic Photographers Guild.)

streams. The Rocky Flats Plant, a facility in Colorado, contaminated the air with radioactive materials and leaked carcinogenic chemicals into groundwater;[19] cleanup workers there were exposed to asbestos, carbon tetrachloride, hexavalent chromium, lead, methylene chloride, and, most heavily, beryllium and beryllium compounds.[20] (See Chapters 5 and 10.)

Nuclear Weapons Testing

From 1945 to 1980, there were 528 atmospheric tests of nuclear weapons worldwide, which created extensive environmental contamination. Testing of nuclear weapons released radioactive and toxic chemicals that contaminated test sites in Nevada, at Semipalatinsk in the Soviet Union, and on atolls and in marine environments in the Pacific Ocean, causing irreversible destruction of indigenous homelands of the Marshallese people and other indigenous Pacific Islander populations. Radioactive isotopes that were released included cesium-137, strontium-90, plutonium-239, plutonium-240, americium-241, and iodine-131. These radionuclides, especially cesium-137 and strontium-90, contaminated the marine environment and bioaccumulated in the food chain. Exposure to iodine-131 increased the incidence of thyroid cancer.[21]

Atmospheric tests of nuclear weapons have been associated with various malignancies. The entire U.S. population had increased rates of leukemia during and for several years after these tests.[22] Some U.S. military personnel exposed to these tests have increased rates of specific malignancies. (See Chapters 10 and 12.)

Atmospheric tests of nuclear weapons in Nevada exposed U.S. children to 15 to 79 times more radiation than previously permitted by the U.S. government. The tests exposed the thyroid glands of some children to 1.1 Gy of ionizing radiation and many million more to more than 0.1 Gy—amounts of radiation exposure that some epidemiologists estimated would cause 10,000 to 75,000 excess thyroid cancers.[22] The National Cancer Institute estimated that up to 212,000 additional cases of thyroid cancer will ultimately occur in the U.S. population due to iodine-131 exposure from nuclear weapons testing.[23]

France conducted 41 nuclear weapons tests between 1966 and 1974, exposing approximately 112,500 residents of French Polynesia to high levels of ionizing radiation.[24] Their incidence of thyroid cancer increased; the highest risk was associated with radiation dose before age 15.[25]

Since the 1950s, human-produced plutonium has been introduced into the Arctic marine environment from detonation of nuclear weapons and planned releases from nuclear power plants. Throughout the world, there is a relatively uniform distribution of plutonium from atmospheric tests of nuclear weapons many years ago.[26] (See Chapter 5.)

WATER CONTAMINATION

War and the preparation for war have contaminated surface water and groundwater. Military forces have destroyed water treatment plants and water distribution systems, often forcing people to use the only available water, which was contaminated with microorganisms (Figure 2-2 in Chapter 2). Provision of safe water during war and its aftermath is essential. (See Profile 13.)

Contamination of Oceans and Other Surface Water

Since its participation in the First World War, the U.S. military has dumped chemical weapons into the Atlantic and Pacific oceans. It dumped large amounts of sulfur mustard, lewisite (an organic arsenic compound), and nerve agents (sarin and tabun), and smaller amounts of other organic arsenic compounds, choking agents, blood agents, and lacrimogenic agents, such as tear gas (Chapter 5). The main risk to human health associated with this dumping has occurred when people have accidentally recovered chemical weapons on fishing boats or when they have touched chemical munitions that had been washed onto beaches.[27]

From 1945 to 1970, the U.S. Army dumped into oceans at least 64 million pounds (32,000 tons) of mustard gas, lewisite, sarin, and tabun as well as bombs, rockets, landmines, and radioactive waste. In 1987, mustard gas was determined to be the likely cause of burns on many dolphins that washed ashore in New Jersey and Virginia. In 2004, a bomb disposal technician was burned by a mustard gas shell that had been inadvertently dredged up in Delaware.[28,29]

Canada also dumped mustard gas into the Atlantic Ocean and chemical weapons into both the Atlantic and the Pacific. Canadian researchers have claimed that risks to humans are negligible because the dumpsites are in a deep-water, static, and near-lifeless environment. This description differs from that of ocean scientists, such as Rachel Carson, the marine biologist who was a founder of the environmental movement, who described the ocean environment, even in deep waters, as full of life and motion.[30]

Ocean dumping finally ended in 1972, when the London Convention, which was established through the United Nations International Maritime Organization, prohibited further dumping of chemical weapons at sea. However, the Convention did not establish methods or criteria to identify or monitor dumpsites and did not require reporting. And, decades later, ocean dumpsites of chemical weapons are still present off the east and west coasts of the United States, off the east coast of Japan, in the Adriatic Sea and the Baltic Sea, and in the Russian Arctic (in the White Sea, Barents Sea, and Kara Sea). Sunken ships off the coast of Italy have been leaking chemical weapons into the Adriatic Sea, adversely affecting the marine ecosystem. In the Pacific Ocean, about 55 miles west of San Francisco, lies the SS *William Ralston*, which sank in 1958 with 1,257 tons of lewisite and 301,000 bombs containing mustard. A barge with a similar cargo also sank at this site.[31]

During the Gulf War, Iraq released approximately 10 million barrels of Kuwaiti oil into the Persian Gulf. This release created substantial stress on the ecosystem, which had already sustained damage from the Iran–Iraq War and from freighter traffic, industrial waste, and oil spills.[32] In the 1990s, after the Gulf War, the Iraqi government conducted a counterinsurgency campaign in the marshes of southern Mesopotamia. In addition to mass killing and forced displacement of the population, the Iraqi government diverted water from these wetlands, permanently desiccating the area and its ecosystem.

Contamination of Groundwater

U.S. military facilities have contaminated soil and groundwater at and near military bases in the United States and elsewhere. For decades at Camp Lejeune, a large U.S. Marine Corps base in North Carolina, toxic chemical dumps and leaks from underground storage tanks contaminated drinking water with industrial solvents, dry-cleaning chemicals, and gasoline.[33] Drinking water from wells there between 1953 and 1987 far exceeded Environmental Protection Agency (EPA) maximum levels for trichloroethylene, perchloroethylene, and benzene. During this 34-year period, more than one million people were stationed there. Toxic and carcinogenic chemicals also contaminated groundwater at Otis Air Force Base in Massachusetts, Picatinny Arsenal in New Jersey, Tinker Air Force Base in Oklahoma, and Hill Air Force Base in Utah.[18,34]

In the 1970s, the U.S. Department of Defense (DoD) started using aqueous film-forming foam (AFFF) because it rapidly extinguishes petroleum-based fires. AFFF contains per- and polyfluoroalkyl substances (PFAS), such as perfluorooctane sulfonate (PFOS) and sometimes perfluorooctanoic acid (PFOA). These chemicals have contaminated drinking water at 126 U.S. military sites above EPA acceptable levels. The DoD has identified 410 military installations in the United States where there had been a known or suspected release of PFAS.[35]

Between 2007 and 2015, the DoD spent approximately $11.5 billion for environmental cleanup at military installations, in its Base Realignment and Closure process, and planned to spend another $3.4 billion to complete this work. Cleanup of environmental contaminants at installations that were closed during this process impeded transfer of property to, and its ultimate reuse by, communities around these bases.[36]

LAND CONTAMINATION

Chemicals and radioactive materials have contaminated land, damaging animal habitats and ecosystems, endangering human health, and making land unusable.

Antipersonnel Landmines and Unexploded Ordnance

Military forces have deployed millions of antipersonnel landmines, which have caused many severe injuries and deaths and made it impossible to use land for any purpose.[37] Landmines and unexploded ordnance can remain in war zones long after combat has ended, creating risks of accidental detonation and leaching of chemicals into soil and groundwater. (See Chapter 4.)

Agent Orange

Agent Orange, a herbicide and defoliant, was used extensively by the U.S. military in the Vietnam War. It contained two active ingredients, 2,4-dichlorophenoxyacetic acid (2,4-D) and 2,4,5-trichlorophenoxyacetic acid (2,4,5-T), as well as traces of 2,3,7,8-tetrachlorodibenzo-p-dioxin (TCDD or dioxin), a potent carcinogen that is a byproduct of herbicide production. From airplanes, helicopters, boats, ground vehicles, and backpack sprayers, the U.S. military sprayed more than 19 million gallons of Agent Orange and other defoliants on more than 6.4 million acres of forests and coastal mangroves in South

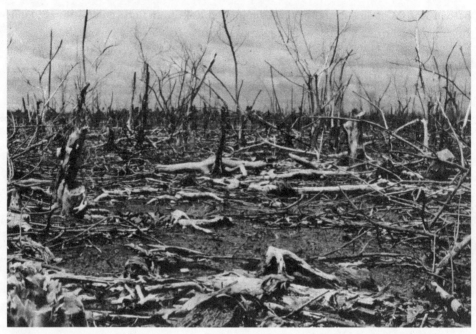

FIGURE 13-3 Mangrove forest destroyed by Agent Orange, Gia Dinh Province, South Vietnam, 1970. (Photograph by Arthur H. Westing.)

Vietnam (Figure 13-3). This spraying was done to remove foliage that provided cover for North Vietnamese soldiers (the Viet Cong) and to damage crops on which they relied. (See Chapters 10 and 12.)

Depleted Uranium

Arms manufacturers have used DU, a radioactive and toxic heavy metal, in producing armor-penetrating bullets and shell casings that were used extensively, mainly by the U.S. military, during the Gulf War and the Iraq War.[38] People were exposed by inhalation, skin contact, and ingestion and by being wounded with DU-containing bullets or shells. The toxic effects of DU include decreased immune responses, damaged cell structure, and cell death.[39] (See Chapters 10 and 12.)

Bombing

Aerial bombardment injures and kills people, destroys urban and rural infrastructure, and displaces people. During the Second World War, about 40,000 people were killed by Germany's bombing of London and nearby areas, at least 80,000 people were killed by the U.S. firebombing of Tokyo, 500,000 people died in Allied fire bombings of 70 cities in Germany, and more than 200,000 died from the acute effects of atomic bomb explosions at Hiroshima and Nagasaki.[2] Bombing also wounded hundreds of thousands of people during the war. Bombing has also caused unexpected adverse consequences; for example, U.S. bombing during the Vietnam

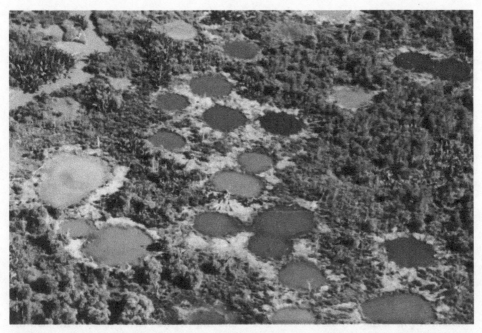

FIGURE 13-4 Mangrove forest damaged by U.S. bombs, Bien Hoa Province, South Vietnam, 1971. (Photograph by Arthur H. Westing.)

War produced craters that filled with water and became breeding ponds for mosquitoes that transmitted malaria (Figure 13-4). (See Chapters 4, 5, and 6.)

Resource Wars

Resource wars occur when countries or groups within a country use military force to acquire or control sources of raw materials, such as oil, water, minerals, and timber (Chapter 1). Resource wars, frequently fought in remote areas populated by Indigenous Peoples, often damage or contaminate the environment. For example, resource wars to control oil include attacks on pipelines, refineries, and other oil infrastructure, causing fires and oil spills.[40,41]

Military forces have funded some wars with illegal logging, mining, and other resource extraction—activities that have contaminated the environment and damaged animal habitats and ecosystems. For example, during civil wars in Liberia and Sierra Leone, military forces extracted and traded timber and diamonds. The Islamic State (ISIS), when it occupied oil-fields in Iraq and Syria from 2014 to 2017, extracted and exported petroleum. During civil wars in several countries in sub-Saharan Africa, insurgent forces have hunted large animals, such as elephants for their ivory;[42] as a result, wars in Africa between 1946 and 2010 were associated with reduced numbers of large mammals in protected areas.[43]

Other Military Impacts on Habitats

Military forces have intentionally destroyed animal habitats.[44] Turkish forces set forest fires to reduce tree cover for Kurdish fighters in their armed conflict with the Kurdish Workers'

Party (1978–1980). During the Second Lebanon War, Israel targeted petroleum storage facilities, creating an oil slick along more than 60 miles of the Lebanon coastline, killing seabirds, invertebrates, and plants.[42]

Military training and testing has contaminated soil and groundwater with radioactive waste, lead and other heavy metals, and chemicals in fuels, explosives, propellants, and solvents. Many of these substances persist for long periods and ultimately affect wildlife and plants. Researchers have documented resultant morbidity and mortality in amphibians, reptiles, birds, fish, and invertebrates.[43] Military training activities, including bombing, shelling, and gunfire, also adversely affect wildlife and plants.[44]

Scorched-Earth Strategies

Military forces have sometimes used *scorched-earth strategies*, aiming to destroy everything that might be useful to the enemy, including weapons, transport vehicles, communication sites, industrial resources, agricultural lands, food storage sites, and water sources—thereby injuring and killing civilians and damaging the environment. Ancient Greek and Roman military forces used scorched-earth strategies. So did General William Tecumseh Sherman in his march to the sea during the U.S. Civil War, Russian troops retreating from the advancing German Army during the First World War,[45] and the German Army when it invaded the Soviet Union during the Second World War.

Intentional Flooding

Intentional flooding has occasionally been used during war to prevent use of land held by enemy forces and civilians and to prevent movement of enemy troops. Direct attacks and sabotage can easily damage dams or dikes, releasing impounded water and causing death and destruction. Recovery from these actions can take decades.[46]

During the Siege of Leiden in 1573 (in what is now The Netherlands), dikes were breached to prevent the advance of the Spanish military. During the Second Sino-Japanese War, China breached dikes on the Yangtze River and the Yellow River to prevent the advance of Japanese troops. The most devastating example of intentional flooding occurred in 1938, when the Chinese Army dynamited the Huayuankou Dike on the Yellow River near Chengchow; several thousand Japanese soldiers and several hundred thousand Chinese civilians drowned, and 11 cities, 4,000 villages, and several million acres of farmland were destroyed.[37,46]

During the Second World War, Allied forces bombed dams on the Eder River and the Sorpe River in Germany, creating a flood that prevented it from manufacturing military equipment.[37,46] In Italy, the German army intentionally flooded the Pontine Marshes south of Rome in an attempt to obstruct the advance of Allied forces; although the army tried to contain increased mosquito breeding from the flooding, Italian civilians returning to this area developed malaria.[47] Military forces also used this tactic in the Korean War and other armed conflicts.[46]

International law has since prohibited intentional flooding and other manipulation of nature as a tactic during war. The Convention on the Prohibition of Military or Any Other Hostile Use of Environmental Modification Techniques—also known as the Environmental

Modification Convention—was approved by the UN General Assembly in 1976 and entered into force in 1978. It prohibits "any technique for changing—through deliberate manipulation of natural processes—the dynamics, composition or structure of the Earth, including its biota, lithosphere [the rigid outer part of the Earth], hydrosphere and atmosphere" such that it would have "widespread, long-lasting or severe effects as the means of destruction, damage or injury to any other State-Party."[48]

Protocol II, which was added in 1977 to the Geneva Conventions, has provided additional protection against the disruption of infrastructure. It states: "Works or installations containing dangerous forces, mainly dams, dykes, and nuclear electrical generating stations, shall not be made the object of attack, even where these objects are military objectives, if such attack may cause the release of dangerous forces and consequent severe losses among the civilian population."[49]

DISPLACEMENT AND THE ENVIRONMENT

Environmental conditions, such as droughts caused by climate change, can forcibly displace populations. And displacement of populations can adversely affect the environment.

Often with no other options, displaced persons may have to cut down trees for firewood. If they do not have adequate sanitation and waste disposal, they may contaminate soil and surface water. Refugee camps in the African Great Lakes Region, Mozambique, Sudan, and Afghanistan–Pakistan border areas have contributed to deforestation, air and water pollution, and adverse effects on vulnerable ecosystems.[50,51]

Displaced persons face many institutional, political, and implementation obstacles for improving their environmental health conditions. For example, laws and policies have prevented developing infrastructure for permanent camps for displaced persons.

Environmental health for displaced populations could be improved by better camp planning, strengthening regulations and guidelines, improving plans for housing and solid waste management, promoting coordination among agencies and organizations, and including displaced persons in planning and decision-making.[52]

FRESHWATER AVAILABILITY AND CLIMATE CHANGE AS POTENTIAL CAUSES OF ARMED CONFLICT

Decreased availability of freshwater can lead to armed conflict. An analysis of a global spatial time series, which looked at renewable freshwater surface water resources and their relationship to armed conflict worldwide for the 1980–2002 period, found at the global level a strong relationship between unusually low rainfall and the probability of a high-intensity intrastate war during the following year.[53]

In addition to climate change, population growth is contributing to water shortages, especially in Africa, the Middle East, and South Asia. Water scarcity affects at least 700 million people globally. Another 1.6 million people face economic water shortages, in which

TABLE 13-1 Water Conflicts, 1800–2019, by Time Period Begun

Time Period	Number	Annual Average
1800–1899	14	0.14
1900–1999	177	1.77
2000–2009	220	22.00
2010–2019	466	46.60

(Source: Gleick PH. The water conflict chronology. 2019. Available at: http://worldwater.org/water-conflict/. Accessed on February 4, 2021.)

countries lack the infrastructure to optimally utilize water from rivers and aquifers.[54] In addition to causing direct health consequences, inadequate access to water can lead to food shortages and armed conflict.

Sharing of water between countries is common; about 60% of water flowing into all rivers is shared by two or more countries. Cooperative agreements have been developed and implemented in many shared river basins.[55] Although water-related armed conflict has occurred infrequently, water-related disputes have been increasing (Table 13-1).[56] In order to prevent water-related armed conflict, high-income countries, in their enlightened self-interest, need to support strategic planning and water resource development in low- and middle-income countries by providing financial resources and technical assistance.[57]

Climate change, resulting from emission of greenhouse gases, is causing changes in precipitation, extreme weather events, and sea-level rise—with many socioeconomic, political,

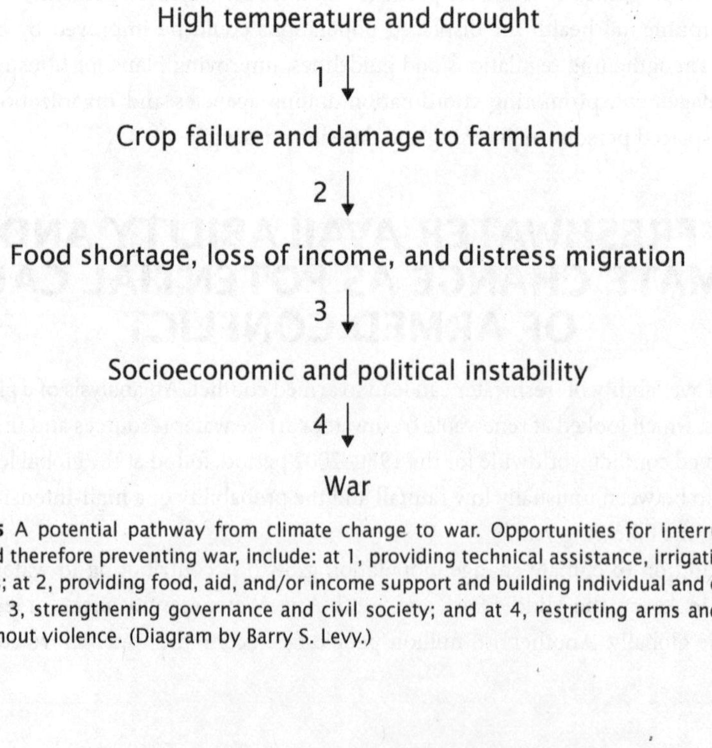

High temperature and drought

1 ↓

Crop failure and damage to farmland

2 ↓

Food shortage, loss of income, and distress migration

3 ↓

Socioeconomic and political instability

4 ↓

War

FIGURE 13-5 A potential pathway from climate change to war. Opportunities for interrupting this pathway, and therefore preventing war, include: at 1, providing technical assistance, irrigation, and resistant seeds; at 2, providing food, aid, and/or income support and building individual and community resilience; at 3, strengthening governance and civil society; and at 4, restricting arms and resolving conflicts without violence. (Diagram by Barry S. Levy.)

and health consequences.[58,59] Since the mid-1800s, ambient temperature has risen about 1.0°C (1.8°F) and it is likely to increase another 1.0°C or substantially more by 2100.[60] Heat waves are hotter, more frequent, and longer lasting.[61] Global warming is increasing rainfall and flooding in some areas, while decreasing rainfall and increasing drought in others. And it is contributing to an increased frequency of severe hurricanes, cyclones, and other extreme weather events.[60]

Climate change is increasing the occurrence of heat-related disorders, respiratory disorders, vector-borne and waterborne infectious diseases, injuries from extreme weather events, and mental disorders.[58] Warmer temperatures and extremes of precipitation are reducing crop production and food security and increasing malnutrition.[62-64] Reduced food security and reduced availability of freshwater are displacing many people; by 2050, climate change could displace 200 million people.[65]

Climate change can contribute to the start or persistence of conflict.[66,67] Two large meta-analyses concluded that deviations from mild ambient temperature and from the normal range of precipitation increase the risk of conflict.[68,69] A potential pathway from climate change to war, including opportunities for interventions, is shown in Figure 13-5.

Climate change contributed to the start of the Syrian Civil War. Between 2006 and 2011, Syria and other countries in the region experienced a severe drought, to which climate change likely contributed (Figure 13-6). About 60% of farmland in Syria became desert

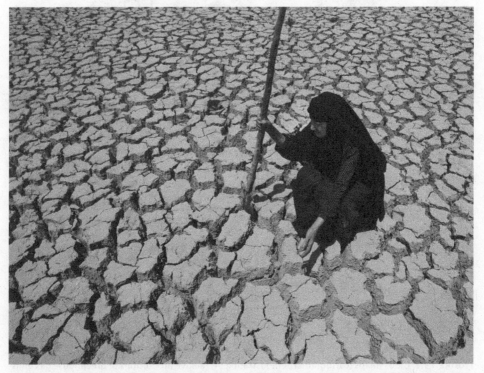

FIGURE 13-6 Woman checks her land in Latifiyah, Iraq, about 20 miles south of Baghdad in 2009. Below-average rainfall and insufficient water in the Euphrates and Tigris rivers left Iraq bone-dry for a second consecutive year. (AP Photo/Hadi Mizban.)

and about 80% of livestock died. More than one million farmers and their family members migrated to urban areas, where they experienced ethnic discrimination. The government, which was already facing serious economic and political challenges and hosting more than one million Iraqi refugees, was overwhelmed and unable to address the basic needs of these displaced people. This situation heightened preexisting political and socioeconomic instability and contributed to the start of the civil war.[70,71]

Climate change has been associated with socioeconomic inequities between countries, which could contribute to armed conflict. In general, the countries that produce the largest amount of greenhouse gases have suffered the fewest health consequences as a result, and those countries that produce the lowest amount—mainly low- and middle-income countries in Africa and South Asia—have suffered the most health consequences (Figure 13-7).[72]

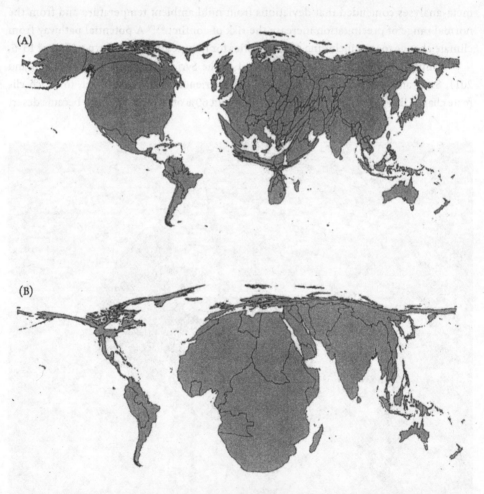

FIGURE 13-7 Global maps (cartograms) demonstrating (A) relative proportions of greenhouse gas emissions, by country; and (B) magnitude and severity of selected health consequences of climate change, by country. (*Source*: Patz JA, Gibbs HK, Foley JA, et al. Climate change and global health: Quantifying a growing ethical crisis. EcoHealth 2007; 4: 397-405. doi.10.1007/s10393-007-0141-1.)

Socioeconomic inequities due to climate change within countries can increase the risk of armed conflict.

Climate change can be addressed through *mitigation measures* implemented to reduce the emission of greenhouse gases, and by *adaptation measures* implemented to reduce the adverse impacts of climate change. Mitigation is achieved largely through policies related to energy use, transportation, agriculture, and land use. Examples of adaptation measures include surveillance for climate-related diseases, preparedness for extreme weather events, and, as shown in Figure 13-5, measures to prevent displacement and war.[58]

PREVENTING THE ENVIRONMENTAL IMPACTS OF WAR

Addressing the environmental impacts of war requires systematically assessing the environmental consequences of war on human health and ecosystems; banning military practices and weapons that have most the devastating impact on the environment; and developing the popular and political will to address these impacts and to prevent war.

Epidemiological, environmental, and ecological surveillance and research need to be improved to better detect and assess the long-term environmental consequences of war and their impact on health. Systematic analyses need to be conducted on exposures to hazardous materials released, especially onto soil and into groundwater, and their impact on human health, animal and plant life, and ecosystems. A major challenge in this work is gaining access to war zones and military bases where hazardous substances have been released.

Existing international conventions and treaties need to be rigorously implemented and new ones need to be developed to prohibit military practices and weapons that adversely affect the environment. These practices include damaging facilities and natural systems that protect the environment and using herbicides, which contaminate farmland and introduce toxic substances into the food chain.

Systematic assessment of the environmental impact of war and prohibition of devastating military practices will require development of the popular and political will to do so. This can be achieved by educating and raising the awareness of the general public and policymakers, advocating for specific policies, and promoting visionary political leadership.

SUMMARY POINTS

- Military forces have contaminated air by use of fossil fuels, chemical releases, and production and testing of nuclear weapons.
- They have dumped chemical weapons into oceans and released chemicals on military bases that have contaminated groundwater.
- They have deployed landmines, sprayed defoliants and other herbicides, used weapons containing depleted uranium, and bombed urban environments.
- Decreased availability of freshwater and climate change can increase the risk of war.

- Preventing the environmental impacts of war requires assessment of these impacts on human health and ecosystems, banning the most devastating military practices and weapons, and developing the popular and political will to address these impacts.

REFERENCES

1. Zwijnenburg W, Hochhauser D, Dewachi O, et al. Solving the jigsaw of conflict-related environmental damage: Utilizing open-source analysis to improve research into environmental health risks. Journal of Public Health 2020; 42: e352-e360.
2. Leaning J. Environment and health: 5. Impact of war. Canadian Medical Association Journal 2000; 163: 1157-1161.
3. Webster D. Aftermath: The Remnants of War. New York: Vintage Books, 1996.
4. Levy BS, Sidel VW. Adverse health consequences of the Iraq War. Lancet 2013; 381: 949-958.
5. Al-Shammari AM. Environmental pollutions associated to conflicts in Iraq and related health problems. Reviews on Environmental Health 2016; 31: 245-250.
6. Stack MK. The soldiers came home sick. The government denied it was responsible. New York Times Magazine, January 11, 2022. Available at: https://www.nytimes.com/2022/01/11/magazine/military-burn-pits.html. Accessed January 24, 2022.
7. Belcher O, Bigger P, Neimark B, Kennelly C. Hidden carbon costs of the "everywhere war": Logistics, geopolitical ecology, and the carbon boot-print of the US military. Transactions of the Institute of British Geographers 2020; 45: 65-80.
8. Heller JM. Oil well fires of Operation Desert Storm—defining troop exposures and determining health risks. Military Medicine 2011; 176: 46-51.
9. Weiler BA, Colby TV, Floreth TJ, Hines SE. Small airways disease in an Operation Desert Storm deployer: Case report and review of the literature on respiratory health and inhalational exposures from Gulf War I. American Journal of Industrial Medicine 2018; 61: 793-801.
10. Lange JL, Schwartz DA, Doebbeling BN, et al. Exposure to the Kuwait oil fires and their association with asthma and bronchitis among Gulf War veterans. Environmental Health Perspectives 2002; 110: 1141-1146.
11. Smith TC, Heller JM, Hooper TI, et al. Are Gulf War veterans experiencing illness due to exposure to smoke from Kuwaiti oil well fires? Examination of Department of Defense hospitalization data. American Journal of Epidemiology 2002; 155: 908-917.
12. Smith B, Wong CA, Smith TC, et al. Newly reported respiratory symptoms and conditions among military personnel deployed to Iraq and Afghanistan: A prospective population-based study. American Journal of Epidemiology 2009; 170: 1433-1442.
13. Falvo MJ, Osinubi OY, Sotolongo AM, Helmer BA. Airborne hazards exposure and respiratory health of Iraq and Afghanistan veterans. Epidemiologic Reviews 2015; 37: 116-130.
14. Szema AM, Peters MC, Weissinger KM, et al. New-onset asthma among soldiers serving in Iraq and Afghanistan. Allergy & Asthma Proceedings 2010; 31: 67-71.
15. Napier BA. Joint U.S./Russian studies of population exposures resulting from nuclear production activities in the southern Urals. Health Physics 2014; 106: 294-304.
16. Balonov M, Alexakhin R, Bouville A, Liljiinzin J-O. Report from the Techa River Dosimetry Review Workshop held on 8–10 December 2003 at the State Research Centre Institute of Biophysics, Moscow, Russia. Health Physics 2006; 90: 97-113.
17. Krestinina L, Preston DL, Davis FG, et al. Leukemia incidence among people exposed to chronic radiation from the contaminated Techa River, 1953–2005. Radiation and Environmental Biophysics 2010; 49: 195-201.
18. Wolbarst AB, Blom PF, Chan D, et al. Sites in the United States contaminated with radioactivity. Health Physics 1999; 77: 247-260.
19. Renner M. "Assessing the Military's War on the Environment" in L Starke (Ed.). State of the World 1991: A WorldWatch Institute Report on Progress Toward a Sustainable Society. New York: W.W. Norton & Company, 1991, pp. 131-152.

20. LaMontagne AD, Van Dyke MV, Martyny JW, Ruttenber AJ. Cleanup worker exposures to hazardous chemicals at a former nuclear weapons plant: Piloting of an exposure surveillance system. Applied Occupational and Environmental Hygiene 2001; 16: 284-290.

21. Prăvălie R. Nuclear weapons tests and environmental consequences: A global perspective. AMBIO 2014; 43: 729-744.

22. Stevens W, Thomas DC, Lyon JL, et al. Leukemia in Utah and radioactive fallout from the Nevada test site: A case-control study. Journal of the American Medical Association 1990; 264: 585-591.

23. Institute of Medicine. Exposure to the American People to Iodine-131 from Nevada Nuclear-bomb Tests: Review of the National Cancer Institute Report and Public Health Implications. Washington, DC: National Academy Press, 1999.

24. Cho A. France grossly underestimated radioactive fallout from atom bomb tests, study finds. Science, March 11, 2021. Available at: https://www.sciencemag.org/news/2021/03/france-grossly-underestima ted-radioactive-fallout-atom-bomb-tests-study-finds. Accessed on April 5, 2021.

25. de Vathaire F, Drozdovitch V, Brindel P, et al. Thyroid cancer following nuclear tests in French Polynesia. British Journal of Cancer 2010; 103: 1115-1121.

26. Skipperud L. Plutonium in the Arctic marine environment: A short review. Scientific World Journal 2004; 4: 460-461.

27. Greenberg MI, Sexton KJ, Vearrier D. Sea-dumped chemical weapons: Environmental risk, occupational hazard. Clinical Toxicology 2016; 54: 79-91.

28. Li C, Srivastava RK, Athar M. Biological and environmental hazards associated with exposure to chemical warfare agents: Arsenicals. Annals of the New York Academy of Sciences 2016; 1378: 143-157. doi: 10.1111/nyas.13214.

29. Smith SL. Toxic legacy: Mustard gas in the sea around us. Journal of Law and Medical Ethics 2011; 39: 34-40.

30. Carson R. The Sea Around Us. New York: Oxford University Press, 1951.

31. Brewer P, Nakayama N. What lies beneath: A plea for complete information. Environmental Science & Technology 2008. Available at: https://pubs.acs.org/doi/pdf/10.1021/es087088h?rand=9rc300rr. Accessed on November 2, 2020.

32. United Nations Environment Programme. Introductory report of the Executive Director: Environmental consequences of the armed conflict between Iraq and Kuwait. New York: UNEP, May 10, 1991.

33. Hamilton JW. Contamination at U.S. military bases: Profiles and responses. Stanford Environmental Law Journal 2016; 35: 223-249.

34. Air Force Center for Engineering and the Environment. Groundwater Plume Mass & Information Booklet. Massachusetts Military Reservation, Cape Cod, Massachusetts, 2010.

35. Copp T. DoD: At least 126 bases report water contaminates linked to cancer, birth defects. Military Times, April 26, 2018. Available at: https://www.militarytimes.com/news/your-military/2018/04/ 26/dod-126-bases-report-water-contaminants-harmful-to-infant-development-tied-to-cancers/. Accessed on April 13, 2020.

36. United States Government Accountability Office. Military Base Realignments and Closures: DOD Has Improved Environmental Cleanup Reporting but Should Obtain and Share More Information (GAO-17-151). Washington, DC: GAO, January 2017.

37. Westing AH. "The Impact of War on the Environment" in BS Levy, VW Sidel (eds.). War and Public Health (2d ed.). New York: Oxford University Press; 2008, pp. 69-84.

38. Edwards R. US fired depleted uranium at civilian areas in 2003 Iraq war, report finds. The Guardian, June 19, 2014. Available at: https://www.theguardian.com/world/2014/jun/19/us-depleted-uranium-weapons-civilian-areas-iraq. Accessed on January 11, 2021.

39. Asic A, Kurtovic-Kozaric A, Besic L, et al. Chemical toxicity and radioactivity of depleted uranium: The evidence from in vivo and in vitro studies. Environmental Research 2017; 156: 665-673.

40. Klare MT. Resource Wars: The New Landscape of Global Conflict. New York: Henry Holt and Company, 2001.

41. Klare MT, Levy BS, Sidel VW. Public health implications of resource wars. American Journal of Public Health 2011; 101: 1615-1619. doi: 10.2105/AJPH.2011.300267.

42. Dudley JP, Ginsberg JR, Plumptre AJ, et al. Effects of war and civil strife on wildlife and wildlife habitats. Conservation Biology 2002; 16: 319-329.

43. Hanson T. Biodiversity conservation and armed conflict: A warfare ecology perspective. Annals of the New York Academy of Sciences 2018; 1429: 50-65.

44. Daskin JH, Pringle RM. Warfare and wildlife declines in Africa's protected areas. Nature 2018; 553: 328-332.

45. Hochschild A. To End All Wars: A Story of Loyalty and Rebellion, 1914–1918. New York: Houghton Mifflin Publishing Company, 2011.

46. Westing AH. "Environmental Hazards of War in an Industrializing World" in AH Westing (ed.). Environmental Hazards of War: Releasing Dangerous Forces in an Industrialized World. London: Sage Publications Ltd., 1990, pp. 1-9.

47. Geissler E, Guillemin J. German flooding of the Pontine Marshes in World War II. Politics and the Life Sciences 2010; 29: 2-23.

48. United Nations. Convention on the Prohibition of Military or Any Other Hostile Use of Environmental Modification Techniques. Signed in 1977, entered into force in 1978. Available at: https://treaties.un.org/doc/Treaties/1978/10/19781005%2000-39%20AM/Ch_XXVI_01p.pdf. Accessed on November 5, 2020.

49. United Nations Human Rights Office of the High Commissioner. Protocol Additional to the Geneva Conventions of 12 August 1949, and Relating to the Protection of Victims of Non-International Armed Conflicts (Protocol II). Available at: https://www.ohchr.org/Documents/ProfessionalInterest/protocol2.pdf. Accessed on November 6, 2020.

50. United Nations High Commissioner for Refugees, International Organization for Migration and Refugee Policy Group. Environmentally-induced population displacements and environmental impacts resulting from mass migrations. In: International Symposium Report, April 21-24, 1996. Geneva: International Organization for Migration, 1996. Available at: https://publications.iom.int/system/files/pdf/environmentally_induced.pdf. Accessed on August 26, 2020.

51. Kibreab G. Environmental causes and impacts of refugee movements: A critique of the current debate. Disasters 1997; 21: 20-38.

52. Behnke NL, Cronk R, Shackelford BB, et al. Environmental health conditions in protracted displacement: A systematic scoping review. Science of the Total Environment 2020; 726: 138234. doi: https://doi.org/10.1016/j.scitotenv.2020.138234.

53. Levy MA, Thorkelson C, Vörösmarty C, et al. Freshwater Availability, Anomalies and Outbreak of Internal War: Results from a Global Spatial Time Series Analysis. Human Security and Climate Change: An International Workshop, Asker, Norway, June 2005. Available at: https://www.ciesin.columbia.edu/pdf/waterconflict.pdf. Accessed on May 14, 2021.

54. United Nations. Water scarcity. Available at: http://www.unwater.org/water-facts/scarcity/. Accessed on September 29, 2020.

55. Levy BS. "Water and Armed Conflict" in JMH Selendy (ed.). Water and Sanitation-Related Diseases and the Changing Environment: Challenges, Interventions, and Preventive Measures. Hoboken, NJ: John Wiley & Sons, Inc., 2019, pp. 53-57.

56. Gleick PH. The water conflict chronology. Available at:https://www.worldwater.org/water-conflict/. Accessed on February 4, 2021.

57. Greenberg MR. Water, conflict, and hope. American Journal of Public Health 2009; 99: 1928-1930.

58. Levy BS, Patz JA (eds.). Climate Change and Public Health. New York: Oxford University Press, 2015.

59. Lemery J, Knowlton K, Sorensen C (eds.). Global Climate Change and Human Health: From Science to Practice (Second Edition). San Francisco: Jossey-Bass, 2021.

60. Stocker TF, Qin D, Plattner G-K, et al. (eds.). Climate change 2013: The Physical Science Basis. Contribution of Working Group 1 to the Fifth Assessment of the Intergovernmental Panel on Climate Change; 2013. Available at: https://www.ipcc.ch/report/ar5/wg1/. Accessed on May 25, 2020.

61. Basu R. "Disorders Related to Heat Waves" in BS Levy, JA Patz (eds.). Climate Change and Public Health. New York: Oxford University Press, 2015, pp. 87-103.

62. Myers SS, Smith MR, Guth S, et al. Climate change and global food systems: Potential impacts on food security and undernutrition. Annual Review of Public Health 2017; 38: 259-277.

63. Porter JR, Xie L, Challinor AJ, et al. "Food Security and Food Production Systems" in CB Field, VR Barros, DJ Dokken, et al. (eds.). Climate Change 2014: Impacts, Adaptation, and Vulnerability. Part A: Global and Sectoral Aspects. Contribution of Working Group II to the Fifth Assessment Report of the Intergovernmental Panel on Climate Change. Cambridge, United Kingdom, and New York: Cambridge University Press, 2014, pp. 485-533.

64. Phalkey RK, Aranda-Jan C, Marx S, et al. Systematic review of current efforts to quantify the impacts of climate change on undernutrition. Proceedings of the National Academy of Sciences USA 2015; 112: E4522-E4529.

65. Swing WL. "Foreword" in IOM International Organization for Migration. Migration, Environment and Climate Change: Assessing the Evidence. Geneva, Switzerland: International Organization for Migration, 2009, pp. 5-6. Available at: https://publications.iom.int/system/files/pdf/migration_and_environment.pdf. Accessed on November 2, 2020.

66. Levy BS, Sidel VW, Patz JA. Climate change and collective violence. Annual Review of Public Health 2017; 38: 241-257.

67. Levy BS, Sidel VW. Collective violence caused by climate change and how it threatens health and human rights. Health and Human Rights 2014; 16: 1-9.

68. Hsiang SM, Burke M, Miguel E. Quantifying the influence of climate on human conflict. Science 2013; 341: 1235367. doi: 10.1126/science.1235367.

69. Hsiang SM, Burke M. Climate, conflict, and social stability: What does the evidence say? Climatic Change 2014; 123: 39-55.

70. Gleick PH. Water, drought, climate change, and conflict in Syria. Weather, Climate and Society 2014; 6: 331-340.

71. Hurley DM. A sequential relationship: Drought's contribution to the onset of the Syrian Civil War. Sigma Iota Rho Journal of International Relations, December 2, 2018. Available at: http://www.sirjournal.org/research/2018/12/12/a-sequential-relationship-droughts-contribution-to-the-onset-of-the-syrian-civil-war. Accessed on May 14, 2021.

72. Patz JA, Gibbs HK, Foley JA, et al. Climate change and global health: Quantifying a growing ethical crisis. EcoHealth 2007; 4: 397-405. doi: 10.1007/s10393-007-0141-1.

Profile 13:
Daniele Lantagne, Ph.D., M.Eng.
Ensuring Access to Safe Water

Human health depends on access to safe water. It takes years for a country to develop its water infrastructure, building water treatment plants and distribution networks and training technical experts to maintain and improve them. But war can destroy much of the infrastructure within minutes and injure or kill technical experts or force them to flee.

Daniele Lantagne has the multidisciplinary expertise and extensive experience that are critical to restoring and maintaining access to safe water—not only in war settings. She earned a master's degree in environmental engineering and a doctoral degree in public health/infectious tropical diseases. Over 9 years, she gained practical field experience—while working with the Centers for Disease Control and Prevention and with Innovations for Poverty Action, a nongovernmental organization—in 70 low- and middle-income countries, including Haiti, Burundi, Rwanda, and Yemen. Much of her field work involved advising and training people at the local level on ways to treat water with locally available materials. She understands that restoring and maintaining access to clean water takes methodical work over time, building trust and relationships with local partners and relying on local people and materials to ensure sustainability.

For almost 10 years, she has been a faculty member at the Tufts University School of Engineering, where she conducts research, consults to ongoing field operations in many countries, and teaches undergraduate and graduate students as well as postdoctoral fellows. She also sends them to low-income countries to perform applied research in real-world settings, and she supervises their work and collaborates with them in writing and widely disseminating reports. Her research focuses on practical field questions: How much chlorine is necessary to kill specific microorganisms in specific settings? How much chlorine could be harmful? How long does the Ebola virus or the COVID-19 virus survive on wood, a tarp, or dirt?

From Horror to Hope. Barry S. Levy, Oxford University Press. © Oxford University Press 2022.
DOI: 10.1093/oso/9780197558645.003.0026

In her academic role, she does much cross-border consulting on water and sanitation issues to people in war zones. For example, teams of water and sanitation workers in Syria and Yemen gather data on access to water and sanitation and then promptly send her the data electronically. She and her colleagues analyze the data and quickly send data analyses to these teams to guide them in maintaining access of war-affected populations to safe water sources and sanitation services. These analyses help the teams answer questions like: Where are water test kits needed? Where do latrines need to be set up? Is the training of local workers effective? How can UNICEF best support a local water trucking network?

Dr. Lantagne points out that technology and engineering represent only 1% of the overall work that needs to be done in war zones and other low-resource settings to restore and improve water and sanitation. Much work is done by anthropologists, sociologists, logistics specialists, and local people themselves. And ultimately countries need to set up training programs and educational institutions, like the new engineering school in Haiti, to ensure that the work is sustainable.

There are lots of challenges in this work: ensuring security to work safely in fragile settings, high turnover of competent local staff members, setbacks resulting from violent attacks on people and facilities. What keeps her going? "Everywhere people are trying to make things better," she observes. "It is invigorating to help them."

Dr. Lantagne is a Professor at the Tufts University School of Engineering.

14

Determining the Health Impacts of War

In war, truth is the first casualty.

AESCHYLUS

INTRODUCTION

Determining the health impacts of war is done to document morbidity and mortality, to assess the needs of affected populations, and to help bring an end to war. Both quantitative and qualitative information can be useful to health professionals, humanitarian aid workers, policymakers, journalists, and the general public.

Quantitative studies can lead to evidence-based recommendations for action. But statistics are just part of the picture; they do not convey the human dimension of the carnage of war. As the late Victor Sidel, my longtime colleague and a leading advocate for health, peace, and social justice, often said: "Statistics are people with the tears washed away."

Qualitative data, such as from focus-group discussions, are needed as well. The personal stories of people affected by war—through words and images—complement statistics in describing the health impacts of war and can help build the popular and political will to protect civilians and end war.

This chapter describes basic approaches to recognizing and assessing the health impacts of war and provides multiple examples of how information can be used to decrease morbidity and mortality, address the needs of affected populations, and help prevent war.

There are at least seven major challenges in accurately determining the health impacts of war:

- Lack of security and stability: Inadequate security and political and socioeconomic instability impede gathering information in war zones.
- Inaccurate reporting: For various reasons, governments, military forces, aid organizations, and individuals may underestimate or overstate morbidity and mortality. Decreased access

From Horror to Hope. Barry S. Levy, Oxford University Press. © Oxford University Press 2022.
DOI: 10.1093/oso/9780197558645.003.0027

to healthcare, cultural and language barriers, and difficulties distinguishing between combatants and civilians contribute to inaccurate reporting.

- Inadequate data systems: Wars often damage systems for collecting, analyzing, and disseminating health data. These systems may have been inadequate before war began, so there may be little or no baseline data for comparison.
- Displaced populations: When people are displaced, especially if they are mobile and dispersed, it is difficult to gather both numerator data (on their injuries, illnesses, and deaths) and denominator data (on the number of people at risk).
- Indirect health impacts: The nature and magnitude of indirect health impacts, which account for most morbidity and mortality during war, are difficult to determine.
- Distant impacts: Fighting often occurs in remote locations. In addition, it is difficult to assess the health consequences of aerial bombing and use of remote-controlled weapons, such as armed drones (unmanned aerial vehicles).
- Delayed impacts: Many impacts of war, including various mental disorders and noncommunicable diseases, such as cancer, tend to occur years after war has ended.

The three basic approaches to recognizing and assessing the health impacts of war are rapid assessments, surveillance, and epidemiological studies. Field epidemiologists and other health professionals play central roles in each of these approaches—in determining the numbers of people affected and at risk, calculating morbidity and mortality rates, assessing and prioritizing the health needs of populations, and monitoring progress and evaluating the impact of interventions.[1]

RAPID ASSESSMENTS

Overview

Rapid assessments are external evaluations that are ideally performed early in a crisis or immediately after a disastrous event, such as a bombing attack on civilians or civilian infrastructure. Rapid assessments collect data from on-the-scene observations; samples of affected people; walkthrough observations; interviews with government officials, community and religious leaders, aid workers, and other key informants; easily available sources of quantitative data; and small-scale surveys. Rapid assessments collect data on population density and composition, vulnerable groups, morbidity and mortality, violations of human rights, food availability, water supply and sanitation, shelter, security, family size, and community organization. Ideally, they use validated assessment tools that incorporate cultural concepts of health and illness of the affected population.

Although they are often done quickly, rapid assessments provide valuable information on the demographics, mobility, health status, and needs of war-affected populations; their health and security risks; and their access to food, water, shelter, and health services. Rapid assessments help ensure that the type and amount of humanitarian aid is appropriate and directed to the most vulnerable people. Provision of aid and other interventions generally need to begin before risk assessments are complete.[1]

Multidisciplinary teams perform rapid assessments. These teams include epidemiologists; specialists in food and nutrition, water and sanitation, logistics, and social and behavioral sciences; and interpreters. These teams often also include representatives of host-country governments, nongovernmental organizations (NGOs), faith community organizations, academic institutions, and human rights groups. Ideally, many team members are fluent in the national language and local dialects.

Challenges in performing rapid assessments include getting access to affected populations and gaining their trust, ensuring security, obtaining relevant and representative health data, coordinating with other organizations, disseminating findings to those who need to know, and ensuring that these findings are not ignored.[1] If a rapid assessment has been sponsored by an international organization or a nongovernmental aid organization, its findings are likely to influence program planning and implementation. Rapid assessments often lead to establishment of surveillance systems for mortality, nutritional status, and incidence of communicable diseases (see next page).

SMART Methodology

SMART is an interagency initiative by a network of NGOs and humanitarian aid organizations that provides a systematic approach for rapid assessments in order to provide reliable information for decision-making and to establish shared resources and systems. The SMART methodology is applicable to war-related humanitarian crises and war-displaced populations.

The SMART methodology recognizes that in order to understand the causes of a crisis and to plan and implement humanitarian assistance, one needs to consider the pre-conflict situation for that population, the evolution of changes, and the context in which the emergency has arisen. Its methodology for household-level surveys focuses on nutritional status of children under 5 years of age and the overall mortality rate of the population in order to assess the magnitude and severity of a humanitarian crisis. Its findings are valuable for prioritizing resources, monitoring how well a relief operation is meeting population needs, and assessing the overall impact of a relief operation.[2]

Example of a Rapid Assessment

Over a 2-week period in March 2013, the Assessment Working Group for Northern Syria, which was composed of a range of humanitarian workers, conducted a rapid assessment in Aleppo, the second-largest city in Syria. It covered 52 (42%) of 125 neighborhoods and represented 70% of the prewar population of the city. It found that there were 2.4 million people in urgent need of humanitarian assistance, 510,000 of whom had been forced from their homes. The rapid assessment determined that 2.4 million people had insufficient access to health services; 2.2 million were "borderline food insecure"; 2.0 million were facing challenges to access adequate shelter and non-food items, such as blankets, water containers, cooking items, and soap; and 240,000 people were lacking sufficient access to water. It identified groups requiring immediate assistance, including internally displaced persons living in vacated buildings, improvised shelters, and collective accommodations. It also identified relief agencies that were already providing health, nutrition, and other assistance.[3]

The rapid assessment made several priority recommendations, including:

- Food security: Provision of basic food items, delivery of wheat flour and fuel support to subsidize bakeries, provision of fuel for cooking, and cash for the most vulnerable groups
- Healthcare: Medicines to treat injuries and diseases, repair of health infrastructure, provision of medical staff, a referral system for critically ill patients, and needed medical equipment
- Nutrition: Nutritional support for vulnerable groups, recruitment and training of breast-feeding counselors and outreach workers to provide women with infant and child feeding support, unconditional cash grants for vulnerable groups, and training for health professionals
- Water, sanitation, and hygiene: Solid waste management and garbage collection, fuel and electricity for generators to ensure an adequate water supply, and provision of insecticides, hygiene kits, and water purification systems and tablets
- Protection: Assistance to protect children and other civilians and to restore law and order.

The assessment also made recommendations for shelter and non-food items and for addressing information gaps and needs.[3]

SURVEILLANCE

Overview

Public health surveillance is "the ongoing, systematic collection, analysis, and the interpretation of health-related data essential to planning, implementation, and evaluation of public health practice, closely integrated with the timely dissemination of these data to those responsible for prevention and control."[4] It typically focuses on vulnerable populations. A wide range of sources can provide surveillance data, including physicians and other healthcare workers, hospitals and clinics, clinical laboratories, death registries, government agencies, NGOs, the news media, and even social media. Although surveillance data are inherently incomplete, they can nevertheless identify outbreaks and significant trends, causes and risk factors for morbidity and mortality, and the needs of affected populations—and help prevent illness, injury, and death.

There are several types of surveillance. *Passive surveillance* relies on existing systems to collect, analyze, and disseminate data. *Active surveillance*, which yields more complete data, relies on encouraging clinicians to report illnesses, injuries, and deaths by providing them with various incentives. *Sentinel surveillance*, which yields even more complete data, relies on a relatively small number of selected clinicians who are known to frequently diagnose specific diseases.

In addition, *syndromic surveillance* relies on reports of groups of symptoms and other pre-diagnostic data to detect public health problems, prompting early interventions and further investigation. Symptoms frequently targeted include:

- Cough and other symptoms of acute respiratory infection (a proxy for pneumonia)
- Acute watery diarrhea (which may represent cholera)

- Acute bloody diarrhea (which may indicate bacillary dysentery, or shigellosis)
- Fever (which may indicate malaria, meningitis, or other communicable diseases)
- Fever in combination with a maculopapular rash and cough, coryza, or conjunctivitis (which may indicate measles).[5]

At an early stage of armed conflict, surveillance can be used to minimize the number of people injured and killed. Even limited surveillance data can help in estimating the health status of a population, identifying vulnerable groups, and choosing initial interventions. Surveillance often leads to epidemiological studies that can investigate morbidity and mortality in greater depth.

Example of Public Health Surveillance

In June 1994, soon after civil war and mass genocide in Rwanda, about one million Rwandan refugees fled to Zaire (now the Democratic Republic of the Congo, or the DRC) and 170,000 fled to Burundi. Surveillance was conducted by home-health visitors, who collected mortality data from reports of family members, grave watchers, and distributors of funeral shrouds. The most frequent cause of mortality was diarrheal disease; the most frequent causes of nonfatal illness were malaria, bloody diarrhea, and acute respiratory infections. NGOs in refugee camps in Burundi performed morbidity surveillance for cholera and other diarrheal diseases, malaria, acute respiratory infections, measles, meningitis, and trauma. Surveillance identified a cholera outbreak in one refugee camp, where prompt chlorination of the water supply, health education, and better maintenance of latrines reduced the weekly incidence of new cases from 980 to 350 per 100,000 population within 5 weeks. Surveillance also identified an outbreak of meningococcal meningitis, which promptly led to an immunization program.[6]

In refugee camps in eastern Zaire, clinics operated by NGOs began surveillance. Mortality surveillance, based on recovered bodies, bodies buried in mass graves, and reports from camp hospitals, indicated that the daily crude mortality rate decreased from 34-55 deaths per 10,000 people to 2.5 per 10,000 in about 6 weeks. More than 90% of all deaths occurred outside of healthcare facilities. The highest morbidity and mortality rates were associated with epidemics of cholera and dysentery.

EPIDEMIOLOGICAL STUDIES

Challenges and Opportunities

During war or its aftermath, epidemiological studies can yield valuable information on the nature, severity, and magnitude of health problems and their determinants. These studies can determine morbidity and mortality rates and can identify vulnerable populations and opportunities for prevention.

To be effective during war, epidemiologists need to be competent in conducting thorough assessments of war settings in order to develop effective public health actions. They also need to be able to communicate effectively to guide the implementation of health programs, advocate for necessary policy changes, and facilitate coordination among agencies and organizations.[7]

During war, epidemiologists often need to adapt plans and protocols because of quickly changing circumstances.[8] For example, in the 1982 Lebanese Civil War, situations often changed dramatically, so it was difficult for epidemiologists to maintain continuity of surveillance. Without a centralized authority, epidemiologists had to obtain permission to conduct interviews from militia groups in each neighborhood. Political polarization made data collection difficult. And epidemiologists often needed to make compromises, such as when they were unable to complete interviews because people fled or were not available.[9] (See Profiles 7 and 14.)

Morbidity Studies

Morbidity studies, usually cross-sectional in design, are used to investigate the prevalence of communicable diseases, malnutrition, and noncommunicable diseases. In conducting these studies, epidemiologists sample subgroups of populations using questionnaires, interviews, and measurements, such as weight and height. These studies need to be based on sample sizes that are representative and large enough to reduce bias and sampling error. And they need to take into account potential confounding factors.

Mortality Studies

Mortality studies aim to determine or estimate the number and rate of excess deaths related to war. *Excess mortality* represents the difference between the crude mortality rate during a war compared with the baseline crude mortality rate before the war began. Given inadequate data systems and the widespread practice of not recording deaths in many countries, the baseline crude mortality rate may be difficult to determine. Excess mortality comprises both *direct deaths* and *indirect deaths*. Direct deaths are caused by combat, whether or not the victims are combatants. Indirect deaths are those that are caused by damage to civilian infrastructure and worsening of living conditions in the area affected by a war (Chapters 1 and 2). The three frequently used methods for estimating indirect deaths are retrospective mortality studies, prospective mortality studies based on health information systems, and analyses based on multiple sources of data before, during, and after a war.[10]

Indirect deaths are challenging to quantify and to attribute to war-related causes because it is difficult to:

- Collect health data because of damage to information systems, loss of human resources, and restriction in movement
- Determine the baseline mortality rate in a country or an area within a country where there has been little or no accurate collection of health data for a long time
- Separate indirect deaths related to war from deaths that would have occurred in the same population without war.[10]

Prospective mortality studies, which are based on "body counts," identify, confirm, and describe the circumstances of direct deaths as they occur. These studies are typically not

designed to identify indirect deaths. Data come from multiple sources, including death cer-
tificates, news reports, clergy, burial sites, and death-benefit programs.[11]

In contrast, retrospective mortality studies yield estimates of previous deaths, potentially including both direct and indirect deaths. These studies are based on interviews of a
member of each selected household to obtain information on deaths (numerator data) and
on household members who were present for some time during the study period (denominator data). They then extrapolate these data to the entire population to estimate total mortality. Frequently, two-stage cluster sampling is performed, in which clusters of households
are randomly selected from the total population, and then, within each cluster, individual
households are randomly selected.

Error not related to sampling is likely to be more important than the disadvantages of
any sampling method. To avoid nonsampling error, interviewers must be trained to admin-
ister surveys appropriately so that collected data are accurate. They need to recognize that
people who have suffered significant losses may provide answers that they think the interviewers want to hear, resulting in biased findings. In a retrospective mortality study, potential
sources of bias include failing to recall deaths during the recall period or reporting deaths
that did not occur during the period, reluctance of respondents to discuss deaths, respondents' deliberate provision of misleading or inaccurate information, errors in translation, and
errors in administering a questionnaire. Bias can be minimized by writing clear questions,
standardizing and pilot-testing survey instruments, and providing quality training of interviewers and translators.

There are several ethical issues in performing an epidemiological study during war, the
most important of which is whether the perceived benefits of the study outweigh the risks
of performing it. (See the section on "Ethical Issues in Research" in Chapter 3.) Researchers
need to obtain without coercion the approval of the studied community and participating
individuals. And they need to perform the study in the safest, least intrusive way possible.

Limitations of epidemiological studies during war include inadequate security, insufficient human and financial resources, transportation and communication breakdowns, and
changing conditions. Another limitation is that epidemiological studies may not able to establish cause-and-effect relationships between interventions and health outcomes. Therefore,
epidemiologists often need to resist pressures from government agencies and NGOs that may
want them to demonstrate beneficial impacts of specific interventions.

Determining deaths and the death rate during or after a war is often politically contentious, especially when combatants attribute civilian deaths to an adversary for partisan
reasons. Both overestimation and underestimation of total deaths and the mortality rate frequently occur. Estimated death tolls from several recent wars are still debated.[12]

Some practical suggestions for performing epidemiological research in war and postwar
settings include the following:

- Rely on local partners in developing and implementing a research study
- Undertake contingency planning for unanticipated circumstances
- Understand available resources, local culture, and political considerations
- Use facility-based data, if possible

- Recognize that political obstacles may occur not only during the planning and implementation of a study, but also in the dissemination of results
- Recognize differences in cultural practices and norms
- Use key-informant interviews and focus-group discussions to help understand local power dynamics and social hierarchies
- Recognize that timely dissemination of results is critically important.[13]

Examples of Epidemiological Studies

The Democratic Republic of the Congo

After the Democratic Republic of the Congo Civil War, a cluster survey of 19,500 households, performed between April and July 2004, found that the crude mortality rate was 40% higher than that in the overall sub-Saharan region. The study estimated that 600,000 excess deaths occurred during the January 2003–April 2004 recall period and 3.9 million people died between 1998 and 2004. Most deaths were from easily preventable and treatable illnesses rather than from violence.[14]

Darfur

Six studies performed during the armed conflict in Darfur, Sudan, were used to estimate the total number of deaths during the first years of the conflict (2003–2005). The most reliable of these studies indicated that more than 107,000 total deaths occurred during a 23-month period between 2003 and 2005, mainly due to violence and increased occurrence of malnutrition and other diseases.[15]

Another study in Darfur, performed in 2008 and 2009, demonstrated the limits of traditional frameworks for classifying armed violence. The study found that there were complex patterns of armed conflict, including battles between the major combatants, battles among subgroups of combatant coalitions that were thought to be allied, intertribal conflict, incidents of one-sided violence against civilians by various parties, and incidents of banditry.[16]

Syria

During the Syrian Civil War, a study found that, between 2011 and 2016, there were 101,453 deaths due to war-related violence among civilians, accounting for about 71% of all conflict-related violent deaths there during this period. Of the 17,401 violent deaths among children during this period, it found that about 80% were due to aerial bombardments or shelling, and the remainder were due to shootings, executions, blasts from ground-level explosives, and use of chemical weapons.[17]

Iraq

Many studies have been performed on the adverse health consequences of the Iraq War.[18] The following paragraphs describe studies among civilians during the Iraq War. (War-related health impacts among U.S. military personnel are described in Chapter 12.)

A review of 13 studies between March 2003, when the United States invaded Iraq, and January 2008 provided estimates of Iraqi deaths based on primary research. The studies had used a wide range of methodologies, varying from sentinel data collection to population-based surveys. Studies assessed as having the highest quality yielded the highest estimates, although the range of estimated deaths was wide (between 48 and 759 per day) and cause-specific mortality rates attributable to violence ranged from 0.64 to 10.25 per 1,000 per year. The review concluded that, despite varying estimates, the mortality burden of the war and its sequelae on Iraq was very large.[19]

The Iraq Body Count, a prospective mortality study based on a register of documented deaths during the Iraq War, used reports of deaths from online English-language media agencies derived from a list that met predetermined baseline standards. Each death was validated by at least two independent reports. Accuracy and completeness of mortality data depended on reports of deaths by the news media and the quality of information from the reporting agency. As of July 2021, the Iraq Body Count reported that there were between 185,724 and 208,831 documented civilian deaths from violence since the 2003 start of the Iraq War. The number of deaths reported has likely been an underestimate of the actual number.[20]

The following four epidemiological studies that estimated mortality among Iraqi civilians were population-based, were reported in peer-reviewed journals, and estimated both the excess number of deaths attributable to all causes since the start of the war and the number of deaths caused by violence:

- In September 2004, researchers performed a cluster sample survey in which they interviewed members of 30 households in each of 33 clusters about household composition and births and deaths since January 2002. They estimated that 98,000 more deaths than expected occurred after the invasion, mainly due to violence, and determined that the risk of violent death since the invasion in mid-March 2003 was 58 times higher than in the period before the war.[21]
- In mid-2006, researchers performed a cross-sectional cohort study of deaths in Iraq during a baseline period between January 2002 and mid-March 2003 and since then. They used a sampling methodology similar to that in the study cited above, with 47 clusters of 40 households each. They estimated that, between mid-March 2003 and mid-2006, there were 655,965 excess post-invasion deaths, 92% of which were due to violence.[22]
- In 2008, researchers performed a nationally representative survey of 9,345 households to obtain information on violence-related deaths from January 2002 through February 2003, and from March 2003 through June 2006 (the study period). They estimated that 151,000 violent deaths occurred during the study period.[23]
- In mid-2011, researchers performed a survey of 100 clusters with a total of 2,000 households. They found that, between March 2003 and June 2011, the crude death rate was more than 50% higher than in the 20 months before the war. They estimated that approximately 405,000 excess deaths attributable to the war occurred during this 8-year period. They found that more than 60% of excess deaths were directly attributable to violence and the rest were associated with collapse of infrastructure and indirect war-related causes.[24]

FORENSIC INVESTIGATIONS

Forensic investigations can help to document torture and other human rights abuse during war and its aftermath. These investigations include physical examinations of torture survivors and the bodies of deceased persons, systematic interviews of witnesses, and other methods.[25] (See Chapter 3 and Profile 3.)

An illustrative forensic investigation was performed in 1999 on 1,180 ethnic Albanian refugees living in 31 refugee camps and collective centers in Macedonia and Albania. Most (68%) of the people who were interviewed reported that their families were expelled from their homes by Serb military forces. In total, 50% of those interviewed saw Serb police or soldiers burning the houses of others, 16% witnessed Serb police or soldiers burn their homes, and 14% saw Serb police or soldiers killing someone. High percentages of participants reported that they observed medical facilities, schools, or mosques that had been destroyed. Among the respondents, 31% reported human rights abuses committed against members of their households, including beatings, killings, torture, forced separation and disappearances, gunshot wounds, and sexual assault.[26]

IMPROVING METHODS TO DETERMINE THE HEALTH CONSEQUENCES OF WAR

Governments and humanitarian aid organizations can improve methods for rapid assessments, public health surveillance, and epidemiological studies by implementing a variety of measures. They can develop and improve ways to better estimate population size and population needs during the emergency phase of operations, develop and maintain surveillance systems for morbidity and mortality (including surveillance for cancer and birth defects), adapt methods to estimate population size, perform surveys in urban settings, and expand the capabilities of government agencies and aid organizations to perform surveillance and epidemiological studies and of policymakers to interpret epidemiological and surveillance data.[27] Areas for improvement of epidemiological studies during war and its aftermath include selecting samples from study populations, estimating the total at-risk population (the denominator), accounting for survival bias in household surveys, identifying war-related nonfatal illnesses and injuries, identifying during war those deaths that are not related to war, and improving the security for field research teams.[28]

Recognizing and documenting the health impacts of war has usually been done with limited human and financial resources, inadequate coordination among various entities, and inadequate ways of preventing bias. There is need for the following:

- An independent, nonpartisan mechanism, which ideally would be established and operated by a UN agency or a multilateral organization, to recognize, investigate, document, and report on the health consequences of war. This mechanism would need to include development, implementation, evaluation, and improvement of methodologies to document these consequences.

- A surveillance mechanism to identify population-based risk factors that indicate the probability of imminent war, which could lead to interventions to prevent that war
- Academic programs to educate and train more individuals in methodologies to determine the health impacts of war.[29]

PEACE EPIDEMIOLOGY

Epidemiology can be applied not only to war and its health impacts, but also to peace. Mohsen Rezaeian, an Iranian epidemiologist, has advanced the concept of *peace epidemiology*, which aims to reinforce peace by primary and/or primordial prevention activities (Chapter 15). Peace epidemiology is designed to focus on the positive impacts of peace on public health, such as increasing life expectancy. Peace epidemiology studies could be performed before a war erupts and could be used to help prevent war and promote peace.[30]

SUMMARY POINTS

- Documenting the health and human rights consequences of war is essential for identifying needs of affected populations.
- Both quantitative data and qualitative information are needed.
- Rapid assessments gather crude data quickly for immediate interventions and further studies.
- Public health surveillance gathers information on disease outbreaks and morbidity and mortality trends.
- Epidemiological studies, which provide detailed information on the distribution and determinants of morbidity and mortality, are critically important for preventing the health impacts of war.

REFERENCES

1. Waldman R. "Natural and Human-Made Disasters" in SA Rasmussen, RA Goodman (eds.). The CDC Field Epidemiology Manual. Atlanta: Centers for Disease Control and Prevention, 2018. Available at: https://www.cdc.gov/eis/field-epi-manual/chapters/Natural-Human-Disasters.html. Accessed on November 11, 2020.
2. SMART, Action Against Hunger Canada, and the Technical Advisory Group. SMART: Standardized Monitoring and Assessment for Relief and Transitions. Manual 2.0, 2017. Available at: https://smartmethodology.org/wp-content/uploads/2018/02/SMART-Manual-2.0_Final_January-9th-2017-for-merge-3.pdf. Accessed on May 7, 2021.
3. Assessment Working Group for Northern Syria. Joint Rapid Assessment of Northern Syria: Aleppo City Assessment (Summary Report), March 2013. Available at: https://reliefweb.int/report/syrian-arab-republic/joint-rapid-assessment-northern-syria-aleppo-city-assessment. Accessed on February 1, 2021.
4. Centers for Disease Control and Prevention. Introduction to Public Health Surveillance (Public Health 101 Series). Available at: https://www.cdc.gov/training/publichealth101/surveillance.html. Accessed on April 2, 2021.

5. Sir-Ond-Enguier PN, Ngoungou EB, Nghomo Y-N, et al. Syndromic surveillance of potentially epidemic infectious diseases: Detection of a measles epidemic in two health centers in Gabon, Central Africa. Infectious Disease Reports 2019; 11: 7701. doi: 10.4081/idr.2019.7701.

6. Centers for Disease Control and Prevention. Morbidity and mortality surveillance in Rwandan refugees—Burundi and Zaire, 1994. Morbidity and Mortality Weekly Report 1996; 45: 104-107.

7. McDonnell SM, Bolton P, Sunderland N, et al. The role of the applied epidemiologist in armed conflict. Emerging Themes in Epidemiology 2004; 1: 4. doi: 10.1186/1742-7622-1-4.

8. Axinn WG, Ghimire D, Williams NE. Collecting survey data during armed conflict. Journal of Official Statistics 2012; 28: 153-171.

9. Armenian HK. Perceptions from epidemiologic research in an endemic war. Social Science and Medicine 1989; 28: 643-647.

10. Ratanayake R, Degomme O, Altare C, Guha-Sapir D. Methods and Tools to Evaluate Mortality in Conflicts: Critical Review, Case-studies, and Applications (CRED Occasional Paper No. 237). Brussels, Belgium: WHO Collaborating Centre for Research on Epidemiology of Disasters, University of Louvain, 2008.

11. Seybolt TB, Aronson JD, Fischhoff B (eds.). Counting Civilian Casualties: An Introduction to Recording and Estimating Nonmilitary Deaths in Conflict. Oxford: Oxford University Press, 2013.

12. Guha-Sapir D, Checchi F. Science and politics of disaster death tools. British Medical Journal 2018; 362: k4005. doi: 10.1136/bmj.k4005.

13. Guha-Sapir D, Scales SE. Challenges in public health and epidemiology research in humanitarian settings: Experiences from the field. BMC Public Health 2020; 20: 1761. https://bmcpublichealth.biomed central.com/articles/10.1186/s12889-020-09851-7.

14. Coghlan B, Brennan RJ. Ngoy P, et al. Mortality in the Democratic Republic of Congo: A nationwide survey. Lancet 2006; 367: 44-51.

15. U.S. Government Accountability Office. Darfur Crisis: Death Estimates Demonstrate Severity of Crisis But Their Accuracy and Credibility Could Be Enhanced. Washington, DC: GAO, 2006. Available at: https://www.gao.gov/assets/260/253101.pdf. Accessed on August 11, 2020.

16. de Waal A, Hazlett C, Davenport C, Kennedy J. The epidemiology of lethal violence in Darfur: Using micro-data to explore complex patterns of ongoing armed conflict. Social Science & Medicine 2014; 120: 368-377.

17. Guha-Sapir D, Schlüter B, Rodriguez-Llanes JM, et al. Patterns of civilian and child deaths due to war-related violence in Syria: A comparative analysis from the Violation Documentation Center dataset, 2011–16. Lancet Global Health 2018; 6: 103-110.

18. Levy BS, Sidel VW. Adverse health consequences of the Iraq War. Lancet 2013; 381: 949-958.

19. Tapp C, Burkle FM Jr, Wilson K, et al. Iraq War mortality estimates: A systematic review. Conflict and Health 2008; 2: 1. doi: 10.1186/1752-1505-2-1.

20. Iraq Body Count. Available at: https://www.iraqbodycount.org/. Accessed on July 3, 2021.

21. Roberts L, Lafta R, Garfield R, et al. Mortality before and after the 2003 invasion of Iraq: Cluster sample survey. Lancet 2004; 364: 1857-1864.

22. Burnham G, Lafta R, Doocy S, Roberts L. Mortality after the 2003 invasion of Iraq: A cross-sectional cluster sample survey. Lancet 2006; 368: 1421-1428.

23. Iraq Family Health Survey Study Group. Violence-related mortality in Iraq from 2002 to 2006. New England Journal of Medicine 2008; 358: 474-493.

24. Hagopian A, Flaxman AD, Takaro TK, et al. Mortality in Iraq associated with the 2003–2011 war and occupation: Findings from a national cluster sample survey by the University Collaborative Iraq Mortality Study. PLoS Medicine 2013; 10: e1001533.

25. Office of the United Nations High Commissioner for Human Rights. Istanbul Protocol: Manual on the Effective Investigation and Documentation of Torture and other Cruel, Inhuman or Degrading Treatment or Punishment. New York and Geneva: United Nations, 2004. Available at: https://www. ohchr.org/documents/publications/training8rev1en.pdf. Accessed on May 14, 2021.

26. Iacopino V, Frank MW, Bauer HM, et al. A population-based assessment of human rights abuses committed against ethnic Albanian refugees from Kosovo. American Journal of Public Health 2001; 91: 2013-2018.

27. Spiegel EB, Checchi F, Colombo S, Paik E. Health-care needs of people affected by conflict: Future trends and changing frameworks. Lancet 2010; 375: 341-345.

28. Hagopian A, Flaxman A, Galway L, et al. How to estimate (and not to estimate) war deaths: A reply to van Weezel and Spagat. Research and Politics 2018; 5. doi: 10.1177/2053168017753901.

29. Levy BS, Sidel VW. Documenting the effects of armed conflict on population health. Annual Review of Public Health 2016; 37: 205-218.

30. Rezaeian M. "War epidemiology" versus "peace epidemiology": A personal view. Archives of Iranian Medicine 2020; 23: S38-S42.

Profile 14:
Leslie (Les) Roberts, Ph.D.
Using Epidemiology to End War

Les Roberts's career is an example of following one's inner compass and seeing where it will take you. As he was growing up, he thought he would become a high school physics teacher or maybe an accountant. But after going in 1984 to teach in Kenya—an experience that opened his eyes to poverty and misogyny in low-income countries—he changed his career goals.

On return to the United States, he earned a master of public health degree and a doctoral degree in environmental engineering. He then served for 2 years in the Epidemic Intelligence Service (EIS) of the CDC. He spent 13 of those 24 months assessing the health of refugees in Bosnia, Malawi, Zimbabwe, Rwanda, and Armenia. Serving in the EIS, he says, was like being thrown into water over your head and learning how to swim—and, in the process, learning how to get things done in challenging situations with limited resources. For example, faced with determining the heating capacity of available biofuels so that Armenians could survive the winter, he drew on his engineering skills and his father's knowledge about furnaces. He stayed on for 2 more years at the CDC, working on problems like nitrite contamination of water by animal waste in the Midwest and cross-contamination of the piped water supply in Tajikistan.

Overall, Dr. Roberts has directed more than 50 epidemiological surveys in 17 countries, mainly on deaths caused by armed conflict. Many of these studies were performed during the course of wars, which provided opportunities for the study findings to be used to help protect civilians and to end these wars.

In 2000, he led a survey for the International Rescue Committee during the seven-nation civil war in the Democratic Republic of the Congo (DRC); the survey estimated that 1.7 million—about 10% of the population—had died as a result of the war. The published report led to a UN resolution calling for all foreign armies to withdraw from the DRC, increased coverage of the war in the Western media, and a dramatic rise in humanitarian funding to

From Horror to Hope. Barry S. Levy, Oxford University Press. © Oxford University Press 2022.
DOI: 10.1093/oso/9780197558645.003.0028

address the crisis. After a second survey in mid-2001 placed the death toll at 2.5 million, a UN-brokered accord led to the withdrawal of foreign troops and an "official" end to the war.

In 2004, he directed a study that found that approximately 100,000 Iraqi civilians had died in Iraq since the 2003 U.S. invasion. And 2 years later, he helped launch a second study, which estimated approximately 650,000 excess deaths in Iraq since the invasion.

Over the years, Dr. Roberts and his colleagues have refined their survey methodologies, not only to estimate overall mortality but also to study mortality of children under age 5, maternal mortality, and the incidence of rape and other human rights violations. These methodologies have been utilized by many other researchers in war-related and other fragile settings. And some of his other contributions have also had long-lasting impacts; for example, since years ago when he reported on his study that water in wide-necked containers was often contaminated by hand contact, use of narrow-necked water containers has been standard practice in relief operations.

One of the most gratifying parts of his career, Dr. Roberts observes, has been teaching more than 3,000 public health students—for 10 years as an Adjunct Professor of Public Health at Johns Hopkins and 15 years as a full-time faculty member at Columbia. He has continued to maintain contact with many students who, over the years, have asked for his advice and guidance.

Les never became a certified public accountant. But he did, in a sense, become an accountant, systematically quantifying the impact of war—and providing the evidence to make those responsible for these impacts accountable.

Dr. Roberts is a Professor in the Program on Forced Migration and Health at the Mailman School of Public Health of Columbia University.

PART V

The Future

15

Preventing War and Promoting Peace

If we don't end war, war will end us.
H. G. WELLS

INTRODUCTION

Previous chapters have described the health impacts of war and specific measures to *reduce* these impacts. However, the only way to *eliminate* the health impacts of war is to prevent war. This chapter presents a public health perspective on preventing war and promoting peace, with the ultimate goal of totally eliminating war.

Despite previous efforts to prevent armed conflicts,[1] wars are occurring in the Middle East, Africa, Asia, and elsewhere. Risks for war appear to be on the rise, including increasing nationalism in many countries, growing availability of lethal weapons, mass displacement of people accompanied by political and socioeconomic instability, and the increasing consequences of climate change.

Seventy-five years ago, Albert Einstein said that "a new type of thinking is essential . . . if mankind is to survive."[2] In order to survive, we, as a global society, will need to transform our thinking about war.

APPLYING BASIC PUBLIC HEALTH FRAMEWORKS

Levels of Prevention

The following four levels of prevention constitute a basic framework of public health practice. *Primordial prevention* identifies and reduces root (underlying) causes of illness or injury. *Primary prevention* reduces the likelihood of illness or injury. *Secondary prevention* reduces the impact of illness or injury once it occurs. And *tertiary prevention*

From Horror to Hope. Barry S. Levy, Oxford University Press. © Oxford University Press 2022.
DOI: 10.1093/oso/9780197558645.003.0029

rehabilitates and restores health. Applying this framework to preventing war and its health impacts:

- Primordial prevention identifies and reduces root causes of war.
- Primary prevention addresses the grievances and other precipitating causes of war and resolves disputes nonviolently.
- Secondary prevention attempts to end war and reduce its health and other impacts.
- Tertiary prevention rehabilitates and restores the health of individuals and communities after war has ended.

Host-Agent-Environment Triangle (Epidemiological Triad)

This framework, which was developed primarily to prevent communicable disease, consists of three components: a susceptible *host*, an external *agent*, and an *environment* in which host and agent are both present. Disease occurs due to host–agent interaction in an environment that supports transmission of the agent to the host.[3] Applying this framework to the prevention of war and its health impacts, host represents people at risk, agent represents military forces and their weapons, and environment represents the situations and conditions in which people live.

Within this framework, three types of strategies can be developed to prevent war and its health impacts:

- *Strategies focused on people at risk*, such as supporting people in resolving disputes without violence, increasing understanding and tolerance among groups, and addressing socioeconomic inequities
- *Strategies addressing military forces and their weapons*, such as reducing availability of weapons, addressing militarism, decreasing military expenditures, and strengthening international conventions and treaties
- *Strategies designed to improve the situations and conditions in which people live*, such as protecting human rights, reducing extreme poverty, improving governance, increasing education and employment opportunities, and addressing environmental stress.

ADVANCING A COMPREHENSIVE FRAMEWORK

The following framework, which builds on the two public health frameworks described above, represents a comprehensive approach to preventing war and promoting peace. As shown in Figure 15-1, it consists of:

- Resolving disputes nonviolently
- Reducing the root causes of war
- Strengthening the infrastructure for peace.

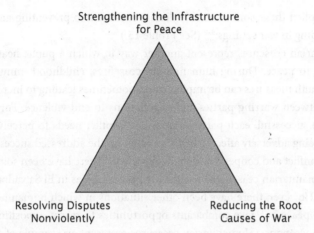

FIGURE 15-1 A comprehensive framework for preventing war and promoting peace. (Diagram by Barry S. Levy.)

Resolving Disputes Nonviolently

Preventing a war is much more desirable than attempting to minimize the health effects of a war that has already begun. Leaders who start a war often discover that they do not have the ability to end it because of major ideological differences, intense ethnic or religious hatred, unwillingness of adversaries to share power or resources, or involvement of other countries.[4]

Diplomacy has been one of the primary approaches to preventing war. Diplomacy, which consists of dialogue in various forms, such as face-to-face negotiations, arbitration and mediation, and conferences, aims to prevent disputes from occurring, to prevent them from evolving into armed conflict, and to end armed conflict that has already begun.

Another primary approach to preventing war has been international *arms control*—limitation on the development, testing, production, stockpiling, deployment, or use of weapons, usually based on collaborative or cooperative efforts of antagonistic or competing countries. It has also been a major strategy in postwar reconstruction and peacebuilding, including programs for former combatants to relinquish their weapons. Arms control is typically done through multilateral or bilateral treaties and other agreements. Several of these treaties and agreements are described in Chapters 4 and 5. Specific information on a wide range of arms control matters can be obtained from the United Nations, government agencies, and nongovernmental organizations, such as the Arms Control Association.

Public health can provide fresh perspectives on preventing war and stopping war that has already begun. For example, because there are similarities in the temporal and spatial patterns of spread of both communicable disease and war (Chapter 1), public health measures to prevent transmission of communicable disease can be applied to prevent war. These measures include interrupting transmission of disease from one person (or group) to another, preventing others in the population from becoming infected and from spreading infection to others, and building group resistance to a disease, such as by changing normative behaviors and developing immunity. Over the past 20 years, Cure Violence Global has successfully applied these communicable disease measures to preventing and interrupting violence, including in war settings.[5-7] (See Profile 15.)

Humanitarian ceasefires represent another way in which a public health perspective can contribute to peace. During humanitarian ceasefires, childhood immunizations and other public health measures can be implemented, sometimes leading to increased trust and cooperation between warring parties and negotiations to end violence. For humanitarian ceasefires to be successful, each party in an armed conflict needs to perceive that its own population is being adversely affected by factors that can be addressed successfully only if it suspends the conflict and cooperates with its opponent.[8] There have been some notable successes with humanitarian ceasefires in achieving peace, such as in El Salvador and Sudan in the late 1980s. However, there have been other situations in which humanitarian ceasefires did not lead to peace but gave combatants opportunities to rearm, reposition their forces, and smuggle in weapons. (Humanitarian ceasefires represent an example of Peace Through Health, as described on page 266.)

Reducing the Root Causes of War

This section discusses reducing five of the root causes of war that were described in Chapter 1: extreme poverty and socioeconomic inequities, militarism and the availability of weapons, poor governance, intergroup animosity, and environmental stress. In addition to addressing these root causes, it is often helpful to search for the underlying causes of root causes by asking such questions as: Why do extreme poverty and socioeconomic inequities exist? Who is promoting militarism and availability of weapons, and why? Why has the quality of governance been allowed to deteriorate? Are there political factors exacerbating intergroup or intragroup animosity? What circumstances are contributing to environmental stress, and why?

Extreme Poverty and Socioeconomic Inequities

Individual poverty and low national income are strongly associated with civil war. The poorest 10% of countries have had a sixfold increased risk of violent civil conflict compared to the richest 10%. Lack of financial resources may make governments more susceptible to rebellion and intrastate war. Many of the poorest countries, such as the Democratic Republic of the Congo, South Sudan, Afghanistan, and Yemen, have recently experienced, or are experiencing, war. Reducing poverty and socioeconomic inequities can help prevent war.[9] For example, leaders of poverty-stricken countries that control abundant oil, minerals, and other resources can utilize these assets to address extreme poverty and socioeconomic inequities.

Militarism and Availability of Weapons

The cultural acceptance of war and violence contributes to a country's willingness to use war in order to achieve its goals.[10] Militarism normalizes war and preparation for war by influencing mass culture and consciousness, politics, and economic priorities. It promotes strong military institutions and resolution of conflicts through force, thereby increasing the probability of war.[11] And it often increases availability of weapons. In the United States, the military-industrial complex has a strong influence on using military power to resolve disputes with other countries and to exert geopolitical influence. (See Chapter 1.) By spreading their work and jobs across many states and congressional districts, defense contractors build and maintain strong public support.[12] As Alain Enthoven, emeritus Stanford economist and a former Deputy Assistant Secretary of Defense, said: "The ideal weapons system is built in 435 congressional districts."[13] Prevention of war needs to include efforts to reduce militarism, availability of weapons, and the influence of the military-industrial complex.

Poor Governance

Improving citizen participation in government through free elections and other democratic processes makes government more accountable. Mechanisms to promote the rule of law and to ensure justice are essential to good governance. Strengthening civil society organizations supports citizen participation and government responsiveness. Improving governance, which is further addressed later in this chapter, helps to reduce the likelihood of war.

Intergroup Animosity

Intergroup animosity can be addressed by efforts to improve understanding and tolerance among people. Bringing adversaries together for intergroup dialogue, active listening, empathy, cooperation, and constructive interactions can build relationships, promote trust and a shared social identity, and instill values supporting nonviolence.[14] When people share experiences, they can relate to others' suffering and be open to peacemaking. Empathy and intergroup understanding can lead to forgiveness and reduce the probability of intergroup violence.[15]

Environmental Stress

Decreased freshwater availability, climate change, and environmental degradation can be causes of, or contributing factors to, war (Chapter 13). As demonstrated in Figure 13-5 in Chapter 13, adaptation measures can reduce the probability of armed conflict due to climate change, such as by providing technical and financial assistance to farmers affected by drought. Efforts to prevent war need to include assessment and reduction of factors that cause environmental stress.

Strengthening the Infrastructure for Peace

Strengthening the infrastructure for peace—peacebuilding—prevents the outbreak, recurrence, or continuation of war by:

- Rehabilitating nations and reintegrating people
- Respecting, protecting, and fulfilling human rights
- Supporting post-conflict reconciliation
- Promoting democracy and the rule of law.

Women have important roles in peacebuilding as well as conflict prevention, conflict resolution, and implementation of measures to protect women against gender-based violence and to uphold women's rights. When women actively participate in a peace process, peace is more sustainable.[16] For example, in Liberia and Sierra Leone, women's networks at the local levels were instrumental in post-conflict reconstruction as women drew on their prewar social networks to mobilize women to demand and foster peace.[17] Zainab Salbi, Iraqi women's rights activist and founder of Women for Women International, advocates that women be fully included in negotiations for ending war and promoting peace: "I find it amazing that the only group of people who are not fighting and not killing and not pillaging and not burning and not raping, and the group of people . . . who are keeping life going in the midst of war are not included [at] the negotiating table."[18]

Rehabilitating Nations and Reintegrating People

Strengthening the infrastructure for peace requires rehabilitating nations damaged by war. Rehabilitation is facilitated by establishing legitimate government in which previous adversaries coexist, establishing security, reorienting the economy to civilian needs and providing jobs for former soldiers, and identifying and addressing perpetrators of abuses.[19] Strengthening the infrastructure for peace also requires reintegrating people who have been traumatized, severely injured, or psychologically impaired by war.

Respecting, Protecting, and Fulfilling Human Rights

Human rights allow people to live with dignity, freedom, equality, justice, and peace. Adherence to the Universal Declaration of Human Rights has helped to protect rights to life, liberty, and security of person; the right to education; the right to freedom of movement; the right to a standard of living adequate for health and well-being, including food, clothing, housing, and medical care and necessary social services; and the right to security in the event of unemployment, sickness, disability, widowhood, old age, or other lack of livelihood in circumstances beyond one's control (Chapter 3).[20]

Supporting Post-Conflict Reconciliation

Survivors of armed conflict often have a desire to seek revenge against adversaries because of the suffering they have experienced.[21] But revenge often leads to more violence. In contrast, post-conflict reconciliation addresses responsibility, blame, and restitution and can lead to peaceful coexistence between previous adversaries.[22]

Truth commissions can facilitate post-conflict reconciliation. Established after more than 35 wars, genocides, and mass killings during the past five decades, they have investigated the causes and consequences of human rights violations, war crimes, and other serious abuses. They have established facts, acknowledged victims, protected survivors, and facilitated changes in public policy and individual behavior.[23-25] Truth commissions have been most effective when integrated into an overall transitional justice strategy that has included criminal prosecutions, reparation policies, and institutional reforms.[23] Although truth commissions can establish the foundation for a culture of peace based on human rights, it is the responsibility of governments, nongovernmental organizations, and individuals to build on this foundation.[26]

Promoting Democracy and the Rule of Law

Strengthening the infrastructure for peace includes ensuring free elections and other processes by which citizens can influence government decisions that affect their lives. Democratization can play an important role in establishing and maintaining peace. However, as foreign policy expert Michael Mandelbaum observed in his book *The Rise and Fall of Peace on Earth*: "Peace comes from democracy, but democracy cannot be installed from the outside."[27]

The *rule of law*—"a durable system of laws, institutions, norms, and community commitment that delivers: accountability, just laws, open government, and accessible and impartial justice"[28]—is basic to peace, security, and political stability. It is essential for protecting human rights and fundamental freedoms, achieving social and economic progress, enabling access to public services, reducing corruption, and preventing abuse of power. It is integral to maintaining the social contract between people and their government.

The rule of law can help to reduce violent conflict by providing legitimate processes to resolve grievances and disincentives for violence. Immediately after a war, accountable justice and corrections institutions as well as police and law enforcement agencies that respect and protect human rights are essential for security, stability, and peace. These institutions and agencies bring to justice perpetrators of crimes and violators of human rights, facilitate nonviolent resolution of disputes, and help establish and maintain trust and social cohesion.[29]

ROLES

Preventing war and promoting peace involve multiple actors and multiple sectors of global society. This section explores the roles of the United Nations, civil society, and health professionals.

Roles of the United Nations

Setting Goals

An important role of the United Nations is setting global goals related to peace, health, development, and other issues. The Sustainable Development Goals (SDGs) were established in 2015 by the UN General Assembly, as targets for 2030. Strengthening the infrastructure for peace is consistent with SDG 16 (Peace, Justice and Strong Institutions), which "aims to promote peaceful and inclusive societies for sustainable development, provide access to justice for all, and build effective, accountable, and inclusive institutions at all levels."[30] The primary target of SDG 16 is to "significantly reduce all forms of violence and related death rates everywhere."[30]

UN Peacekeeping

UN peacekeeping helps war-affected countries create conditions for sustainable peace. UN peacekeepers have reduced the risk of recurrent war by more than 85%, mainly by addressing root causes of war during times of peace. They protect civilians, observe peace processes, and assist former combatants in implementing peace agreements. They strengthen the infrastructure for peace by establishing free elections, maintaining local security, facilitating disarmament, demobilizing troops, and reintegrating rebels—and by strengthening human rights.[31] (Some military forces, including U.S. troops, have also served peacekeeping functions.)

During the past seven decades, more than one million men and women have served in 71 UN peacekeeping operations. As of June 2021, there were 12 active UN peacekeeping operations, mainly in Africa and the Middle East, staffed by about 100,000 UN-uniformed peacekeepers from 125 countries, mainly from Africa and Asia.[32]

Ideally, peacekeepers are deployed before disputes become violent, as was successfully done in Macedonia in 1995–1999, in the Central African Republic in 1998–2000, and in several operations in Haiti since 1993. However, the United Nations focuses almost entirely on crises and emergencies—not prevention of war—and generally becomes engaged only after large-scale violence has occurred. Former UN Secretary-General Kofi Annan observed that the international community has been reluctant to spend the political and financial capital necessary for a peace operation unless war is imminent. He lamented: "Existing problems usually take precedence over potential ones and, while the benefits of prevention lie in the future and are difficult to quantify, the costs must be paid in the present."[33]

The World Health Organization Health & Peace Initiative

Dr. Tedros Adhanom Ghebreyesus, the Director-General of the World Health Organization (WHO), has stated, "There is no peace without health and no health without peace."[34] The WHO Health & Peace Initiative recognizes that conflicts are a major obstacle to health and that lack of access to healthcare and social services can indirectly lead to conflict. Delivering healthcare can help prevent this vicious cycle and provide health benefits and contributions to peace. In its Health & Peace Initiative, the WHO develops innovative ways to address conflict, strengthen resilience to violence, and empower people to (re)build peaceful relations with each other. Health interventions are especially suited for building peace because caring for sick and injured people is generally seen as a neutral activity and a universal good. Health is frequently perceived as a common goal for all sides of a conflict, capable of aligning warring factions toward a shared goal.[35]

In the WHO Health & Peace Initiative, health programs can be used not only to work *in* conflict, but also to work *on* conflict. Health interventions relevant to peace can help improve the possibility of peace by (a) including conflict sensitivity in humanitarian analyses and assessments, recruitment, programming, and monitoring and evaluation; (b) working to improve trust and communication between citizens and the government by making healthcare more accessible and equitable; (c) building collaboration between different sides in a conflict on common topics, such as the delivery of care; and (d) improving social cohesion at the local level through community healing or inclusive health-promotion initiatives.[35]

BOX 15-1 Examples of Measures That Can Be Implemented by Civil Society to Address Violence, Terror, and War

Holding leaders accountable for complying with international law

Speaking truth to power

Protecting children in war-affected areas

Supporting women's values

Speaking for the voiceless

Learning nonviolent conflict resolution

Claiming a great vision

Remembering your humanity

Meeting colleagues on the other side

Rejecting the glorification of war and violence

(Source: Ashford M-W, Dauncey G. Enough Blood Shed: 101 Solutions to Violence, Terror and War. Gabriola Island, BC, Canada: New Society Publishers, 2006.)

Roles of Civil Society

There are many ways that civil society can help prevent war and promote peace. Civil society organizations can identify and investigate disputes and help resolve them nonviolently. They can deescalate violence and promote political stability. They can address the root causes of war. They can foster reconciliation and people-to-people communication, which can re-frame and change perceptions. They can identify and analyze neglected problems and gaps in public policy and recommend -- and advocate for -- solutions. They can mobilize constituencies for peace and increase the possibility of durable peace. And they can transform values and support a culture of peace.[36]

Physician Mary-Wynne Ashford and sustainability consultant Guy Dauncey, in their book *Enough Blood Shed*, address what ordinary citizens can do. They draw on stories from many countries to demonstrate the effectiveness of nonviolence, peacebuilding, conflict resolution, citizen diplomacy, and forgiveness, and they describe 101 solutions to violence, terror, and war that can be implemented by individuals, schools, the media, business and labor, and cities, nations, and the global community. Box 15-1 provides some examples of these solutions.[37]

Roles of Health Professionals

During war, health professionals provide clinical and public health services, treating all in need, regardless of their nationality or affiliation.[38] In the aftermath of war, health professionals help restore healthcare facilities and health services. And health professionals also help to prevent war and promote peace—through education and awareness-raising; through assessment, documentation, and research; and through advocacy.[39,40] Profiles throughout this book provide illustrative examples of the roles of health professionals. Public health professors William H. Wiist and Shelley K. White, in their book *Preventing War and Promoting Peace: A Guide for Health Professionals*, provide much additional valuable information on these roles.[41]

Throughout the world, health professionals address the impact of violence on health. In doing so, they find numerous ways in which they can contribute to the prevention of war and the promotion of peace. *Peace Through Health*, a concept fostered by physicians Neil Arya and Joanna Santa Barbara, has demonstrated and supported ways in which health professionals can advance peace.[42,43] In addition to humanitarian ceasefires described earlier in this chapter, these ways include extending healthcare to opposition groups, healing physical and psychological trauma, improving individual's sense of security, convening groups to achieve superordinate goals, and providing solidarity and support for victims of war.

Education and Awareness-Raising

The role of health professionals in education starts with educating and raising the awareness of other health professionals about the health impacts of war and the prevention of war. Health professionals also educate and raise the awareness of people and organizations in other sectors of society, government policymakers, journalists, and the general public.

A prime example of health professionals' role in education and awareness-raising for the prevention of war has been the work of the International Physicians for the Prevention of Nuclear War (IPPNW) and its country affiliates, including Physicians for Social Responsibility (PSR), its U.S. affiliate, and Medact, its affiliate in the United Kingdom. Starting in 1962, the founders of PSR wrote a series of articles, which were published in the *New England Journal of Medicine*, on the consequences of nuclear weapon attacks on major U.S. cities.[44] These articles and the work of IPPNW and its country affiliates for decades have influenced national and international policy, supporting nuclear weapon treaties and reductions in nuclear weapon arsenals of the United States and the Soviet Union (and Russia).[45,46] IPPNW, along with PSR and its other country affiliates, received the 1985 Nobel Peace Prize. And the International Campaign to Abolish Nuclear Weapons (ICAN), which was launched by IPPNW, received the 2017 Nobel Peace Prize.

In 2009, the American Public Health Association (APHA) adopted a policy statement on the role of public health practitioners, academics, and advocates in relation to war, which included public health competencies for the prevention of war. These competencies focused on militarism, international peace work, peace advocacy, and research on the causes and consequences of war and their relationship to health.[47] The Working Group on the Prevention of War has recommended that schools of public health and public health organizations incorporate these competencies into professional preparation programs, research, and advocacy.[11]

Assessment, Documentation, and Research

By assessing and documenting the health impacts of war and performing research on the causation and prevention of these impacts, health professionals can help protect civilians and help end wars. Clinicians assess and document the health impacts of war affecting their patients and others, and they participate in research on these impacts. Public health professionals and humanitarian aid workers gather relevant information by rapid assessments, public health surveillance, and epidemiological studies, much of it for immediate use in responding to humanitarian needs and reducing the health impacts of war (Chapter 14).

During war and its aftermath, health professionals defend human rights by investigating violations of medical neutrality, assessing damage to healthcare facilities in war zones, obtaining medical data on victims of alleged human rights abuses, and participating in forensic investigations to document torture and other human rights abuses. And health professionals defend other health professionals worldwide who have been imprisoned, tortured, or otherwise abused for performing their duties and adhering to ethical standards (Chapter 3).[48]

For more than 30 years, Physicians for Human Rights has investigated and documented violations of medical neutrality, health crises of displaced populations, use of indiscriminate weapons, torture, deliberate injury and rape, and mass execution. Its current work focuses on torture, asylum and persecution, attacks on healthcare workers and facilities, killings and mass atrocities, sexual violence, prohibited weapons, COVID-19, and health professionals who are complicit in or actively contributing to violations of human rights.[48,49]

Advocacy

Health professionals have relevant knowledge and skills as well as public credibility that enables them to be strong advocates for preventing war and promoting peace. Health professionals are usually most influential when they present factual information and share firsthand observations and experiences. Health professionals shape public opinion on many issues and influence policymakers in governments, nongovernmental organizations, and international organizations. These issues include protection of civilians, access to health services, nonviolent conflict resolution, military spending, the international arms trade, and the health impacts of weapons.

In order to improve the effectiveness of advocacy, health professionals need to improve their advocacy skills for interacting with the news media, using social media and the Internet, influencing government policymakers, conducting advocacy campaigns, and utilizing new advocacy methods.[50] They also need to build broader partnerships with people and organizations in other sectors of society.

Often, health professionals can advocate most effectively by working with or within professional associations, such as APHA, the American Medical Association, the American Nursing Association, Physicians for Human Rights, and PSR, Medact, and other country affiliates of the IPPNW. Over the past five decades, APHA has adopted many policies directly related to war, including opposing specific wars, banning certain classes of weapons, and ending violent attacks on health workers and health facilities in war settings.[51]

TOWARD A WORLD WITHOUT WAR

The ultimate goal of preventing war and promoting peace is abolishing war and establishing a culture of peace. In a world without war, disputes would be settled nonviolently and military resources would be reallocated to health, education, and other societal benefits. A culture of peace would nurture respect for human dignity, highlight the similarities among people, foster social justice, and promote human rights.

Smallpox was, for centuries, a scourge of humanity. In 1797, an effective vaccine was developed. But it was not until almost two centuries later that smallpox was eradicated. More than a vaccine, eradication of smallpox required capabilities and resources as well as the popular and political will to do so.

We, as a global society, have the capabilities and resources to end war.

We can develop the popular and political will to do so.

We can move from horror to hope.

What will you do to end war and promote peace?

SUMMARY POINTS

- A public health approach for preventing war and promoting peace includes resolving disputes nonviolently, reducing the root causes of war, and strengthening the infrastructure for peace.
- Prevention of war can be achieved by interrupting the transmission of violence.
- Prevention of war can be achieved by reducing extreme poverty and socioeconomic inequities, militarism and the availability of weapons, poor governance, intergroup animosity, and environmental stress.
- Prevention of recurrent war can be achieved, post-conflict, by rehabilitating nations and reintegrating people, protecting human rights, supporting reconciliation, and promoting democracy and the rule of law.
- Health professionals can help prevent war and promote peace through education and awareness-raising; assessment, documentation, and research; and advocacy.

REFERENCES

1. United Nations. Peace and Security. Available at: https://www.un.org/en/global-issues/peace-and-security. Accessed on November 19, 2021.
2. Atomic education urged by Einstein. New York Times, May 25, 1946. Available at: https://timesmachine.nytimes.com/timesmachine/1946/05/25/100998236.html. Accessed on July 2, 2021.
3. Centers for Disease Control. Principles of Epidemiology in Public Health Practice (3rd edition). Available at: https://www.cdc.gov/csels/dsepd/ss1978/ss1978.pdf. Accessed on July 6, 2021.
4. Pettersson T, Högbladh S, Öberg M. Organized violence, 1989–2018 and peace agreements. Journal of Peace Research 2019; 56: 589-603.
5. Slutkin G. "Violence Is a Contagious Disease" in Institute of Medicine and National Research Council. Contagion of Violence: Workshop Summary. Washington, DC: The National Academies Press, 2013. Available at: https://doi.org/10.17226/13489. Accessed at June 27, 2021.
6. Slutkin G, Ransford C, Zvetina D. How the health sector can reduce violence by treating it as contagion. AMA Journal of Ethics 2018; 20: 47-55.
7. Cure Violence Global. Our impact. Available at: https://cvg.org/impact. Accessed on July 5, 2021.
8. Santa Barbara J, MacQueen G. Peace through health: Key concepts. The Lancet 2004; 364: 384-386.
9. Braithwaite A, Dasandi N, Hudson D. Does poverty cause conflict? Isolating the causal origins of the conflict trap. Conflict Management and Peace Science 2016; 33: 45-66.

10. Hauerwas S, Hogan L, McDonagh E. The case for abolition of war in the twenty-first century. Journal of the Society of Christian Ethics 2005; 25: 17-35.

11. Wiist WH, Barker K, Arya N, et al. The role of public health in the prevention of war: Rationale and competencies. American Journal of Public Health 2014; 104: e34-e47.

12. Pemberton M. "The War Profiteers: Defense Contractors Driving the Permanent War Economy" in WH Wiist, SK White (eds.). Preventing War and Promoting Peace: A Guide for Health Professionals. Cambridge, UK: Cambridge University Press, 2017, pp. 116-128.

13. Dickson P. "Enthoven's Discovery" in The Official Rules: 5,427 Laws, Principles, and Axioms to Help You Cope with Crises, Deadlines, Bad Luck, Rude Behavior, Red Tape, and Attacks by Inanimate Objects. Mineola, NY: Dover Publications, 2013, p. 99.

14. Christie DJ, Montiel CJ. Contributions of psychology to war and peace. American Psychologist 2013; 68: 502-513.

15. Leidner B, Tropp LR, Lickel B. Bringing science to bear—on peace, not war. American Psychologist 2013; 68: 514-526.

16. Krause J, Krause W, Bränfors T. Women's participation in peace negotiations and the durability of peace. International Interactions 2018; 44: 985-1016.

17. Gizelis T-I. A country of their own: Women and peacebuilding. Conflict Management and Peace Science 2011; 28: 522-542. doi: 10.1177/0738894211418412.

18. Salbi Z. Women, wartime, and the dream of peace. TED Talk, TEDGlobal 2010. Available at: https://www.ted.com/talks/zainab_salbi_women_wartime_and_the_dream_of_peace?language=su. Accessed on July 7, 2021.

19. Doyle MW, Sambanis N. Making War & Building Peace: United Nations Peace Operations. Princeton, NJ: Princeton University Press, 2006.

20. United Nations. The Universal Declaration of Human Rights. Proclaimed by the United Nations General Assembly, Paris, December 10, 1948. Available at: https://www.un.org/en/universal-declaration-human-rights/. Accessed on October 8, 2020.

21. Hassan G, Ventevogel P, Jefee-Bahloul H, et al. Mental health and psychosocial wellbeing of Syrians affected by armed conflict. Epidemiology and Psychiatric Sciences 2016; 25: 129-141.

22. Summerfield D. Effects of war: Moral knowledge, revenge, reconciliation, and medicalised concepts of "recovery." British Medical Journal 2002; 325: 1105-1107.

23. González E, Varney H. Truth Seeking: Elements of Creating an Effective Truth Commission. Amnesty Commission of the Ministry of Justice of Brazil; New York: International Center for Transitional Justice, 2013. Available at:https://www.ictj.org/sites/default/files/ICTJ-Book-Truth-Seeking-2013-English.pdf. Accessed on April 20, 2021.

24. Bakiner O. Truth Commissions: Memory, Power, and Legitimacy. Philadelphia: University of Pennsylvania Press, 2016.

25. Hayner PB. Truth commission. Available at: britannica.com/topic/truth-commission. Accessed on July 28, 2020.

26. Borer TA. Gendered war and gendered peace: Truth commissions and postconflict gender violence: Lessons from South Africa. Violence Against Women 2009; 15: 1169-1193.

27. Mandelbaum M. The Rise and Fall of Peace on Earth. New York: Oxford University Press, 2019.

28. World Justice Project. What is the Rule of Law? Available at: https://worldjusticeproject.org/about-us/overview/what-rule-law. Accessed on January 23, 2022.

29. United Nations and the Rule of Law. Rule of Law and Peace and Security. Available at: https://www.un.org/ruleoflaw/rule-of-law-and-peace-and-security/. Accessed on February 5, 2021.

30. United Nations and the Rule of Law. Sustainable Development Goal 16. Available at: https://www.un.org/ruleoflaw/sdg-16/. Accessed on February 5, 2021.

31. Sandler T. International peacekeeping operations: Burden sharing and effectiveness. Journal of Conflict Resolution 2017; 61: 1875-1897.

32. United Nations Peacekeeping. Available at: peacekeeping.un.org/en. Accessed on June 25, 2021.

33. Goldstein JS. Winning the War on War: The Decline of Armed Conflict Worldwide. London: Plume, a Member of Penguin Group, 2011.

34. Director-General's Opening Remarks at the World Health Assembly. Geneva, May 24, 2021. Available at: https://www.who.int/director-general/speeches/detail/director-general-s-opening-remarks-at-the-world-health-assembly---24-may-2021. Accessed on July 10, 2021.

35. World Health Organization. Health & Peace Initiative. Available at: https://apps.who.int/iris/handle/10665/332938. Accessed on July 10, 2021.

36. Barnes C. Agents for Change: Civil Society Roles in Preventing War & Building Peace. Den Haag, The Netherlands: European Centre for Conflict Prevention/International Secretariat of the Global Partnership for the Prevention of Armed Conflict, 2006. Available at: https://www.gppac.net/files/2018-11/Agents%20for%20Change.pdf. Accessed on July 9, 2021.

37. Ashford M-W, Dauncey G. Enough Blood Shed: 101 Solutions to Violence, Terror and War. Gabriola Island, BC, Canada: New Society Publishers, 2006.

38. Sidel VW, Levy BS. "Physician-Soldier: A Moral Dilemma?" in TE Beam, LR Sparacino (Specialty Editors). Military Medical Ethics: Volume 1 (Textbooks of Military Medicine). Falls Church, VA: Office of the Surgeon General, United States Army; Washington, DC: Borden Institute, Walter Reed Army Medical Center; and Bethesda, MD: Uniformed Services University of the Health Sciences; 2003, pp. 293-312.

39. Yusuf S, Anand S. Can medicine prevent war? Imaginative thinking shows that it might. British Medical Journal 1998; 317: 1669-1670.

40. Buhmann C, Santa Barbara J, Arya N, Melf K. The roles of the health sector and health workers before, during and after violent conflict. Medicine, Conflict and Survival 2010; 26: 4-23.

41. Wiist WH, White SK. Preventing War and Promoting Peace: A Guide for Health Professionals. Cambridge, UK: Cambridge University Press, 2017.

42. Arya N, Santa Barbara J (eds.). Peace Through Health: How Health Professionals Can Work for a Less Violent World. Sterling, VA: Kumarian Press, 2008.

43. Arya N. Approaching Peace Through Health with a critical eye. Peace Review: A Journal of Social Justice 2019; 31: 131-138. doi: 10.1080/10402659.2019.1667560.

44. Sidel VW, Geiger HJ, Lown B. The physician's role in the postattack period. New England Journal of Medicine 1962; 266: 1137-1145.

45. Physicians for Social Responsibility. Available at: https://www.psr.org/. Accessed on July 12, 2021.

46. International Physicians for the Prevention of Nuclear War. Available at: https://www.ippnw.org/. Accessed on July 12, 2021.

47. American Public Health Association. The Role of Public Health Practitioners, Academics, and Advocates in Relation to Armed Conflict and War (Policy Statement 20095), adopted November 10, 2009. Available at: https://www.apha.org/policies-and-advocacy/public-health-policy-statements/policy-database/2014/07/22/13/29/the-role-of-public-health-practitioners-academics-and-advocates-in-relation-to-armed-conflict. Accessed on July 9, 2021.

48. Geiger HJ, Cook-Deegan RM. The role of physicians in conflicts and humanitarian crises: Case studies from the field missions of Physicians for Human Rights, 1988 to 1993. Journal of the American Medical Association 1993; 270: 616-620.

49. Physicians for Human Rights. Available at: phr.org. Accessed on January 17, 2022.

50. Galer-Unti RA. "Advocacy Skills for the Primary Prevention of War" in WH Wiist, SK White (eds.). Preventing War and Promoting Peace: A Guide for Health Professionals. Cambridge, UK: Cambridge University Press, 2017, pp. 257–269.

51. American Public Health Association. Policy Statement Database. Available at: https://www.apha.org/Policies-and-Advocacy/Public-Health-Policy-Statements/Policy-Database. Accessed on July 8, 2021.

Profile 15:
Gary Slutkin, M.D.
Treating Violence as Epidemic Disease

Gary Slutkin's career trajectory demonstrates how a health professional, using well-established methods of infectious disease control, can stop the transmission of violence and possibly help to transform violence prevention.

Dr. Slutkin is an infectious disease physician and epidemiologist. After completing his training in internal medicine and infectious disease, he worked as director of the tuberculosis (TB) control program of the San Francisco Department of Public Health, where he controlled a major epidemic of TB using community health workers. In 1985, he moved to Somalia, where he developed a TB control program and helped investigate and control a large epidemic of cholera. After 3 years in Somalia, he was recruited by the World Health Organization (WHO) Global Programme on AIDS to guide its work in Central and East Africa. He then became director of the WHO Intervention Development Department.

After almost 10 years of work in Africa, Dr. Slutkin moved to Chicago, where the epidemic of lethal community violence captured his attention. Soon, he noted epidemiological similarities between community violence and communicable diseases. He then applied the tools of infectious disease epidemiology to investigate community violence. Mapping the incidence of violence, he noticed the same type of clustering that he had seen when he investigated cholera in Somalia and AIDS in Uganda. As he developed epidemic curves (graphic representation of new cases over time) of the incidence of homicides in Chicago and other U.S. cities, he noticed the same wave-upon-wave pattern of new cases that he had seen with epidemics of infectious diseases in Africa and elsewhere. And as he investigated risk factors for lethal violence, he discovered that the greatest predictor of a violent incident was a

From Horror to Hope. Barry S. Levy, Oxford University Press. © Oxford University Press 2022.
DOI: 10.1093/oso/9780197558645.003.0030

previous violent incident or previous exposure to violence—just as the greatest risk factor for many infectious diseases is previous exposure to someone with that disease. Dr. Slutkin concluded that violence meets the criteria and the dictionary definitions of communicable epidemic disease.

In 2000, Dr. Slutkin established Cure Violence Global, a nongovernmental organization that uses science-based methods to investigate violent behavior, interrupt its transmission, prevent its spread, and change group behavioral norms. Cure Violence Global has recruited "violence interrupters," who have credibility and trust in their communities, and has trained them to detect and prevent imminent violence. It also recruited and trained outreach workers and others in methods of detection, persuasion, cooling of emotions, perspective shifting, individual behavioral change, and changing group norms on using violence. By interrupting violence, Cure Violence Global has prevented many shootings and spread of violence.

Outreach workers work together with violence interrupters, mentoring high-risk clients to help them achieve long-term behavioral change, supporting clients with job training and support, and addressing other life needs. To change group norms, Cure Violence Global implements public education campaigns, community events, and responses to acts of violence until local social pressure brings about "herd immunity" to violence in a community.

As of September 2021, there had been 20 studies and eight fully independent evaluations of Cure Violence Global programs by U.S. government and international agencies and universities, which have demonstrated 40% to 70% decreases in community violence in cities in the United States, Latin America, and elsewhere. The Cure Violence Global epidemic model has been adopted by many public health departments in the United States. It has been implemented in Mexico, Honduras, Colombia, Jamaica, the United Kingdom, and South Africa, and has been accompanied by similar reductions in violence. And it has been used to reduce violence during the Syrian Civil War and in Iraq and the West Bank.

Dr. Slutkin is the Founder and Chief Executive Officer of Cure Violence Global.

Profile 16:
Amy Hagopian, Ph.D.,
and Evan Kanter, M.D., Ph.D.
Teaching About War and Health

Amy Hagopian and Evan Kanter direct the "War & Health" course at the University of Washington (UW), one of the few courses on war in schools of public health.

During the 1990s, Dr. Hagopian was employed by the UW School of Medicine to support rural hospitals in the five-state region served by the school. Over time, she became increasingly involved with workforce development and wrote her doctoral thesis on migration of health workers from low-income to high-income countries. In 2008, she collaborated with Iraqi epidemiologists and others on a study to characterize the increasing rate of childhood leukemia in Basra between 1993 and 2007. A few years later, she directed a large-scale study to estimate Iraqi mortality associated with the U.S. invasion in 2003. She describes her research and practice work as addressing the maldistribution of political and economic power in society.

Dr. Kanter is a psychiatrist and neuroscientist who, early in his career, performed basic and clinical research on traumatic memory. Since completing a psychiatry residency 30 years ago, he has treated, at Veterans Health Administration facilities, many military veterans with posttraumatic stress disorder and other conditions related to war trauma. For the past 10 years, he has worked in community mental health settings, treating refugees and other civilians adversely affected by war, including torture survivors, suffering from similar disorders. Dr. Kanter has worked to promote peace for many years. In medical school, he organized Soviet-American student and faculty exchanges. He has participated in peacebuilding initiatives in the Middle East, especially in Iraq. He is especially interested in nuclear weapons issues and, in 2009, served as national president of Physicians for Social Responsibility.

From Horror to Hope. Barry S. Levy, Oxford University Press. © Oxford University Press 2022.
DOI: 10.1093/oso/9780197558645.003.0031

In 2010, Dr. Hagopian and Dr. Kanter co-directed a major conference at UW on framing war as a public health problem, which served as a springboard for their "War & Health" course. Because war is not widely appreciated as a legitimate area of scholarship in public health, they initially faced opposition to establishing a course. But, over the next few years, the need to expand course offerings to undergraduate students created an enthusiastic market.

Their four-credit "War & Health" course, taught annually at UW since 2015 to a class of more than 50 students, meets for 1½-hour lectures on Mondays and Wednesdays, and 1-hour discussions on Fridays. As students enter the course, each selects a "study war" for the quarter and is assigned to a small group, which includes a student from each study war. Approximately 10 graduate students in the course moderate the Friday discussions. Study wars include the Second World War, the Vietnam War, the Mexican drug wars, and wars in Iraq, Afghanistan, Rwanda, Syria, and Yemen. On Thursdays, students post three-paragraph essays on the relationship of their specific wars to the topic for the week, such as the role of health workers in mitigating their war. Students read each other's essays prior to the Friday discussions so they are familiar with each other's work before the discussion takes place. Students' midcourse papers address the health effects of study wars. Students also participate in a role-play exercise in which they represent various stakeholder organizations at a House Armed Services Committee hearing that is considering the future of the intercontinental ballistic missile system. Students also participate in an "activism exercise" in which they watch a film or attend a demonstration and then write a paper about the experience.

Dr. Hagopian and Dr. Kanter pose questions to students about their study wars, including: What health problems were caused? What structural violence factors, such as racism, oppression, and poverty, were related? How might health professionals or others have intervened?

These are questions for all of us to address about war.

Dr. Hagopian is a Professor at the University of Washington School of Public Health and Vice Chair of the Global Alliance on War, Conflict and Health. Dr. Kanter is a Clinical Assistant Professor in the Department of Health Services at the University of Washington School of Public Health and Medical Director of the Asian Counseling and Referral Service in Seattle.

Index